Neuroanatomy

An Atlas of Structures, Sections, and Systems

EIGHTH EDITION

Neuroanatomy

An Atlas of Structures, Sections, and Systems

EIGHTH EDITION

Duane E. Haines, Ph.D.
**Professor Emeritus, Department of Anatomy
and Professor of Neurology and Professor of
Neurosurgery at the University of Mississippi
Medical Center**

Illustrators: M. P. Schenk, BS, MSMI, CMI, FAMI
W. K. Cunningham, BA, MSMI
Computer Graphics: C. P. Runyan, BS
Photographer: G. W. Armstrong, RBP
Typist: L. K. Boyd

. Wolters Kluwer | Lippincott Williams & Wilkins
Health
Philadelphia · Baltimore · New York · London
Buenos Aires · Hong Kong · Sydney · Tokyo

Acquisitions Editor: Crystal Taylor
Product Manager: Catherine Noonan
Marketing Manager: Joy Fisher-Williams
Vendor Manager: Bridgett Dougherty
Manufacturing Manager: Margie Orzech
Designer: Doug Smock
Compositor: Aptara, Inc.

First Edition, 1983   Portuguese Translation, 1991
Second Edition, 1987   Chinese Translation (Taiwan), 1997
Third Edition, 1991   Japanese Translation, 1996, 2000
Fourth Edition, 1995   Chinese (Bejing) Translation, 2001
Fifth Edition, 2000   Chinese (Nanjing) Translation, 2002
Sixth Edition, 2004   Brazilian Translation, 2007
Seventh Edition, 2008   Korean and Russian Translations, 2008

351 West Camden Street   Two Commerce Square, 2001 Market Street
Baltimore, MD 21201   Philadelphia, PA 19103

Printed in China

9 8 7 6 5 4 3 2 1

Library of Congress Cataloging-in-Publication Data

Haines, Duane E.
  Neuroanatomy : an atlas of structures, sections, and systems / Duane
E. Haines. – 8th ed.
    p. ; cm.
  Includes bibliographical references and index.
  ISBN 978-1-60547-653-7 (alk. paper)
  1. Neuroanatomy–Atlases. I. Title.
  [DNLM: 1. Central Nervous System–anatomy & histology–Atlases. WL 17]
  QM451.H18 2012
  611'.8—dc22

                              2011004726

DISCLAIMER

To purchase additional copies of this book, call our customer service department at (800) 638-3030 or fax orders to (301) 223-2320. International customers should call (301) 223-2300.

Visit Lippincott Williams & Wilkins on the Internet: http://www.lww.com. Lippincott Williams & Wilkins customer service representatives are available from 8:30 am to 6:00 pm, EST.

Preface to the Eighth Edition

This new edition of *Neuroanatomy, An Atlas of Structures, Sections, and Systems* has endeavored to: 1) continue to provide a sound anatomical base for correlating structure and function; 2) introduce new information in the form of new MRIs, CTs, text, and artwork that integrates and explains concepts that will be encountered in the clinical setting; 3) emphasize contemporary clinical and basic science terminology; and 4) expand the treatment of neuroscience as seen in clinical medicine through additional examples, text revisions, and a more comprehensive overview of systems neurobiology. Understanding systems neurobiology is the key element in the successful diagnosis of the neurologically compromised patient.

I have received suggestions and comments from my basic science and clinical colleagues and from medical students, residents, and graduate students that have been factored into this new edition. These insights have been quite helpful in deciding what new images and text would be appropriate in the face of a changing educational environment.

Modifications, improvements, and label corrections have been made in existing illustrations and many portions of the text have been revised. The major changes or new information introduced in the Eighth Edition of *Neuroanatomy* are as follows:

First, the cranial nerve chapter (Chapter 3) has been revised, additional clinical information added, and cross-references included to figures in other chapters where cranial nerve information is discussed and/or illustrated. This will allow the user to quickly identify the location of key information relating to cranial nerves throughout the book when using this particular chapter. In addition, all cranial nerves that appear in drawings in Chapter 2 are highlighted in yellow to emphasize their positions and relationships to adjacent structures more clearly.

Second, a number of new images, with accompanying text, have been added to demonstrate examples of clinical conditions that have important anatomical correlates. These include, for example, meningitis and meningiomas, which relate to the structure of the meninges, and tumors of the choroid plexus, which nicely illustrate the relationship between ventricular shape and size and the effects of blockage of cerebrospinal fluid flow. The text describing the causative agents of meningitis has also been revised and expanded. A persistent fetal posterior cerebral artery (commonly called a fetal PCA) is seen in about 25% of individuals. Examples of this developmental finding, as well as examples of aberrant anterior cerebral artery development, are also new to this edition.

Third, a major change in Chapter 6 is the replacement of all black-and-white stained sections with color versions of the same sections. This provides an excellent level of anatomical detail, especially in the brainstem, of many nuclei and tracts that have important clinical implications. In addition, revisions have been made in the descriptions of the "Vascular Syndromes" throughout this chapter and modifications of some labels on the line drawings.

Fourth, in like manner, all of the black-and-white versions of the stained sections in Chapter 7 have also been replaced with color versions. This enhances the clarity and visual impact of these images and allowed the labeling to be modified, as needed, to identify several additional and important structures. In addition, some MRIs accompanying the stained sections have been moved or replaced.

Fifth, Chapter 8, which is a broad-based consideration of neural systems directly applicable to clinical neuroscience, has been revised and upgraded in several ways. First, the text accompanying each figure has been modified with an eye toward enhancing clinical information and applicability. Second, a new series of 10 illustrations showing representative spinal and cranial nerve reflexes, each with an accompanying description, has been added. These new images and text immediately follow the sections on sensory pathways, motor pathways, and efferents of the cranial nerves. This is the most appropriate location in this chapter for these reflexes, because it follows the major pathways and cranial nerve projections that are all essential parts of reflexes. In addition, a table summarizes other reflexes that are part of the neurological examination or are commonly encountered in clinical situations. Third, another new section has been added to this chapter that details the structure and connections of the hypothalamus, the pituitary, the organization of fibers traversing the internal capsule, and the topography of thalamocortical projections. These six illustrations are accompanied by explanatory text that, in most cases, also includes clinically relevant information. The addition of this material offers relevant basic science and clinical information that was not available in earlier editions, and it is also in response to suggestions from my colleagues that inclusion of this material would enhance the educational value of this Atlas.

Sixth, the questions and explained answers that constitute Chapter 10 have been revised and new ones added. These new Q&As reflect the new information (clinical and basic science) introduced with the new images now included in Chapters 2–4 and 8.

Two further issues figured prominently in this new edition. First, the question of whether, or not, to use eponyms in their possessive form. To paraphrase one of my clinical colleagues, "Parkinson did not die of his disease (so-called "Parkinson's" disease); he died of a stroke. It was never his own personal disease." There are rare exceptions, such as Lou Gehrig's disease, but the point is well taken. McKusick (1998a,b) also has made compelling arguments in support of using the nonpossessive form of eponyms. However, it is acknowledged that views differ on this question-much like debating how many angels can dance on the head of a pin. Consultation with my neurology and neurosurgery colleagues, the style adopted by *Dorland's Illustrated Medical Dictionary* (2007) and *Stedman's Medical Dictionary* (2008), a review of some of the more comprehensive neurology texts (e.g., Rowland, 2005; Victor and Ropper, 2001), the standards established in the *Council of Biology Editors Manual for Authors, Editors, and Publishers* (1994), and the

American Medical Association's Manual of Style (1998) clearly indicate an overwhelming preference for the nonpossessive form. Recognizing that many users of this book will enter clinical training, it was deemed appropriate to encourage a contemporary approach. Consequently, the nonpossessive form of the eponym is used.

The second issue concerns use of the most up-to-date anatomical terminology. With the publication of *Terminologia Anatomica* (Thieme, New York, 1998), a new official international list of anatomical terms for neuroanatomy is available. This new publication, having been adopted by the International Federation of Associations of Anatomists, supersedes *all* previous terminology lists. Every effort has been made to incorporate any applicable new or modified terms into this book. The number of changes is modest and related primarily to directional terms: "posterior" for "dorsal," "anterior" for "ventral," and so on. In most cases, the previous term appears in parentheses following the official term (i.e., *posterior [dorsal] cochlear nucleus*). In addition, a new terminology is adopted for the *Edinger-Westphal nuclei* (Kozic et al., 2011) that accommodates contemporary discoveries in systems neurobiology.

Lastly, but certainly not least, the Eighth Edition is about 15 pages shorter than the Seventh Edition, despite of the fact that a number of new illustrations and related text were added. This is due to the fact that many of the Q&As are now available as an online resource through thePoint. A sampling of these Q&As is provided in the print version, while the majority is available online as Bonus Material. The decision to make this design change, with the resulting decrease in page numbers, seems justified by the significant added value of the new clinical information, MRIs and CTs, pathway drawings, and new text.

Duane E. Haines
Jackson, Mississippi

References

Council of Biology Editions Style Manual Committee. *Scientific Style and Format—The CBE Manual for Authors, Editors, and Publishers,* 6th Ed. Cambridge: Cambridge University Press, 1994.

Dorland's Illustrated Medical Dictionary, 31st ed. Philadelphia: Saunders/Elsevier, 2007.

Federative Committee on Anatomical Terminology. *Terminologia Anatomica.* New York: Thieme, 1998.

Iverson C, et al. *American Medical Association Manual of Style—A Guide for Authors and Editors,* 10th ed. New York: Oxford University Press, 2007.

Kozicz T, Bittencourt JC, May PJ, Reiner A, Gamlin PDR, Palkovits M, Horn AKE, Toledo CAB, Ryabinin AE. The Edinger-Westphal nucleus: A historical, structural and functional perspective on a dichotomous terminology. *J Comp Neurol* (in press, January 2011).

McKusick VA. On the naming of clinical disorders, with particular reference to eponyms. *Medicine* 1998a;77: 1–2.

McKusick VA. *Mendelian Inheritance in Man, A Catalog of Human Genes and Genetic Disorders,* 12th ed. Baltimore: The Johns Hopkins University Press, 1998b.

Rowland LP. *Merritt's Neurology,* 11th ed. Baltimore: Lippincott Williams & Wilkins, 2005.

Stedman's Medical Dictionary, 28th ed. Philadelphia: Lippincott Williams & Wilkins, 2006.

Victor M, Ropper AH. *Adams and Victor's Principles of Neurology,* 7th ed. New York: McGraw-Hill, Medical Publishing Division, 2001.

Acknowledgments

My clinical and basic science colleagues, medical and graduate students, and residents (especially those in Neurology and Neurosurgery) have been very gracious in offering comments and suggestions regarding this new edition. In fact, they were most patient with my numerous and incessant questions, both great and small. The goal has always been to create a useful educational document.

The modifications in this Eighth Edition were broad based and affected every chapter in one way or another. While new anatomical and clinical information was introduced, a special effort was made to focus on improving clinical relevance and applicability throughout the book. To both of these ends, the following individuals have offered especially insightful suggestions and have been particularly helpful: Drs. Paul May and James Lynch (Anatomy); Drs. Andy Parent, Gustavo Luzardo, James Walker, Jared Marks (for his excellent efforts to get many of the images I needed), Louis Harkey, and Razvan Buciuc (Neurosurgery); Drs. Allissa Willis and Hartmut Uschman (Neurology); Dr. Bob Wineman (Radiology); Ms. Emily Young, Mr. Matt Rhinewalt, and Mr. Joey Verzwyvelt (Medical Students); all of the aforementioned individuals are at the University Of Mississippi Medical Center. Other individuals who have offered important suggestions include: Dr. Barbara Puder (Samuel Merritt University), Dr. Ann Butler (George Mason University), Dr. George Martin (Ohio State University), and Dr. Cristian Stefan. The reviewers commissioned by LWW were: Dr. Patricia A. Brewer, Phil DeVasto, Lauren Ehrlichman, Dr. Erica M. Fallon; Dr. Charles H. Hubscher, Dr. Julie A. Kmiec, Dr. George F. Martin, Ahmed Miam, Brent G. Mollon, Asheer Singh, Dr. Cristian Stefan, and Dr. Maria Thomadaki.

Many interactions bring ideas to mind that have certainly become part of this new edition. Sometimes these are casual conversations in passing in the hallway, a point made during a grand round presentation, or a comment during a review session with residents. Consequently, the specific origin of the comment may have faded. Recognizing this fact, I would like to express my sincere appreciation to my faculty colleagues at the University Of Mississippi Medical Center in the Departments of Anatomy, Neurology (Dr. Alec Auchus, Chairman), Neurosurgery (Dr. Louis Harkey, Chairman), Radiology (Dr. Tim McCowan, Chairman), and the residents in Neurology and Neurosurgery, for comments and suggestions that have certainly been included herein. The excellent cooperation and fruitful interactions between the Department of Anatomy and these clinical departments has always been absolutely outstanding. I would also like to thank Mr. W. (Eddie) Herrington and Mr. Joe Barnes who were the Chief CT/MRI Technologist and Senior MRI Technologist, respectively, during the preparation of this edition, for their unfailing cooperation; Mr. David Case currently occupies the Chief CT/MRI Technologist position. A special thanks is due Ms. Madelene Hyde for allowing me to steal a great idea.

Modifications, both great and small, to the existing artwork and labeling scheme, as well as the generation of many new renderings and tables, were the work of Michael Schenk (Director of Biomedical Illustration Services) and Walter (Kyle) Cunningham (Medical Illustrator). Mr. Chuck Runyan (Biomedical Photography) patiently scanned and cleaned the sections used to produce the color images of the stained sections in Chapters 6 and 7. Mr. Bill Armstrong (Director of Biomedical Photography) developed preliminary versions of a number of images for this edition. I am enormously appreciative of their time, energy, dedication, and professionalism to create the best possible images, photographs, and artwork for this new edition. Their interest in going the extra mile to "get it perfect," and their outstanding cooperation (and, I might add, patience) with the author, is greatly appreciated. Ms. Lisa Boyd, my secretary of many years, did all of the typing for the Eighth Edition. I greatly appreciate her patience, cooperation, and good-natured approach, especially with all the tedious details. She was one essential element in getting the final draft done in a timely manner.

Over the years, many colleagues, friends, and students (now faculty or medical/dental practitioners) have made many helpful comments. They are again acknowledged here, because these earlier suggestions continue to influence this book: Drs. A. Agmon, A. Alqueza, B. Anderson, C. Anderson, R. Baisden, S. Baldwin, R. Borke, A. S. Bristol, Patricia Brown, Paul Brown, T. Castro, B. Chronister, C. Constantinidis, A. Craig, J. L. Culberson, V. Devisetty, E. Dietrichs, J. Evans, B. Falls, C. Forehand, R. Frederickson, G. C. Gaik, E. Garcis-Rill, G. Grunwald, B. Hallas, T. Imig, J. King, P. S. Lacy, A. Lamperti, G. R. Leichnetz, E. Levine, R. C. S. Lin, J. C. Lynch, T. McGraw-Ferguson, G. F. Martin, G. A. Mihailoff, M. V. Mishra, R. L. Norman, R. E. Papka, A. N. Perry, K. Peusner, C. Phelps, H. J. Ralston, J. Rho, L. T. Robertson, D. Rosene, A. Rosenquist, I. Ross, J. D. Schlag, M. Schwartz, J. Scott, V. Seybold, L. Simmons, K. L. Simpson, D. Smith, S. Stensaas, C. Stefan, D. G. Thielemann, S. Thomas, M. Tomblyn, J. A. Tucker, D. Tolbert, F. Walberg, S. Walkley, M. Woodruff, M. Wyss, R. Yezierski and A. Y. Zubkov. I have greatly appreciated their comments and suggestions. The stained sections used in this Atlas are from the teaching collection in the Department of Anatomy at West Virginia University School of Medicine; the author was on the faculty at WVU from 1973 to 1985.

This Eighth Edition would not have been possible without the interest and support of the publisher, Lippincott Williams & Wilkins. I want to express thanks to my editors, Crystal Taylor (Acquisitions Editor), Catherine Noonan (Associate Product Manager), Joy Fisher-Williams (Marketing Manager), Bridgett Dougherty (Vendor Manager), Amanda Ingold (Editorial Assistant), and especially Kelly Horvath (Freelance Editor) for their encouragement, continuing interest, and confidence in this project. Their cooperation has given me the opportunity to make the improvements seen herein.

Lastly, but clearly not least, I want to express a special thanks to my wife, Gretchen. The significant changes made in this edition required attention to many, and multiple, details. She carefully and critically reviewed all of the text, patiently listened to more neurobiology than she could have ever imagined, and gleefully informed me about rules of grammar and punctuation that I am not sure I even knew existed. I gladly dedicate this Eighth Edition to Gretchen.

Table of Contents

Duane E. Haines, Ph.D.

Recipient of the 2008 Henry Gray/Elsevier Distinguished Educator Award from The American Association of Anatomists

Elected a Fellow of the American Association of Anatomists and a Fellow of the American Association for the Advancement of Science

Recipient of the 2010 Alpha Omega Alpha Robert J. Glaser Distinguished Teacher Award from AOA and The Association of American Medical Colleges

Neuroanatomy Consultant for Stedman's Medical Dictionary and for Dorland's Illustrated Medical Dictionary

1

Introduction and Reader's Guide

The new edition of this atlas continues the tradition of emphasizing the anatomy of the central nervous system (CNS) in a clinically relevant format. It offers an initial learning opportunity that is as directly relevant, as reasonably possible, to how the same information will be applied in the clinical years. This approach includes, but is not limited to, 1) correlating CNS anatomy with what is seen in magnetic resonance imaging (MRI) and computer tomography (CT) and using these images to teach basic concepts; 2) introducing, at the appropriate times, literally hundreds of clinical terms, phrases, and examples that are in the proper anatomical and clinical context; 3) highlighting cerebrovascular anatomy with clinical examples; 4) developing the skills and understanding of the basic concepts that will expedite diagnosis of the neurologically compromised patient; 5) focusing on closely related topics in concise chapters; and 6) emphasizing the structure and function of pathways, and their corresponding deficits when lesions appear therein, in a clinical orientation.

Understanding central nervous system structure is the basis for learning pathways, neural function, and developing the skill to diagnose the neurologically impaired patient. Following a period devoted to the mastery of CNS morphology, a significant portion of most courses is spent learning functional systems in their clinical context. This learning opportunity may take place in a laboratory setting or as a self-directed, independent learning experience. This atlas continues to offer a *comprehensive and integrated guide*—one that correlates: 1) external brain anatomy with MRI and blood supply; 2) meninges and ventricles with examples of meningeal infections, meningeal hemorrhage, tumors, and ventricular blood; 3) internal brain anatomy in *Clinical* and *Anatomical Orientations* with MRI, blood supply, including the organization of tracts and nuclei and many clinical examples; 4) summaries of clinically relevant pathways in both *Anatomical* and *Clinical Orientations* with neurotransmitters, numerous clinical correlations, and the essential concept of laterality; and (5) a large variety of images, such as angiogram, CT, MRI, magnetic resonance angiography (MRA), and magnetic resonance venography (MRV). All of this is in a convenient and informative format in which related information is located on facing pages.

The goal of this atlas is to show how essential a sound knowledge of anatomical information is to the clinical experience, to emphasize the clinical application of this information, and to provide many clinical examples in their proper context. The format is dynamic, flexible, and it emphasizes structure/function and lesion/deficit concepts, and makes the learning (or review) experience an interesting and rewarding exercise.

Recognizing that about 50% of intracranial events that result in neurological deficits are vascular related, vascular anatomy and territories are emphasized. Vascular patterns, both superficial and deep, are correlated with external spinal cord and brain anatomy (Chapter 2) and internal structures, such as tracts and nuclei (Chapter 6); reviewed in each pathway drawing (Chapter 8); and shown in angiograms, MRAs, and MRVs (Chapter 9). This approach has several advantages: 1) the vascular pattern is *immediately* related to the structures just learned; (2) vascular patterns are shown in the sections of the atlas in which they belong and *in their proper context*; (3) the reader cannot proceed from one part of the atlas to the next without being reminded of blood supply; and (4) the conceptual importance of the distribution pattern of blood vessels in the CNS is repeatedly reinforced.

A thorough knowledge of systems (pathways and reflexes), including their blood supply, is essential to diagnosis the neurologically compromised patient. To this end, Chapter 8 provides a series of semi-diagrammatic illustrations of various clinically relevant

pathways in both *Anatomical* and *Clinical Orientations*. New to this chapter is an extensive series of *spinal cord and brainstem reflexes* that includes the afferent limb and its fiber type, the circuit within the CNS, the efferent limb, and the functional characteristics of the reflex. These images of pathways and reflexes show: 1) the trajectory of fibers that comprises the entire reflex or pathway; 2) the laterality of fibers comprising the reflex or pathway, this being an extremely important concept in diagnosis; 3) the positions and somatotopy of fibers comprising each pathway at representative levels; (4) a review of the blood supply to the entire pathway; 5) important neurotransmitters associated with fibers of the pathway; 6) examples of deficits seen following lesions of the pathway at various levels throughout the neuraxis; and 7) functional correlates of normal and damaged reflexes. The pathway illustrations in *Clinical Orientation* emphasize the location of tracts in MRI, thereby placing the tract in its proper clinical context. These figures also provide numerous representative examples of lesions, and the corresponding deficits, at different levels of the tract as it passes through the CNS. This approach allows the user maximum latitude in learning the organization of pathways and reflexes, but emphasizes this information in an orientation that will be most useful in the clinical setting. This chapter is designed to be used by itself or integrated with other sections of the atlas; to provide the reader with the structural and clinical essentials of a given pathway in sets of illustrations in both *Anatomical* and *Clinical Orientations*, and to accommodate a variety of instructional approaches.

The advent and common use of imaging methods (MRI, CT, MRA, and MRV) mandates that such images become integral parts of the educational process when teaching and/or learning clinically applicable neuroscience. To this end, this book contains about 260 MRI, CT, MRA, and MRV, plus a variety of angiograms. Most of these images are *directly* correlated with external brain anatomy, such as gyri and sulci, internal structures, including pathways and nuclei, cranial nerves and adjacent structures, or they demonstrate examples of hemorrhages related to the meninges and ventricles or the parenchyma of the brain.

Imaging the Brain (CT and MRI)

Imaging the brain *in vivo* is now commonplace for the patient with neurological deficits. Even most rural hospitals have, or have easy access to, CT or MRI. With this in mind, it is appropriate to make a few general comments on these imaging techniques and what is routinely seen, or best seen, in each. For details of the methods and techniques of CT and MRI, consult sources such as Grossman (1996), Lee et al. (1999), Osborn (1994, 2008), or Buxton (2002).

Computed Tomography (CT)

In CT, the patient is passed between a source of x-rays and a series of detectors. Tissue density is measured by the effects of x-rays on atoms within the tissue as these x-rays pass through the tissue. Atoms of higher number have a greater ability to attenuate (stop) x-rays, whereas those with lower numbers are less able to attenuate x-rays. The various attenuation intensities are computerized into numbers (Hounsfield units or CT numbers). Bone is given the value of $+1,000$ and is white, whereas air is given a value of $-1,000$ and is black. In this respect, a lesion or defect in a CT that is *hyperdense* is shifted toward the appearance of bone; it is more whiter. For example, acute subarachnoid blood in CT is *hyperdense* to the surrounding brain; it is more whiter than the brain and is shifted more to the appearance of bone (Figure 1-1). A lesion in CT that is *hypodense* is shifted toward the appearance of air or cerebrospinal fluid; it is more blacker than the surrounding brain (Figure 1-2). In this

Table 1-1 The Brain and Related Structures in CT

STRUCTURE/FLUID/SPACE	GRAY SCALE
Bone, acute blood	Very white
Enhanced tumor	Very white
Subacute blood	Light gray
Muscle	Light gray
Gray matter	Light gray
White matter	Medium gray
Cerebrospinal fluid	Medium gray to black
Air, fat	Very black

1-1 CT in the axial plane of a patient with subarachnoid hemor-rhage. Bone is white, acute blood (white) outlines the sub-arachnoid space, brain is gray, and cerebrospinal fluid in third and lateral ventricles is black.

example, the territory of the middle cerebral artery is *hypodense* (Figure 1-2). *Isodense* in CT refers to a condition in which the lesion and the surrounding brain have textures and/or shades of gray that are essentially the same. *Iso-* is Greek for equal: "equal density." Extravascular blood, an enhanced tumor, fat, the brain (gray and white matter), and cerebrospinal fluid form an interven-ing continuum from white to black. A CT image of a patient with subarachnoid hemorrhage illustrates the various shades seen in a CT (Figure 1-1). In general, Table 1-1 summarizes the white to black intensities seen for selected tissues in CT.

The advantages of CT are: 1) it is done rapidly, which is espe-cially important in trauma; 2) it clearly shows acute and subacute hemorrhages into the meningeal spaces and brain; 3) it is especially useful for children in trauma cases; 4) it shows bone (and skull frac-tures) to advantage; and 5) it is less expensive than MRI. The disad-

vantages of CT are: 1) it does not clearly show acute or subacute infarcts or ischemia, or brain edema; 2) it does not clearly differenti-ate white from gray matter within the brain nearly as well as MRI, and 3) it exposes the patient to ionizing radiation.

Magnetic Resonance Imaging (MRI)

The tissues of the body contain proportionately large amounts of protons (hydrogen). Protons have a positive nucleus, a shell of neg-ative electrons, and a north and south pole; they function like tiny spinning bar magnets. Normally, these atoms are arranged ran-domly in relation to each other because of the constantly changing magnetic field produced by the electrons. MRI uses this characteris-tic of protons to generate images of the brain and body.

When radio waves are sent in short bursts into the magnet contain-ing the patient, they are called a radiofrequency pulse (RP). This pulse may vary in strength. When the frequency of the RP matches the fre-quency of the spinning proton, the proton will absorb energy from the radio wave (resonance). The effect is twofold. First, the magnetic effects of some protons are canceled out; second, the magnetic effects and energy levels in others are increased. When the RP is turned off, the relaxed protons release energy (an "echo") that is received by a coil and computed into an image of that part of the body.

The two major types of MRI images (MRI/T1 and MRI/T2) are related to the effect of RP on protons and the reactions of these pro-tons (relaxation) when the RP is turned off. In general, those can-celled out protons return slowly to their original magnetic strength. The image constructed from this time constant is called T1 (Figure 1-3). On the other hand, those protons that achieved a higher energy level (were not cancelled out) lose their energy more rapidly as they return to their original state; the image constructed from this time constant is T2 (Figure 1-4). The creation of a T1-weighted

1-2 Axial CT showing a hypodense area within the territory of the middle cerebellar artery on the right side of the patient. This is indicative of a lesion in this region which would result in substantive deficits.

1-3 A sagittal T1-weighted MRI. Brain is gray, and cerebrospinal fluid is black.

1-4 A sagittal T2-weighted MRI. Brain is gray, blood vessels frequently appear black, and cerebrospinal fluid is white.

Table 1-2 The Brain and Related Structures in MRI

NORMAL	T1	T2
Bone	Very black	Very black
Air	Very black	Very black
Muscle	Dark gray	Dark gray
White matter	Light gray	Dark gray
Gray matter	Dark gray	Light gray
Fat	White	Gray
Cerebrospinal fluid	Very black	Very white

ABNORMAL	T1	T2
Edema	Dark gray	Light gray to white
Tumor	Variable	Variable
Enhanced tumor	White	(Rarely done)
Acute infarct	Dark gray	Light gray to white
Subacute infarct	Dark gray	Light gray to white
Acute ischemia	Dark gray	Light gray to white
Subacute ischemia	Dark gray	Light gray to white

image versus a T2-weighted image is based on a variation in the times used to receive the "echo" from the relaxed protons.

The terms *hyperintense, hypointense,* and *isointense* apply to T1- and T2-weighted MRI. *Hyperintense* in T1 is a shift toward the appearance of fat, which is white in the normal patient; a hyperintense lesion in T1 is more whiter than the surrounding brain (Figure 1-5A; Table 1-2). In this example, the tumor (a meningioma) and the surrounding edematous areas are *hyperintense*: more whiter than the surrounding brain (Figure 1-5A). In T2, *hyperintense* is a shift toward

the appearance of cerebrospinal fluid which is also white in the normal individual (Figure 1-4); a hyperintense condition in T2 is also more whiter than the surrounding brain (Table 1-2). *Hypointense* in both T1 and T2 is a shift toward the appearance of air or bone in the normal patient; this is a shift to more black than the surrounding brain. In this example of a T1 MRI, there are *hypointense* areas (*arrows*) adjacent to the lateral ventricles in frontal and occipital areas (Figure 1-5B); these are darker than the surrounding brain. *Isointense* refers to a situation in which a lesion and the surrounding brain have shades of gray and/or textures that are basically the same. In this example of a pituitary tumor in a T2 MRI, the color and texture of the tumor is essentially the same as the surrounding brain; it is *isointense* (Figure 1-5C). *Iso-* is Greek for equal: "equal intensity."

Table 1-2 summarizes the white to black intensities seen in MRI images that are T1-weighted versus T2-weighted. It should be emphasized that a number of variations on these two general MRI themes are routinely seen in the clinical environment.

The advantages of MRI are: 1) it can be manipulated to visualize a wide variety of abnormalities or abnormal states within the brain; and 2) it can show great detail of the brain in normal and abnormal states. The disadvantages of MRI are: 1) it does not show acute or subacute subarachnoid hemorrhage or hemorrhage into the substance of the brain in any detail; 2) it takes much longer to do and, therefore, is not useful in acute situations or in some types of trauma; 3) it is comparatively more expensive than CT; and 4) the scan is extremely loud and may require sedation in children.

The ensuing discussion briefly outlines the salient features of individual chapters. In some sections, considerable flexibility has been designed into the format; at these points, some suggestions are made as to how the atlas can be used. In addition, new clinical correlations and examples have been included, and Chapter 10, which contains questions in the style of the U.S. Medical Licensing Examination, has been revised and enlarged.

■ Chapter 2 ■

This chapter presents: 1) the gross anatomy of the spinal cord and its principal arteries; and 2) the external morphology of the brain from all views, including the insular cortex, accompanied by MRIs and drawings of the vasculature patterns from the same perspective. In this revised/reorganized chapter, emphasis is placed on correlating

1-5 Axial MRIs showing a hyperintense lesion, meningioma, and edema (**A**), hypointense areas in the white matter of the hemisphere (**B, arrows**), and a pituitary tumor (PT) that is isointense (**C**).

external brain and spinal cord anatomy with their respective vascular patterns. Clinical terminology, of the type encountered in the clinical setting, for the major branching patterns of the anterior, middle, and posterior cerebral arteries is emphasized (A_1–A_5, M_1–M_4, and P_1–P_4, respectively).

■ Chapter 3 ■

This chapter focuses on: 1) the relationships of cranial nerves; 2) their exits from the brainstem; 3) their appearance in representative MRI; and 4) examples of cranial nerve deficits seen in cases with lesions of the brainstem. Most pages in this chapter are laid out such that a gross view of one or more cranial nerves appears in a photograph at the top of the page followed by several MRIs of the same nerve(s). Also included is a new Table that summarizes many structural and functional points related to cranial nerves. In addition, there is also a detailed cross-reference to other sections of the Atlas where cranial nerve information is found.

■ Chapter 4 ■

This revised chapter focuses on four issues essential to clinical medicine as related to the nervous system: first, the structure of the meninges, with examples of tumors, infections, and hemorrhages related thereto; second, cisterns, their relationships to the brainstem, and examples of subarachnoid hemorrhages (which is, simply put, blood in the cisterns); third, the shape and relationships of the ventricles, with examples of blood in the ventricular system; and fourth, the locations of the choroid plexus within the ventricular system and examples of tumors of this important structure. Important new clinical information and concepts are introduced in this chapter.

■ Chapter 5 ■

The study of general morphology of the hemisphere and brainstem is continued in the two sections of Chapter 5. The first section contains a representative series of coronal slices of brain, each of which is accompanied, *on the same page*, by MRIs. The brain slice is labeled by complete names, some with abbreviations, and the MRIs are labeled with abbreviations that correspond to those on the brain slice. The second section contains a series of brain slices cut in the axial plane, each of which is accompanied, again *on the same page*, by MRIs. Labeling of the axial slices is done the same way as for the coronal slices.

The similarities between the brain slices and the MRIs are remarkable, and this style of presentation closely integrates anatomy in the slice with that as seen in the corresponding MRI. Because the brain, as sectioned at autopsy or in clinical pathological conferences, is viewed as an unstained specimen, the preference here is to present the material in a format that will most closely parallel what is seen in these clinical situations.

■ Chapter 6 ■

This new edition improves on the innovation of illustrating images in their classic *Anatomical Orientation* and providing for their conversion to the *Clinical Orientation* on each set of facing pages. The *Clinical Orientation* is universally recognized in the clinical setting and clinical imaging techniques.

The previous edition of this atlas offered numerous online extras including gross brain dissections, approximately 38 color brain slices in axial, coronal, and sagittal planes, and the capability to flip selected axial images of the brainstem from an *Anatomical Orientation* to a *Clinical Orientation*. This third option is especially applicable to clinical medicine. Flipping an image from *Anatomical Orientation* to *Clinical Orientation* places everything in the image (be it a line drawing or stained section) into a clinical format: 1) the image shape directly matches a corresponding MRI or CT, 2) the image now has right and left sides—remember, it matches MRI and CT and, 3) all tracts in the image match exactly their position, topography, etc, as it appears in the clinical setting. Images in Chapter 6 that can be flipped to a *Clinical Orientation* are identified by this symbol in the lower left of the image.

Clinical Orientation
Image Image
Online

All stained sections and line drawings with this symbol can be flipped, using online resources, from Anatomical to Clinical Orientations by clicking on the curved arrow (place the cursor on this arrow and it says 'Flip the image') at the lower right margin of the screen. All labels will follow the flip, so all internal structures can be identified, or used in other formats (such as labels on/off), in the Clinical Orientation. An especially poignant example of the importance of the Clinical Orientation: the face is represented upside down in the spinal trigeminal tract and nucleus in the Anatomical Orientation, but is represented right side up in the Clinical Orientation. The value of the Clinical Orientation is intuitively obvious.

Chapter 6 consists of six sections covering, in sequence, the spinal cord, medulla oblongata, cerebellar nuclei, pons, midbrain, and diencephalon and basal nuclei, all with MRI. In this format, the right-hand page contains a complete image of the stained section. The left-hand page contains a labeled line drawing of the stained section, accompanied by a figure description, and a small orientation drawing. In this new edition, *all stained sections of the CNS in cross section (spinal cord through forebrain) in Chapter 6 now appear in full color*.

Beginning with the first spinal cord level (sacral, Figure 6-1), the long tracts most essential to understanding how to diagnose the neurologically impaired patient are colored. These are the posterior column–medial lemniscus system, the lateral corticospinal tract, and the anterolateral system. In the brainstem, these tracts are joined by the colorized spinal trigeminal tract, the ventral trigeminothalamic tract, and all of the motor and sensory nuclei of cranial nerves. This scheme continues rostrally into the caudal nuclei of the dorsal thalamus and the posterior limb of the internal capsule. Each page has a color key that specifies the structure and function of each colored structure. This approach emphasizes anatomical–clinical integration.

Semi-diagrammatic representations of the internal blood supply to the spinal cord, medulla, pons, midbrain, and forebrain follow each set of line drawings and stained sections. This allows the immediate, and convenient, correlation of structure with its blood supply as one is studying the internal anatomy of the neuraxis. In addition, *tables that summarize the vascular syndromes or lesions of the spinal cord, medulla, pons, midbrain, and forebrain* are located on the pages facing each of these vascular drawings. This approach allows for an easy correlation between which vessel may be occluded, the structures located within this vascular territory, and the deficits that may result. Successful diagnosis requires excellent knowledge of what structure is served by what vessel.

The internal anatomy of the brainstem is commonly taught in an *Anatomical Orientation*. That is, posterior structures, such as the vestibular nuclei and colliculi, are "up" in the image, whereas anterior structures, such as the pyramid and crus cerebri, are "down" in the image. However, when the brainstem is viewed in the clinical setting, as in CT or MRI, this orientation is reversed. In the *Clinical Orientation*, posterior structures (4th ventricle, colliculi) are "down" in the image, whereas anterior structures (pyramid, basilar pons, crus cerebri) are "up" in the image.

Recognizing that many users of this book are pursuing a health care career, it is essential to correlate brainstem anatomy with MRI and CT. This allows correlation of the size, shape, and configuration of brainstem sections (line drawings and stained slices) with MRI and CT at comparable levels. It also offers the user the opportunity to visualize how nuclei, tracts (and their somatotopy) and vascular territories are represented in MRI and CT. Understanding the brain in the *Clinical Orientation* (as seen in MRI or CT) is absolutely essential to diagnosis.

The continuum from *Anatomical Orientation* to *Clinical Orientation* is achieved by: 1) placing a small version of the colorized line drawing on the facing page (page with the stained section) in *Anatomical Orientation*; 2) showing how this image is flipped top to bottom into a *Clinical Orientation*; and 3) following this flipped image with (usually) T1 and T2 MRIs at levels comparable to the accompanying line drawing and stained section (Figure 1-6). The internal structures outlined *on each T1-weighted MRI*

1-7 CT of a patient following injection of a radiopaque contrast media into the lumbar cistern. In this example, at the medullary level (a cisternogram), neural structures appear gray and the subarachnoid space appears light.

Anatomical orientation   Clinical orientation

Py
ML
PO
ALS
SpTTr + SpTNu
NuCu
NuGr
HyNu

MRI, T1-weighted image

MRI, T2-weighted image

CT cisternogram

1-6 An example of the brainstem showing anatomical and clinical orientations at about the caudal one-third of the medulla and the corresponding T1-weighted MRI (with especially important structures labeled), T2-MRI, and CT-cisternogram. The abbreviations are keyed to the full label on the facing page in Chapter 6. For additional examples and details of brainstem and spinal cord, see Chapter 6.

(brainstem) and CT (spinal cord) image at levels corresponding with the stained section and line drawing are those fundamental to understanding the neurologically compromised patient. This approach clearly illustrates how anatomical information and concepts are arranged, and used, in images (MRI and CT) that are commonplace in the clinical environment.

Every effort has been made to use MRI and CT that match, as closely as possible, the line drawings and stained sections in the spinal cord and brainstem portions of Chapter 6. Recognizing that this match is subject to the vicissitudes of angle and individual variation, special sets of images were used in Chapter 6. The first set consisted of T1- and T2-weighted MRI generated from the same individual. The second set consisted of CT images from a patient who had an injection of the radiopaque contrast medium Isovue-M 200 (iopamidol injection 41%) into the lumbar cistern. This contrast medium diffused throughout the spinal and cranial subarachnoid spaces, outlining the spinal cord and brainstem (Figure 1-7). Images at spinal levels show neural structures as gray surrounded by a light subarachnoid space; this is a "CT myelogram." A comparable image at brainstem levels is a "CT cisternogram."

The juxtaposition of MRI to stained section extends into the forebrain section of Chapter 6. Many anatomical features seen in the forebrain stained sections are easily identified in the adjacent MRI. These particular MRIs are not labeled so as to allow the user to develop and practice his or her interpretive skills. The various subsections of Chapter 6 can be used in a variety of ways and will accommodate a wide range of student and/or instructor preferences.

■ Chapter 7 ■

The photographs of stained axial and sagittal sections in Chapter 7 *are now presented in full color*, are still accompanied with their respective MRIs, and are organized to provide four important levels of information. First, the *general* internal anatomy of brain structures can be identified in each photograph. Second, axial photographs are on left-hand pages and arranged from dorsal to ventral (Figures 7-1 to 7-9), whereas sagittal photographs are on right-hand pages and arranged from medial to lateral (Figures 7-2 to 7-10). This provides complete representation of the brain in *both* planes for use as independent study sets (axial only, sagittal only) or as integrated/correlated sets (compare facing pages). Third, because axial and sagittal sections are on facing pages *and* the plane of each section is indicated on its companion by a heavy line, the user can easily visualize the positions of internal structures in more than one plane and develop a clear concept of three-dimensional topography. In other words, one can identify structures dorsal or ventral to the axial plane by comparing them with the sagittal, and structures medial or lateral to the sagittal plane by comparing them with the axial. Fourth, the inclusion of MRIs with representative axial and sagittal stained sections provides excellent examples of the fact that structures seen in stained sections are easy to recognize in clinical images.

▪ Chapter 8 ▪

This chapter contains summaries of a variety of clinically relevant CNS tracts and/or pathways in both *Anatomical and Clinical Orientations* and introduces *a new series of circuit drawings and flow-charts that details pathways for spinal and brainstem/cranial nerve reflexes.* This chapter has four features that enhance the user's understanding of facts that are especially relevant to the clinical setting. First, the inclusion of pathway information in atlas format broadens the basis one can use to teach functional neurobiology. This is especially the case when pathways are presented in a style that enhances the development of diagnostic skills. Second, each figure, either in *Anatomical or Clinical Orientation*, illustrates a particular pathway in its entirety by showing: 1) its origins, longitudinal extent, course throughout the neuraxis and termination; 2) its laterality—an all-important issue in diagnosis; 3) its point of decussation, if applicable; 4) its position in representative cross sections of the brainstem and spinal cord; and 5) the somatotopic organization of fibers within the pathway, if applicable. The blood supply to each pathway is also reviewed. Third, a brief summary mentions the main neuroactive substances associated with cells and fibers composing particular segments of the pathway under consideration. The action of the substance, if widely agreed on, is indicated as excitatory (+) or inhibitory (−). *This allows the reader to correlate closely a particular neurotransmitter with a specific population of projection neurons and their terminals.* The limits of this approach, within the confines of an atlas format, are self-evident: transmitters associated with some pathways are not well-known; colocalized substances are not identified; and transmitter synthesis and degradation are not discussed. Fourth, *the clinical correlations that accompany each pathway drawing provide examples of deficits resulting from lesions, at various levels in the neuraxis, of the fibers composing that specific pathway.* Also, examples are given of syndromes or diseases in which these deficits are seen. The drawings in this section were designed to provide the maximal amount of information, to keep the extraneous points to a minimum, and to do it all in a single, easy-to-follow illustration.

Interspersed within the pathway drawings in *Anatomical Orientation* are 13 sets of facing pages (a total of 26 pages) of pathways in a *Clinical Orientation* (Figures 1-8, 1-9). These are spaced so as to immediately follow, and complement, the corresponding pathway presented in an *Anatomical Orientation*. These *Clinical Orientation* pathways focus on cranial nerves and on those long tracts that are especially important to the diagnosis of the impaired patient. Lesions at representative levels, and their corresponding deficits, are also a feature of these pathways in *Clinical Orientation* (Figure 1-9). This approach recognizes that in some educational settings the pathways are taught Anatomically, whereas in others the emphasis is on Clinical Orientation; both approaches are accommodated in this atlas. However, it is appropriate to emphasize that when viewing the MRI of patients who are neurologically compromised by lesion or disease, *all of the internal anatomy and tracts are*

1-8 The medulla, pons, and midbrain portions of the posterior column–medial lemniscus pathway (see Figure 8-5A for the entire pathway) superimposed on MRI and shown in a *Clinical Orientation*. For convenience only, this example from Figure 8-5A is reduced here to fit in a single column.

in a Clinical Orientation. It is essential that students *recognize and understand* this fact of clinical reality.

Because it is not possible to anticipate *all* pathways that may be taught in a wide range of neurobiology courses, flexibility has been designed into Chapter 8. The last figure in each section is a blank master drawing that follows the same general format as the preceding figures. Photocopies of these blank master drawings can be used by the student for learning and/or reviewing any pathway and by the instructor to teach additional pathways not included in the atlas or to use as a substrate for examination questions.

1-9 The medulla, pons, and midbrain portions of the posterior column-medial lemniscus pathway (see Figure 8-5B for the entire pathway) superimposed on MRI in a *Clinical Orientation*, with lesions and corresponding deficits at representative levels. For convenience only, this example from Figure 8-5B is reduced here to fit in a single column.

■ Chapter 9 ■

This chapter contains a series of angiograms (arterial and venous phases), magnetic resonance angiography (MRA) images, and magnetic resonance venography (MRV) images. The angiograms are shown in lateral and anterior–posterior projections—some as standard views with corresponding digital subtraction images. MRA and MRV technology are noninvasive methods that allow for the visualization of arteries (MRA) and veins and venous sinuses (MRV). However, there are many situations when both arteries and veins are seen with either method. Use of MRA and MRV is commonplace, and this technology is an important diagnostic tool.

■ Chapter 10 ■

A primary goal in the study of functional human neurobiology is to become a competent health care professional. Another, and equally significant, goal is to pass examinations. These may be course examinations, the National Board Subject Examination (many courses require these); or standardized tests, such as the USMLE Step 1 and Step 2, given at key intervals and taken by all students.

The questions comprising Chapter 10 were generated in the recognition that examinations are an essential part of the educational process. Whenever possible, and practical, these questions are in the USMLE Step-1 style (single best answer). These questions emphasize: 1) anatomical and clinical concepts and correlations; 2) the application of basic human neurobiology to medical practice; and 3) how neurological deficits and diseases relate to damage in specific parts of the nervous system. In general, the questions are grouped by chapter. However, in some instances, questions draw on information provided in more than one chapter. This is sometimes essential in an effort to make appropriate structural/functional/clinical correlations. At the end of each group of questions the correct answers are provided, explained, and referenced to a page (or pages) in which further information may be found. Although not exhaustive, this list of questions should provide the user with an excellent opportunity for self-assessment covering a broad range of clinically relevant topics.

■ References ■

1. Bruxton RB. *Introduction to Functional Magnetic Resonance Imaging, Principles and Techniques*. Cambridge, UK: Cambridge University Press, 2002.
2. Grossman CB. Magnetic *Resonance Imaging and Computed Tomography of the Head and Spine*. 2nd Ed. Baltimore: Williams & Wilkins, 1996.
3. Lee SH, Roa KCVG, Zimmerman RA. *Cranial MRI and CT*. 4th Ed. New York, NY: McGraw-Hill Health Professions Division, 1999.
4. Osborn AG. *Diagnostic Neuroradiology*. St. Louis: Mosby, 1994.
5. Osborn AG. *Year Book of Diagnostic Radiology*. St. Louis: Mosby, 2008.

2

External Morphology of the Central Nervous System

Posterior View

C2 Posterior root (PR)

Dura

Arachnoid

C3 PR

Posterior spinal
artery

Denticulate
ligament

C4 PR

Posterior spinal
medullary artery

C5 PR

Anterior View

C2 Anterior root (AR)

Dura

Denticulate
ligament

C3 AR

Arachnoid

Anterior spinal
medullary artery

C4 AR

Anterior spinal
artery

C5 AR

2-1 Posterior (upper) and anterior (lower) views showing the general features of the spinal cord as seen at levels C2–C5. The dura and arachnoid are reflected, and the pia is intimately adherent to the spinal cord and rootlets. Posterior and anterior spinal medullary arteries (see also Figure 2-3 on facing page) follow their respective roots. The posterior spinal artery is found medial to the entering posterior rootlets (and the dorsolateral sulcus), whereas the anterior spinal artery is in the anterior median fissure (see also Figure 2-2, facing page).

Radiculopathy results from spinal nerve root damage. The most common causes are *intervertebral disc disease/protrusion* or *spondylolysis*, and the main symptoms are *pain radiating in a root or dermatomal distribution*, and *weakness*, and *hyporeflexia* of the muscles served by the affected root. The discs most commonly involved at cervical (C) and lumbar (L) levels are C6–C7 (65%–70%), C5–C6 (16%–20%), L4–L5 (40%–45%), and L5–S1 (35%–40%). Thoracic disc problems are rare, well under 1% of all disc protrusions.

Posterior View

Sulci:
- Posterior median
- Posterior intermediate
- Posterolateral

C7 Posterior root

Spinal (posterior root) ganglion

Fasciculus gracilis
Fasciculus cuneatus

Anterior View

Anterior spinal artery

Anterior radicular artery

C7 Anterior root

Anterior funiculus

Anterior median fissure

2-2 Posterior (upper) and anterior (lower) views showing details of the spinal cord as seen in the C7 segment. The posterior (dorsal) root ganglion is partially covered by dura and connective tissue.

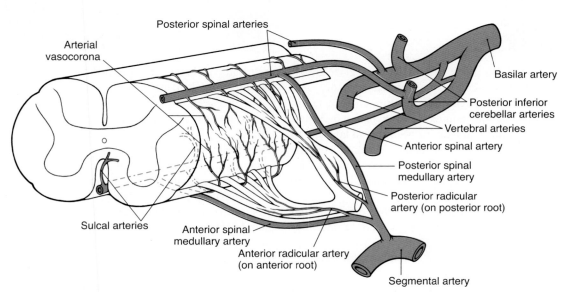

Posterior spinal arteries

Arterial vasocorona

Basilar artery

Posterior inferior cerebellar arteries

Vertebral arteries

Anterior spinal artery

Posterior spinal medullary artery

Posterior radicular artery (on posterior root)

Sulcal arteries

Anterior spinal medullary artery

Anterior radicular artery (on anterior root)

Segmental artery

2-3 Semi-diagrammatic representation showing the origin and general location of principal arteries supplying the spinal cord. The *anterior and posterior radicular arteries* arise at every spinal level and serve their respective roots and ganglia. The *anterior and posterior spinal medullary arteries* (also called **medullary feeder arteries** or **segmental medullary arteries**) arise at intermittent levels and serve to augment the blood supply to the spinal cord. The **artery of Adamkiewicz** is an unusually large spinal medullary artery arising usually on the left in low thoracic or upper lumbar levels (T9–L1). The arterial vasocorona is a diffuse anastomotic plexus covering the cord surface.

A   B   C

Thoracic
cord

T9

Dura and
arachnoid

Lumbar and
sacral cord
(LuSaCd)

LuSaCd

L1

Sacral and
coccygeal
cord
(SaCoCd)

SaCoCd

Conus
medullaris

Lumbar
cistern

Filum
terminale
internum
(FTInt)

FTInt

Cauda
equina
(CaEq)

CaEq

L5

Posterior
root
ganglion

S1

Dura and
arachnoid

2-4 Overall posterior (**A,B**) and sagittal MRI (**C**, T2-weighted) views of the lower thoracic, lumbar, sacral, and coccygeal spinal cord segments and the cauda equina. The dura and arachnoid are retracted in **A** and **B**. The cauda equina is shown in situ in **A**, and in **B** the nerve roots of the cauda equina have been spread laterally to expose the conus medullaris and filum terminale internum. This latter structure is also called the pial part of the filum terminale. See Figures 6-1 and 6-2 on pp. 94–97 for cross-sectional views of the cauda equina.

In the sagittal MRI (**C**), the lower portions of the cord, the filum terminale internum, and cauda equina are clearly seen. In addition, the intervertebral discs and the bodies of the vertebrae are clear. The *lumbar cistern* is an enlarged part of the subarachnoid space caudal to the end of the spinal cord. This space contains the anterior and posterior roots from the lower part of the spinal cord that collectively form the *cauda equina*. The filum terminale internum also descends from the conus medullaris through the lumbar cistern to attach to the inner surface of the dural sac. The dural sac ends at about the level of the S2 vertebra and is attached to the coccyx by

the filum terminale externum (also see Figure 4-1 on p. 57). A *lumbar puncture* is made by inserting a large-gauge needle (18–22 gauge) between the L4 and L5 (preferred) vertebrae or the L3 and L4 vertebrae and retrieving a sample of cerebrospinal fluid from the lumbar cistern. This sample may be used for a number of diagnostic procedures.

A *cauda equina syndrome* may be seen in an extruded disc (L4–L5 more common level) that impinges on the cauda equina and in patients with tumor, trauma, or other conditions that damage these nerve roots. The symptoms are usually bilateral and may include: 1) significant *weakness* (paraplegia is a possible outcome) and hypo- or areflexia of the lower extremity; 2) *saddle anesthesia* (commonly seen), which presents as sensory deficits on the buttocks, medial and posterior aspects of thighs, genitalia and anus, and perineum; 3) *urinary retention* (commonly seen) or *incontinence*, decreased sphincter tone, and fecal incontinence; and 4) *decrease in sexual function* (may appear later if cause is left untreated). Although sensory loss is common, these patients may or may not experience low back pain or *sciatica*.

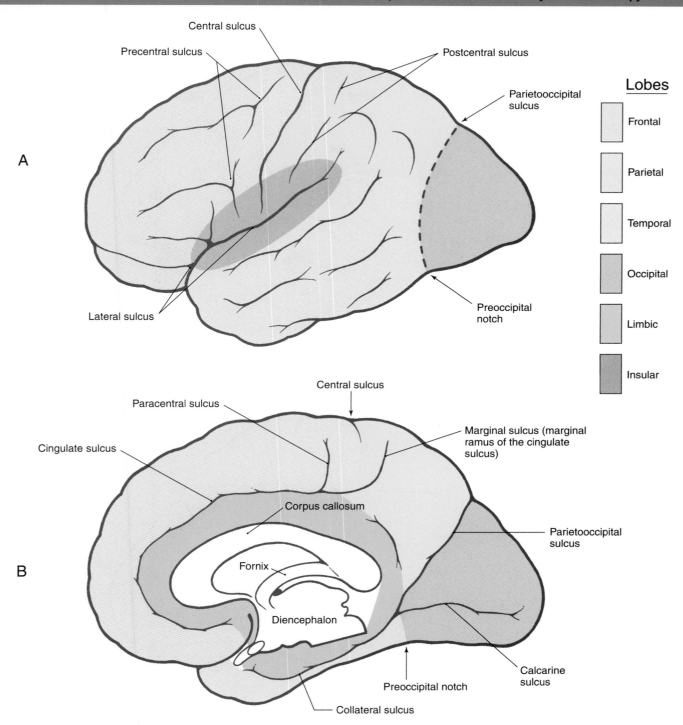

2-5 Lateral (**A**) and medial (**B**) views of the cerebral hemisphere showing the landmarks used to divide the cortex into its main lobes.

On the lateral aspect, the central sulcus (of Rolando) separates frontal and parietal lobes. The lateral sulcus (of Sylvius) forms the border between frontal and temporal lobes. The occipital lobe is located caudal to an arbitrary line drawn between the terminus of the parieto-occipital sulcus and the preoccipital notch. A horizontal line drawn from approximately the upper two-thirds of the lateral fissure to the rostral edge of the occipital lobe represents the border between parietal and temporal lobes. The insular cortex (see also Figures 2-39 to 2-41 on pp. 38 and 39) is located internal to the lat-

eral sulcus. This part of the cortex is made up of long and short gyri that are separated from each other by the central sulcus of the insula. The insula, as a whole, is separated from the adjacent portions of the frontal, parietal, and temporal opercula by the circular sulcus.

On the medial aspect, the cingulate sulcus separates medial portions of frontal and parietal lobes from the limbic lobe. An imaginary continuation of the central sulcus intersects with the cingulate sulcus and forms the border between frontal and parietal lobes. The parieto-occipital sulcus and an arbitrary continuation of this line to the preoccipital notch separate the parietal, limbic, and temporal lobes from the occipital lobe.

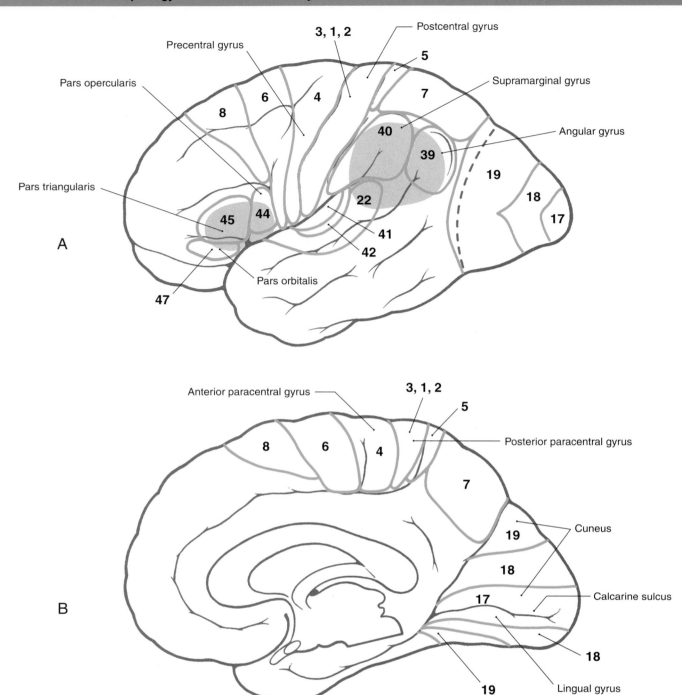

2-6 Lateral (**A**) and medial (**B**) views of the cerebral hemisphere showing the more commonly described Brodmann areas. In general, area 4 comprises the primary somatomotor cortex, areas 3, 1, and 2 the primary somatosensory cortex, and area 17 the primary visual cortex. Area 41 is the primary auditory cortex, and the portion of area 6 in the caudal part of the middle frontal gyrus is generally recognized as the frontal eye field.

The inferior frontal gyrus has three portions: a pars opercularis, pars triangularis, and a pars orbitalis. A lesion that is located primarily in areas 44 and 45 (shaded) will give rise to what is called a *Broca aphasia*, also called *motor, expressive,* or *nonfluent aphasia*. These patients do not have paralysis of the vocal apparatus, but rather have great difficulty turning ideas into meaningful speech. These patients may have *mutism* or slow, labored speech that consists of familiar single words or short phrases with words left out (*telegraphic speech*). These patients are well aware of their deficits.

The inferior parietal lobule consists of supramarginal (area 40) and angular (area 39) gyri. Lesions in this general area of the cortex (shaded), and sometimes extending into area 22, will give rise to what is known as *Wernicke aphasia*, also sometimes called *sensory, receptive,* or *fluent aphasia*. Patients with a sensory aphasia speak freely and without hesitation, but what is said may make little sense due to the use of inappropriate words at inappropriate places in the sentences (*paraphasia,* or sometimes called *word salad*). These patients may be unaware of their deficits.

2-7 Lateral (**A**) and medial (**B**) views of the cerebral hemisphere showing the somatotopic organization of the primary somatomotor and somatosensory cortices. The lower extremity and foot areas are located on medial aspects of the hemisphere in the anterior paracentral (motor) and the posterior paracentral (sensory) gyri. The remaining portions of the body extend from the margin of the hemisphere over the convexity to the lateral sulcus in the precentral and postcentral gyri.

An easy way to remember the somatotopy of these important cortical areas is to divide the precentral and postcentral gyri generally into thirds: a lateral third that represents the face area, a middle third that represents the upper extremity and hand with particular emphasis on the hand, and a medial third that represents the trunk and hip. The rest of the body representation, lower extremity and foot, is on the medial aspect of the hemisphere in the anterior (motor) and posterior (sensory) paracentral gyri. Lesions of the somatomotor cortex result in motor deficits on the contralateral side of the body, whereas lesions in the somatosensory cortex result in a loss of sensory perception from the contralateral side of the body.

The medial surface of the right hemisphere (**B**) illustrates the position of the left portions of the visual field. The inferior visual quadrant is located in the primary visual cortex above the calcarine sulcus, whereas the superior visual quadrant is found in the cortex below the calcarine sulcus.

Longitudinal fissure

Superior frontal gyrus (SFGy)

Middle frontal gyrus (MFGy)

Superior frontal sulcus (SFSul)

Precentral sulcus (PrCSul)

Precentral gyrus (PrCGy)

Central sulcus (CSul)

Postcentral gyrus (PoCGy)

Postcentral sulcus

Precentral gyrus (PrCGy)

Central sulcus (CSul)

Supramarginal gyrus

Superior parietal lobule

Occipital gyri

Anterior cerebral arteries

MFGy

SFGy

SFSul

PrCSul

PrCGy

CSul

PoCGy

Falx cerebri

ACA territory

2-8 Superior (dorsal) view of the cerebral hemispheres showing the main gyri and sulci and an MRI (inverted inversion recovery—lower left) and a CT (lower right) identifying structures from the same perspective. Note the area of infarction representing the territory of the anterior cerebral artery (ACA). The infarcted area involves lower extremity, hip, and, possibly, lower trunk cortical areas; because the lesion is in the left hemisphere, the deficits are on the patient's right side.

Frontopolar branches of ACA

Orbitofrontal branches of MCA (M₄)

Callosomarginal branches (from ACA)

Branches of MCA (M₄)
Prerolandic

Rolandic

Parietal

Paracentral branches (from ACA)

Internal parietal branches (from ACA)

Angular branches of MCA (M₄)

Parieto-occipital sulcus

Branches of PCA
Parieto-occipital (P₄)

Calcarine (P₄)

2-9 Superior (dorsal) view of the cerebral hemispheres showing the location and general branching patterns of the anterior (ACA), middle (MCA), and posterior (PCA) cerebral arteries.

Compare the distribution of ACA branches with the infarcted area in Figure 2-8 on the facing page.

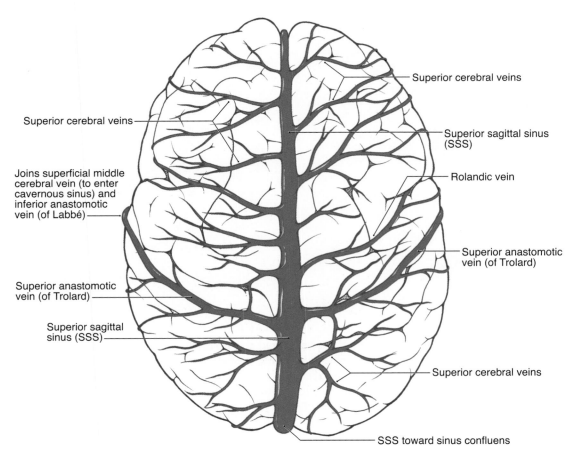

Superior cerebral veins

Superior cerebral veins

Superior sagittal sinus (SSS)

Joins superficial middle cerebral vein (to enter cavernous sinus) and inferior anastomotic vein (of Labbé)

Rolandic vein

Superior anastomotic vein (of Trolard)

Superior anastomotic vein (of Trolard)

Superior sagittal sinus (SSS)

Superior cerebral veins

SSS toward sinus confluens

2-10 Superior (dorsal) view of the cerebral hemispheres showing the location of the superior sagittal sinus and the locations and general branching patterns of veins. See Figures 9-4 and

9-5 (pp. 297–298) for comparable angiograms (venous phase) of the superior sagittal sinus.

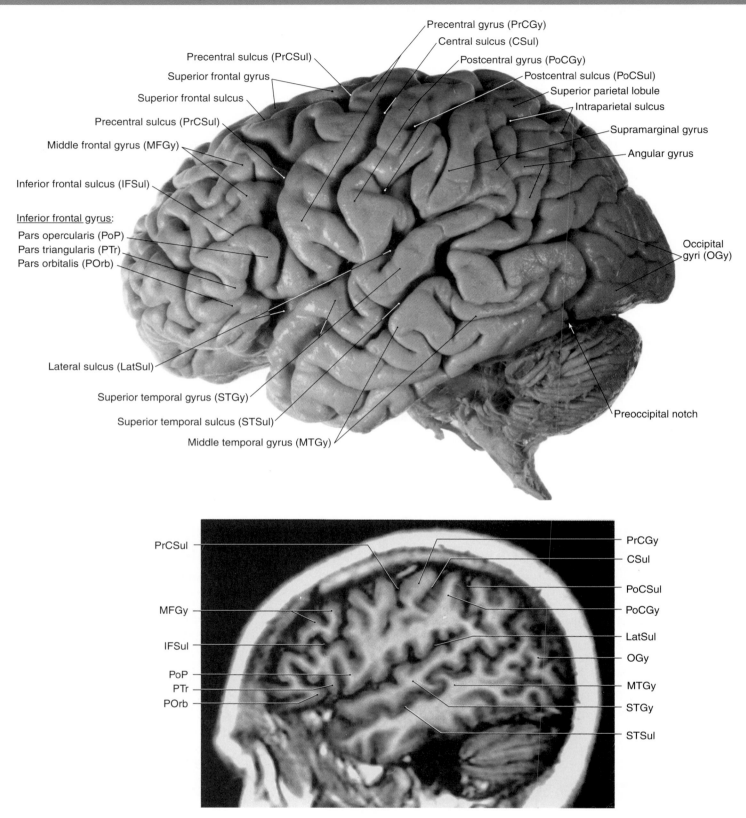

2-11 Lateral view of the left cerebral hemisphere showing the principal gyri and sulci and an MRI (inversion recovery) identifying many of these structures from the same perspective. Especially important cortical areas are the precentral and postcentral gryi (primary *somatomotor* and *somatosensory* cortex, respectively, for the body, excluding the lower extremity), the parts of the inferior frontal gyrus (partes opercularis, triangularis, and orbitalis), and the supramarginal and angular gyri that collectively form the inferior parietal lobule. The *frontal eye field* is located primarily in the caudal area of the middle frontal gyrus adjacent to the precentral gyrus.

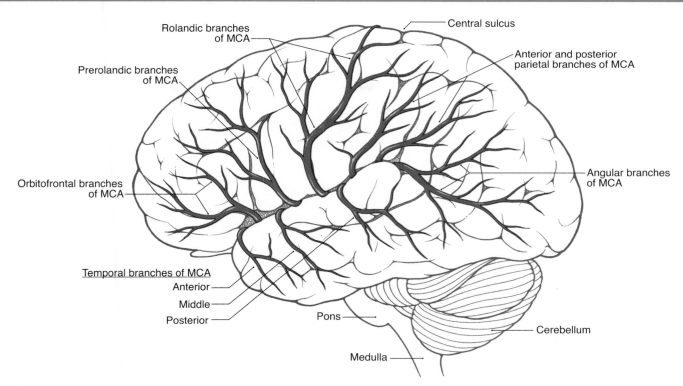

2-12 Lateral view of the left cerebral hemisphere showing the branching pattern of the middle cerebral artery. The middle cerebral artery initially branches in the depths of the lateral sulcus (as M_2 and M_3 segments: see Figures 2-40 and 2-41 on p. 39); these branches, when seen on the surface of the hemisphere, represent the M_4 segment. The individual branches of the overall M_4 segment are named usually according to their relationship to gyri, sulci, or position on a lobe. Terminal branches of the posterior and anterior cerebral arteries course over the edges of the temporal and occipital lobes, and parietal and frontal lobes, respectively (see Figure 2-9 on p. 17). See Figure 9-1 (p. 294) for a comparable angiogram of the middle and anterior cerebral arteries.

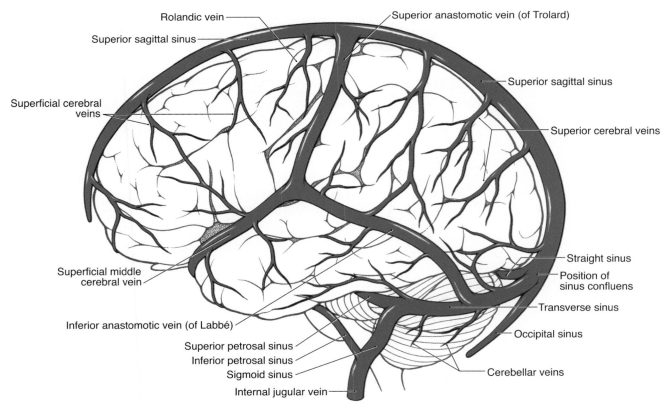

2-13 Lateral view of the left cerebral hemisphere showing the locations of sinuses and the locations and general branching patterns of veins. Communication between veins and sinuses or between sinuses also is indicated. See Figures 9-2 (p. 295) and 9-11 (p. 304) for comparable angiogram and MRV of the sinuses and superficial veins.

2-14 Inferior (ventral) view of the cerebral hemispheres and diencephalon with the brainstem caudal to midbrain removed and two MRIs (inversion recovery—lower left; T2-weighted—lower right) showing many structures from the same perspective. Note the relationships of the midbrain to surrounding structures (cerebellum, medial aspect of the temporal lobe, uncus [as related to *uncal herniation*], and hypothalamus and optic tract) and to the cisterns.

Orbital branches of ACA

Anterior cerebral
artery (ACA, A₂)

Internal carotid
artery

Posterior communicating
artery

Anterior temporal
branch of PCA
(P₃ segment)

P₃ segment of PCA

Posterior temporal
branch of PCA
(P₃ segment)

Orbitofrontal branches
of MCA (M₄)

Internal carotid
artery

Superior
trunk of MCA

M₁ segment of MCA

Inferior
trunk of MCA

Lenticulostriate
arteries

Posterior
communicating artery

Quadrigeminal
artery

Parieto-occipital branch
of PCA (P₄ segment)

Calcarine branch of
PCA (P₄ segment)

2-15 Inferior (ventral) view of the cerebral hemisphere, with the brainstem removed, showing segments P₁–P₄ of the posterior cerebral artery (PCA), a small portion of the anterior cerebral artery, and the initial branching of the M₁ segment of the middle cerebral artery into superior and inferior trunks. The correlation between the superior and inferior trunks of the MCA and segments M₂–M₄ are shown in Figure 2-41 on p. 39. There are four segments of the PCA, P₁–P₄.

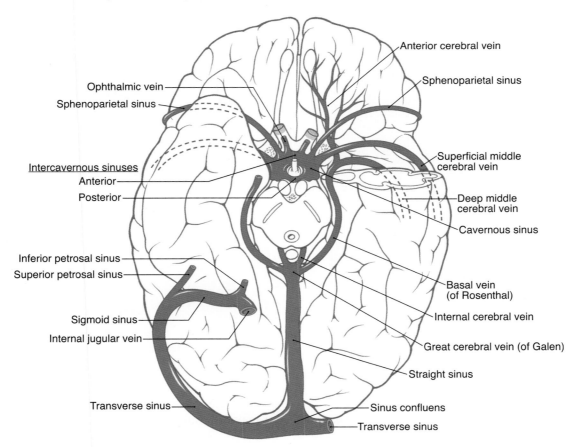

Ophthalmic vein

Sphenoparietal sinus

Intercavernous sinuses
Anterior
Posterior

Inferior petrosal sinus
Superior petrosal sinus

Sigmoid sinus

Internal jugular vein

Transverse sinus

Anterior cerebral vein

Sphenoparietal sinus

Superficial middle
cerebral vein

Deep middle
cerebral vein

Cavernous sinus

Basal vein
(of Rosenthal)

Internal cerebral vein

Great cerebral vein (of Galen)

Straight sinus

Sinus confluens

Transverse sinus

2-16 Inferior (ventral) view of the cerebral hemisphere, with the brainstem removed, showing the relationships of the main sinuses and the anterior cerebral vein, the deep middle cerebral vein, and the superficial middle cerebral vein. See Figures 9-5 (p. 298), 9-9 (p. 302), and 9-11 (p. 304) for comparable views of these veins and sinuses.

Frontal pole
Longitundinal fissure
Olfactory bulb
Orbital sulci
Olfactory sulcus (OlfSul)
Orbital gyri (OrbGy)
Gyrus rectus (GyRec)
Olfactory tract
Temporal pole (TPole)
Basilar pons (BP)
Uncus
Occipitotemporal sulcus
Parahippocampal gyrus
Occipitotemporal gyri
Collateral sulcus
Glossopharyngeal nerve
Middle cerebellar peduncle (MCP)
Flocculus
Facial nerve
Vagus nerve
Vestibulocochlear nerve
Abducens nerve
Medulla
Olive (inferior); olivary eminence
Decussation of pyramids
Cerebellum (Cbl)

GyRec
OlfSul
OrbGy
Tpole
Trigeminal nerve
BP
MCP
Fourth ventricle
Cbl
BP

2-17 Inferior (ventral) view of the cerebral hemispheres, dien-cephalon, brainstem, and cerebellum, and two MRIs (both T1-weighted images) that show structures from the same perspective. Note the slight differences in the sizes of the fourth ventricle. The larger space seen in the right MRI is representative of a slightly lower axial plane through the pons when compared to the left MRI, which represents a slightly more superior plane. The latter is bordered by the superior cerebellar peduncles. A detailed view of the inferior (ventral) aspect of the brainstem is seen in Figure 2-20 on p. 24.

A₂ segment of ACA
A₁ segment of ACA
Posterior communicating artery
Superior cerebellar artery
Basilar artery
Anterior spinal artery
Posterior spinal artery

Anterior communicating artery
Ophthalmic artery
Internal carotid artery
Anterior, polar temporal, and uncal branches of M₁
Superior trunk of MCA
M₁ segment of MCA
Inferior trunk of MCA
Lenticulostriate arteries
Posterior cerebral artery
Anterior inferior cerebellar artery
Posterior inferior cerebellar artery
Vertebral artery

2-18 Inferior (ventral) view of the cerebral hemispheres, diencephalon, brainstem, and cerebellum, which shows the arterial patterns created by the internal carotid and vertebrobasilar systems. Note the cerebral arterial circle (of Willis). Details of the cerebral arterial circle and the vertebrobasilar arterial pattern are shown in Figure 2-21 on p. 25. See Figure 9-9 and 9-10 (pp. 302–303) for comparable MRAs of the cerebral arterial circle and its major branches.

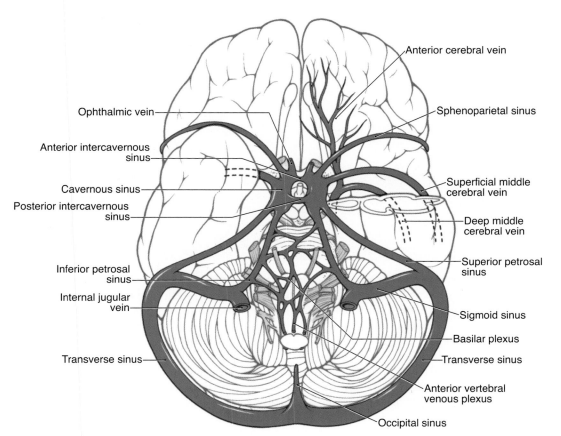

Ophthalmic vein
Anterior intercavernous sinus
Cavernous sinus
Posterior intercavernous sinus
Inferior petrosal sinus
Internal jugular vein
Transverse sinus

Anterior cerebral vein
Sphenoparietal sinus
Superficial middle cerebral vein
Deep middle cerebral vein
Superior petrosal sinus
Sigmoid sinus
Basilar plexus
Transverse sinus
Anterior vertebral venous plexus
Occipital sinus

2-19 Inferior (ventral) view of the cerebral hemispheres, diencephalon, brainstem, and cerebellum showing the locations and relationships of principal sinuses and veins. Compare this figure with Figure 2-16 (p. 21).

Gyrus rectus   Olfactory tract

CN II

CN III

Optic nerve (cranial nerve II)

Optic chiasm

Optic tract

Infundibulum

Oculomotor nerve (cranial nerve III)

Mammillary body

Uncus

Interpeduncular fossa

Crus cerebri

Trochlear nerve (cranial nerve IV)

Basilar pons

Parahippocampal gyrus

Trigeminal nerve (cranial nerve V)

Abducens nerve (cranial nerve VI)

Middle cerebellar peduncle (brachium pontis)

Facial nerve (cranial nerve VII)

Intermediate nerve

Flocculus

Vestibulocochlear nerve (cranial nerve VIII)

Olive (inferior); olivary eminence

Glossopharyngeal nerve (cranial nerve IX)

Choroid plexus

Retroolivary sulcus (postolivary sulcus)

Vagus nerve (cranial nerve X)

Hypoglossal nerve (cranial nerve XII)

Preolivary sulcus (exit of twelfth nerve)

Pyramid

Brs of posterior inferior cerebellar artery

Anterior median fissure

Accessory nerve (cranial nerve XI)

Motor decussation (decussation of pyramids)

2-20 Detailed view of the inferior (ventral) aspect of the diencephalon and brainstem with particular emphasis on the points at which cranial nerves exit/enter the brainstem (CNs III–XII) and the general relationships of the optic nerve, chiasm, and tract. The inset (upper left) illustrates an important relationship: *the oculomotor nerve exits between the superior cerebellar and the posterior cerebral (P₁ segment of PCA) arteries.* In this location, it is susceptible to damage from *aneurysms arising from the basilar bifurcation or from the posterior communicating artery/PCA intersection.* Such lesions give rise to deficits (seen individually or in combinations) characteristic of third nerve injury, such as *dilated pupil, loss of most eye movement,* and *diplopia.* Other important relationships also include the cranial nerves of the pons–medulla junction (VI, VII, VIII) and the cranial nerves associated with the *cerebellopontine angle* (VII, VIII, IX, X). In this view, it is easy to appreciate the fact that cranial nerves VI–XII occupy a compact area at the caudal aspect of the pons and lateral medulla. Lesions in this area may result in a variety of cranial nerve, and potentially additional, deficits.

Vessels   ## Structures

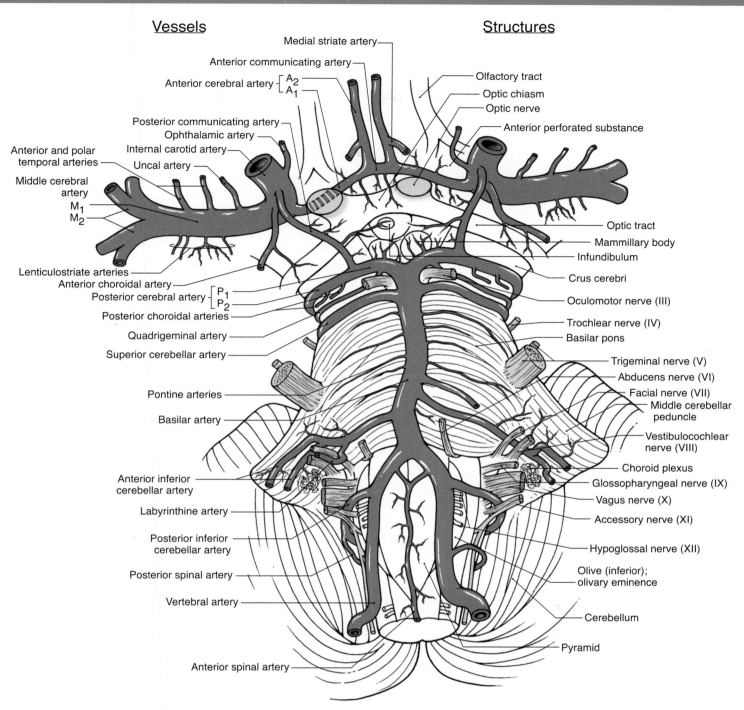

Medial striate artery
Anterior communicating artery
Anterior cerebral artery $\begin{bmatrix} A_2 \\ A_1 \end{bmatrix}$
Posterior communicating artery
Ophthalamic artery
Anterior and polar temporal arteries
Internal carotid artery
Uncal artery
Middle cerebral artery
M_1
M_2
Lenticulostriate arteries
Anterior choroidal artery
Posterior cerebral artery $\begin{bmatrix} P_1 \\ P_2 \end{bmatrix}$
Posterior choroidal arteries
Quadrigeminal artery
Superior cerebellar artery
Pontine arteries
Basilar artery
Anterior inferior cerebellar artery
Labyrinthine artery
Posterior inferior cerebellar artery
Posterior spinal artery
Vertebral artery
Anterior spinal artery

Olfactory tract
Optic chiasm
Optic nerve
Anterior perforated substance
Optic tract
Mammillary body
Infundibulum
Crus cerebri
Oculomotor nerve (III)
Trochlear nerve (IV)
Basilar pons
Trigeminal nerve (V)
Abducens nerve (VI)
Facial nerve (VII)
Middle cerebellar peduncle
Vestibulocochlear nerve (VIII)
Choroid plexus
Glossopharyngeal nerve (IX)
Vagus nerve (X)
Accessory nerve (XI)
Hypoglossal nerve (XII)
Olive (inferior); olivary eminence
Cerebellum
Pyramid

2-21 Inferior (ventral) view of the brainstem showing the relationship of brain structures and cranial nerves to the arteries forming the vertebrobasilar system and the cerebral arterial circle (of Willis). The posterior spinal artery usually originates from the posterior inferior cerebellar artery (left), but it may arise from the vertebral (right). Although the labyrinthine artery may occasionally branch from the basilar (right), it most frequently originates from the anterior inferior cerebellar artery (left). Many vessels that arise ventrally course around the brainstem to serve dorsal structures. The anterior cerebral artery consists of A_1 (between the internal carotid bifurcation and the anterior communicating artery) and segments A_2–A_5, which are distal to the anterior communicating artery (see Figure 9-3 on p. 296 for details).

Lateral to the internal carotid bifurcation is the M_1 segment of the middle cerebral artery (MCA), which usually divides into superior and inferior trunks that continue as the M_2 segments (branches) on the insular cortex. The M_3 branches of the MCA are those located on the inner surface of the opercula, and the M_4 branches are located on the lateral aspect of the hemisphere (see Figure 2-41 on p. 39). Between the basilar bifurcation and the posterior communicating artery is the P_1 segment of the posterior cerebral artery; P_2 is between the posterior communicator and the first temporal branches. See Figures 9-9, 9-10, and 9-12 (pp. 302, 303, and 305) for comparable MRA of the cerebral arterial circle and vertebrobasilar system. See Figure 4-10 on p. 62 for the blood supply of the choroid plexus.

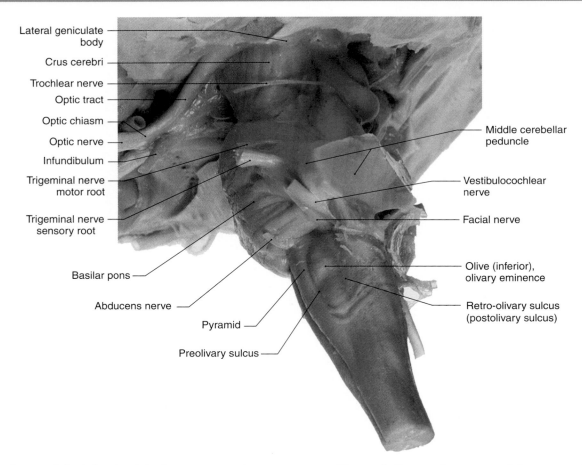

Lateral geniculate body
Crus cerebri
Trochlear nerve
Optic tract
Optic chiasm
Optic nerve
Infundibulum
Trigeminal nerve motor root
Trigeminal nerve sensory root
Basilar pons
Abducens nerve
Pyramid
Preolivary sulcus

Middle cerebellar peduncle
Vestibulocochlear nerve
Facial nerve
Olive (inferior), olivary eminence
Retro-olivary sulcus (postolivary sulcus)

2-22 Lateral view of the left side of the brainstem emphasizing structures and cranial nerves on the ventral aspect of the thalamus and brainstem. Compare with Figure 2-24 on the facing page. The cerebellum and portions of the temporal lobe have been removed.

Anterior cerebral artery
Optic nerve
Optic chiasm
Optic tract
Posterior perforated substance
Trochlear nerve
Lateral geniculate body
Medial geniculate body
Middle cerebellar peduncle
Vestibulocochlear nerve

Olfactory tract
Medial olfactory stria
Lateral olfactory stria
Anterior perforated substance
Infundibulum
Mammillary body
Crus cerebri
Basilar pons
Trigeminal nerve
Abducens nerve
Facial nerve
Pyramid

2-23 View of the inferior (ventral) aspect of the diencephalon and part of the brainstem with the medial portions of the temporal lobe removed. Note structures of the hypothalamus, cranial nerves, and optic structures, including the lateral geniculate body. Also note the intimate relationship between the optic tract and the crus cerebri; vascular lesions to these structures at this point result in an *anterior choroidal artery syndrome*. For an added perspective, compare this view with those in Figures 2-20 and 2-21 on pp. 24 and 25.

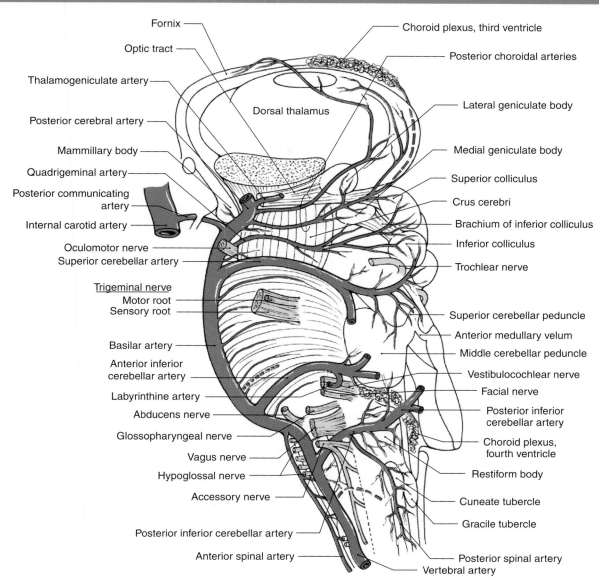

Fornix
Optic tract
Thalamogeniculate artery
Posterior cerebral artery
Mammillary body
Quadrigeminal artery
Posterior communicating artery
Internal carotid artery
Oculomotor nerve
Superior cerebellar artery
Trigeminal nerve
Motor root
Sensory root
Basilar artery
Anterior inferior cerebellar artery
Labyrinthine artery
Abducens nerve
Glossopharyngeal nerve
Vagus nerve
Hypoglossal nerve
Accessory nerve
Posterior inferior cerebellar artery
Anterior spinal artery

Dorsal thalamus

Choroid plexus, third ventricle
Posterior choroidal arteries
Lateral geniculate body
Medial geniculate body
Superior colliculus
Crus cerebri
Brachium of inferior colliculus
Inferior colliculus
Trochlear nerve
Superior cerebellar peduncle
Anterior medullary velum
Middle cerebellar peduncle
Vestibulocochlear nerve
Facial nerve
Posterior inferior cerebellar artery
Choroid plexus, fourth ventricle
Restiform body
Cuneate tubercle
Gracile tubercle
Posterior spinal artery
Vertebral artery

2-24 Lateral view of the left side of the brainstem and thalamus showing the relationship of structures and cranial nerves to arteries. Arteries that serve dorsal structures originate from ventrally located parent vessels. The approximate positions of the posterior spinal and labyrinthine arteries, when they originate from the vertebral and basilar arteries, respectively, are shown as dashed lines. Compare with Figure 2-22 on the facing page. See Figure 9-7 (p. 300) for comparable angiogram of the vertebrobasilar system. See Figure 4-10 on p. 66 for another view of the blood supply to the choroid plexus of the third and fourth ventricles.

Anterior communicating artery
Hypothalamus
Crus cerebri
Red nucleus

Anterior cerebral artery
A_2
A_1
Middle cerebral artery (M_1)
Posterior communicating artery
Posterior cerebral artery
P_2
P_1
Cerebral aqueduct
Cortical branches of posterior cerebral artery

2-25 A proton density axial MRI through basal regions of the hemisphere and through the midbrain showing several major vessels that form part of the cerebral arterial circle (of Willis). Compare to Figure 2-21 on p. 25. See Figures 9-9 and 9-10 (pp. 302, 303) for comparable MRAs of the cerebral arterial circle.

2-26 Midsagittal view of the right cerebral hemisphere and diencephalon, with brainstem removed, showing the main gyri and sulci and two MRIs (both T1-weighted images) showing these structures from the same perspective. The lower MRI is from a patient with a small *colloid cyst* in the interventricular foramen. When compared with the upper MRI, note the *enlarged lateral ventricle* with resultant *thinning of the corpus callosum*.

A *colloid cyst* (*colloid tumor*) is a congenital growth usually discovered in adult life once the flow of CSF through the interventricular foramina is compromised (*obstructive hydrocephalus*). The patient may have *headache, unsteady gait, weakness of the lower extremities*, visual or somatosensory disorders, and/or personality changes or *confusion*. Treatment is usually by surgical removal.

Internal frontal branches

Callosomarginal branch of ACA

A₃ segment of ACA

Frontopolar branches of ACA

Orbital branches of ACA

A₂ segment of ACA
Anterior communicating artery
A₁ segment of ACA
Internal carotid artery
Posterior communicating artery

Paracentral branches (of ACA)

Internal parietal branches (of ACA)

Parieto-occipital branches of PCA (P₄)

Pericallosal branch of ACA

Calcarine branches of PCA (P₄)
Posterior temporal branches of PCA (P₃)
Anterior temporal branch of PCA (P₃)
Posterior cerebral artery (PCA)
Anterior temporal branch of PCA

2-27 Midsagittal view of the right cerebral hemisphere and diencephalon showing the locations and branching patterns of anterior (ACA) and posterior (PCA) cerebral arteries. The positions of gyri and sulci can be extrapolated from Figure 2-26 (facing page). Terminal branches of the anterior cerebral artery arch laterally over the edge of the hemisphere to serve medial regions of the frontal and parietal lobes, and the same relationship is maintained for the occipital and temporal lobes by branches of the posterior cerebral artery. The ACA is made up of segments A₁ (precommunicating), A₂ (infracallosal), A₃ (precallosal), and A₄ + A₅ (supracallosal + postcallosal). See Figures 9-1 (p. 294) and 9-7 (p. 300) for comparable angiograms of anterior and posterior cerebral arteries.

Inferior sagittal sinus
Superior thalamostriate vein

Posterior vein of the corpus callosum

Superior sagittal sinus

Veins of the caudate nucleus and septum pellucidum

Venous angle

Septal veins

Inferior sagittal sinus

Superior sagittal sinus

Internal occipital veins

Straight sinus

Anterior cerebral vein

Superior cerebellar vein

Great cerebral vein (of Galen)

Transverse sinus

Basal vein (of Rosenthal)

Occipital sinus

Internal cerebral vein

2-28 Midsagittal view of the right cerebral hemisphere and diencephalon showing the locations and relationships of sinuses and the locations and general branching patterns of veins. The continuation of the superior thalamostriate vein (also called the terminal vein due to its proximity to the stria terminalis) with the internal cerebral vein is the *venous angle*. See Figures 9-2 (p. 295) and 9-11 (p. 304) for comparable angiogram (venous phase) and MRV showing veins and sinuses.

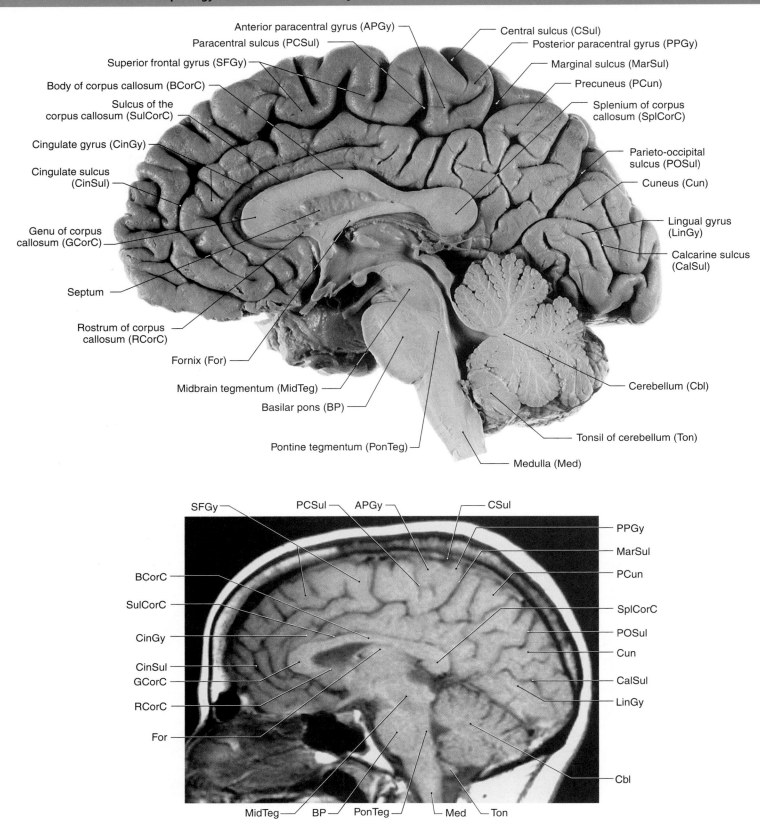

Anterior paracentral gyrus (APGy)
Paracentral sulcus (PCSul)
Superior frontal gyrus (SFGy)
Body of corpus callosum (BCorC)
Sulcus of the corpus callosum (SulCorC)
Cingulate gyrus (CinGy)
Cingulate sulcus (CinSul)
Genu of corpus callosum (GCorC)
Septum
Rostrum of corpus callosum (RCorC)
Fornix (For)
Midbrain tegmentum (MidTeg)
Basilar pons (BP)
Pontine tegmentum (PonTeg)

Central sulcus (CSul)
Posterior paracentral gyrus (PPGy)
Marginal sulcus (MarSul)
Precuneus (PCun)
Splenium of corpus callosum (SplCorC)
Parieto-occipital sulcus (POSul)
Cuneus (Cun)
Lingual gyrus (LinGy)
Calcarine sulcus (CalSul)
Cerebellum (Cbl)
Tonsil of cerebellum (Ton)
Medulla (Med)

SFGy   PCSul   APGy   CSul
BCorC
SulCorC
CinGy
CinSul
GCorC
RCorC
For
MidTeg   BP   PonTeg   Med   Ton

PPGy
MarSul
PCun
SplCorC
POSul
Cun
CalSul
LinGy
Cbl

2-29 A midsagittal view of the right cerebral hemisphere and diencephalon with the brainstem and cerebellum in situ. The MRI (T1-weighted image) shows many brain structures from the same perspective. Important cortical relationships in this view include the cingulate, parieto-occipital, and calcarine sulci; the *primary visual cortex* is located on either bank of the calcarine sulcus. The cingulate gyrus, medial aspect of the superior frontal gyrus, and precuneus occupy much of the medial surface of the hemisphere. Note that the medial terminus of the central sulcus is above the splenium of the corpus callosum. This clearly illustrates the fact that the primary somatomotor (anterior paracentral gyrus) and somatosensory (posterior paracentral gyrus) cortices for the lower extremity are located somewhat caudally on the medial aspect of the hemisphere.

Body of fornix (For)
Septum pellucidum (Sep)
Interventricular foramen
Column of fornix
Anterior commissure (AC)
Lamina terminalis
Supraoptic recess
Optic chiasm (OpCh)
Optic nerve
Massa intermedia
Dorsal thalamus (DorTh)
Choroid plexus of third ventricle
Stria medullaris thalami
Habenula
Suprapineal recess
Posterior commissure
Pineal (P)
Superior colliculus (SC)
Quadrigeminal cistern (QCis)
Inferior colliculus (IC)
Cerebral aqueduct (CA)
Anterior medullary velum (AMV)
Fourth ventricle (ForVen)
Hyth
Infundibulum (In)
Infundibular recess
Mammillary body (MB)
Hypothalamic sulcus
Oculomotor nerve
Interpeduncular fossa (IpedFos)
Basilar pons (BP)
Posterior inferior cerebellar artery
Medulla

For
DorTh
Sep
Internal cerebral vein
AC
P
Hypothalamus
Tentorium cerebelli
OpCh
QCis
In
SC
Pituitary gland
IC
MB
AMV
ForVen
IpedFos   BP   CA

2-30 A midsagittal view of the right cerebral hemisphere and diencephalon with the brainstem in situ focusing on the details primarily related to the diencephalon and third ventricle. The MRI (T1-weighted image) shows these brain structures from the same perspective. Note the recesses of the third ventricle in the vicin- ity of the hypothalamus, the position of the lamina terminalis, and the general relationships of the ventricular system in the midsagittal plane. These relationships are important to understanding images of patients with *subarachnoid hemorrhage* (see Figure 4-5 on p. 61 for examples). Hyth = hypothalamus.

Inferior colliculus (IC)

Pineal

Internal cerebral vein
Frenulum

Superior colliculus (SC)

Pulvinar nuclear
complex (PuNu)

Medial
geniculate
body (MGB)

PulNu

SC

MGB

LGB

Brachium of
superior
colliculus

Lateral
geniculate
body (LGB)

IC

Brachium of
inferior
colliculus

Crus cerebri

Crus cerebri

Trochlear nerve
(cranial nerve IV)

Trochlear nerve
(cranial nerve IV)

Anterior medullary velum

Superior cerebellar
peduncle

Facial colliculus

Sulcus limitans

Middle cerebellar
peduncle

Superior fovea

Striae medullares of
fourth ventricle

Inferior cerebellar peduncle
(juxtarestiform body and
restiform body)

Lateral recess of
fourth ventricle

Vestibular area

Restiform body

Tela choroidea (cut edge)

Inferior fovea

Vagal trigone

Level of obex

Hypoglossal trigone

Tuberculum cuneatum (cuneate tubercle)

Tuberculum gracile
(gracile tubercle)

Posterolateral sulcus

Posterior intermediate sulcus

Trigeminal tubercle (tuberculum cinereum)

Cuneate fasciculus

Gracile fasciculus

Posterior median sulcus

2-31 Detailed superior (dorsal) view of the brainstem, with cerebellum removed, providing a clear view of the rhomboid fossa (and floor of the fourth ventricle) and contiguous parts of the caudal diencephalon. The dashed line on the left represents the position of the sulcus limitans and the area of the inferior cerebellar peduncle is shown on the right. This structure is composed of the restiform body plus the juxtarestiform body, the latter of which contains fibers interconnecting the vestibular area in the lateral floor of the fourth ventricle and cerebellar structures (cortex and

nuclei). The tuberculum cinereum is also called the trigeminal tubercle (tuberculum trigeminale) because it is the surface representation of the spinal trigeminal tract and its underlying nucleus on the lateral aspect of the medulla just caudal to the level of the obex (see also Figure 2-32 on the facing page). The facial colliculus is formed by the underlying abducens nucleus and internal genu of the facial nerve, the hypoglossal trigone by the underlying hypoglossal nucleus, and the vagal trigone by the dorsal motor nucleus of the vagal nerve. Also see Figure 2-34 on p. 34.

Vessels   Structures

Thalamogeniculate arteries

Choroid plexus, third ventricle
Pineal
Habenula
Medial thalamus
Superior colliculus

Brachium of superior colliculus
Lateral thalamus
Pulvinar nucleus
Internal capsule

Choroid plexus, lateral ventricle

Medial and lateral posterior choroidal arteries
Quadrigeminal artery

Superior cerebellar artery:
Medial branch
Lateral branch

Lateral geniculate body
Medial geniculate body
Brachium of inferior colliculus
Crus cerebri
Trochlear nerve (IV)
Inferior colliculus
Superior cerebellar peduncle
Anterior medullary velum
Facial colliculus
Vestibular area
Inferior cerebellar peduncle
Middle cerebellar peduncle
Choroid plexus, fourth ventricle
Hypoglossal trigone

Anterior inferior cerebellar artery

Posterior inferior cerebellar artery

Glossopharyngeal nerve (IX)
Vagal nerve (X)
Accessory nerve (XI)
Restiform body
Vagal trigone
Trigeminal tubercle (tuberculum cinereum)
Cuneate tubercle
Gracile tubercle

Posterior spinal artery

Gracile fasciculus

Cuneate fasciculus

2-32 Superior (dorsal) view of the brainstem and caudal diencephalon showing the relationship of structures and some of the cranial nerves to arteries. The vessels shown in this view have originated ventrally and wrapped around the brainstem to gain their dorsal positions. In addition to serving the medulla, branches of the posterior inferior cerebellar artery also supply the choroid plexus of the fourth ventricle. The tuberculum cinereum is also called the trigeminal tubercle. For an additional perspective on the blood supply to the choroid plexus of the third and fourth ventricles see Figure 4-10 on p. 66.

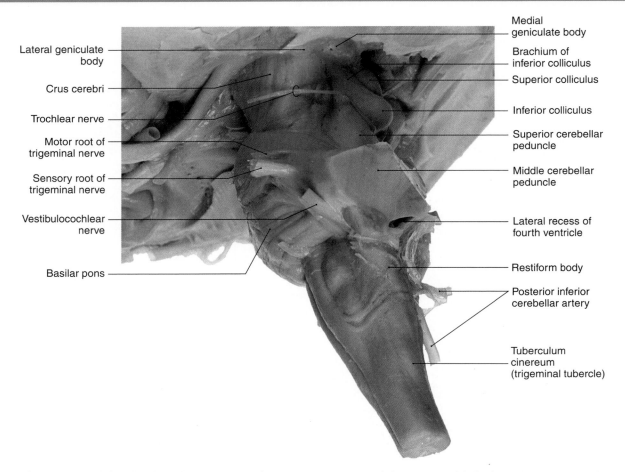

Lateral geniculate body

Crus cerebri

Trochlear nerve

Motor root of trigeminal nerve

Sensory root of trigeminal nerve

Vestibulocochlear nerve

Basilar pons

Medial geniculate body

Brachium of inferior colliculus

Superior colliculus

Inferior colliculus

Superior cerebellar peduncle

Middle cerebellar peduncle

Lateral recess of fourth ventricle

Restiform body

Posterior inferior cerebellar artery

Tuberculum cinereum (trigeminal tubercle)

2-33 Lateral view of the left side of the brainstem emphasizing structures that are located dorsally. The cerebellum and portions of the temporal lobe have been removed. Compare with Figure 2-35 on the facing page.

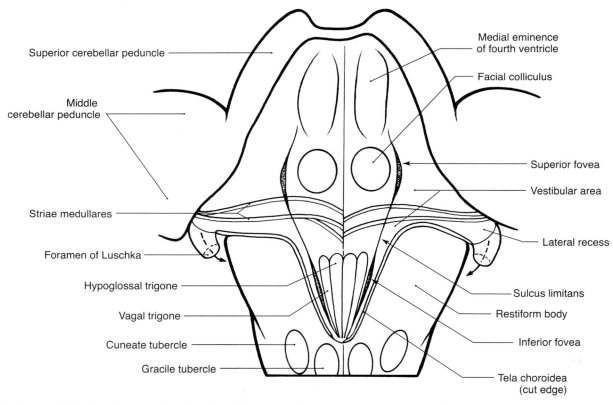

Superior cerebellar peduncle

Middle cerebellar peduncle

Striae medullares

Foramen of Luschka

Hypoglossal trigone

Vagal trigone

Cuneate tubercle

Gracile tubercle

Medial eminence of fourth ventricle

Facial colliculus

Superior fovea

Vestibular area

Lateral recess

Sulcus limitans

Restiform body

Inferior fovea

Tela choroidea (cut edge)

2-34 The floor of the fourth ventricle (rhomboid fossa) and immediately adjacent structures. The signs and symptoms of lesions in this ventricle may present as deficits representing damage to the facial colliculus (VIth nucleus, internal genu of VII), hypoglossal trigone (XIIth nucleus), or vestibular and possibly cochlear nuclei, or may be more global reflecting injury to medullary and pontine centers. Also compare with Figure 2-31 on p. 32.

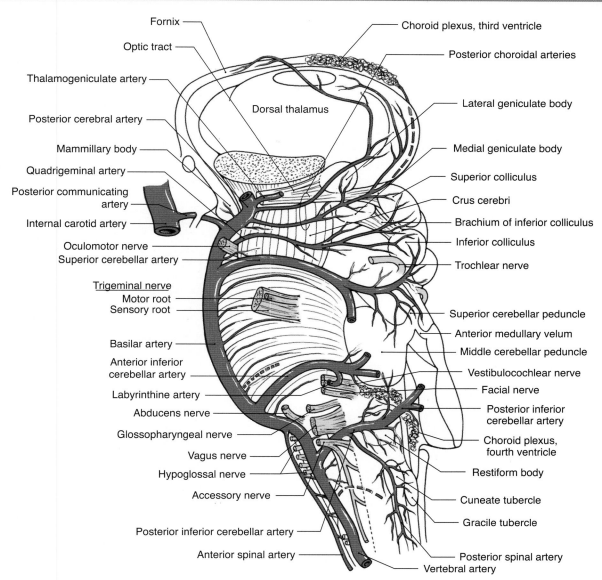

Fornix

Optic tract

Thalamogeniculate artery

Posterior cerebral artery

Mammillary body

Quadrigeminal artery

Posterior communicating artery

Internal carotid artery

Oculomotor nerve

Superior cerebellar artery

<u>Trigeminal nerve</u>
Motor root
Sensory root

Basilar artery

Anterior inferior cerebellar artery

Labyrinthine artery

Abducens nerve

Glossopharyngeal nerve

Vagus nerve

Hypoglossal nerve

Accessory nerve

Posterior inferior cerebellar artery

Anterior spinal artery

Dorsal thalamus

Choroid plexus, third ventricle

Posterior choroidal arteries

Lateral geniculate body

Medial geniculate body

Superior colliculus

Crus cerebri

Brachium of inferior colliculus

Inferior colliculus

Trochlear nerve

Superior cerebellar peduncle

Anterior medullary velum

Middle cerebellar peduncle

Vestibulocochlear nerve

Facial nerve

Posterior inferior cerebellar artery

Choroid plexus, fourth ventricle

Restiform body

Cuneate tubercle

Gracile tubercle

Posterior spinal artery

Vertebral artery

2-35 Lateral view of the brainstem and thalamus, which shows the relationship of structures and cranial nerves to arteries. The approximate positions of the labyrinthine and posterior spinal arteries, when they originate from the basilar and vertebral arteries, respectively, are shown as dashed lines. Arteries that distribute to posterior/dorsal structures originate from the vertebral, basilar, and initial segments of the posterior cerebral arteries and arch around the brainstem, or caudal thalamus, to access their targets. From this view, notice the compact nature of the cranial nerves at the pons–medulla junction and the lateral and ventral aspect of the medulla (CNs VI–XII). Compare with Figure 2-33 on the facing page.

2-36 Rostral (**A**, superior surface), caudal (**B**, inferior surface), and an inferior view (**C**, inferior aspect) of the cerebellum. The view in **C** shows the aspect of the cerebellum that is continuous into the brainstem via cerebellar peduncles. The view in **C** correlates with the superior surface of the brainstem (and middle superior cerebellar peduncles) as shown in Figure 2-31 on p. 32.

Note that the superior view of the cerebellum (**A**) correlates closely with cerebellar structures seen in axial MRIs at comparable

levels (**D, E**). Structures seen on the inferior surface of the cerebellum, such as the tonsil (**F**), correlate closely with an axial MRI at a comparable level. In **G**, note the appearance of the margin of the cerebellum, the general appearance and position of the lobes, and the obvious nature of the middle cerebellar peduncle. All MRI images are T1-weighted.

2-37 A median sagittal view of the cerebellum (**A**) showing its relationships to the midbrain, pons, and medulla. This view of the cerebellum also illustrates the two main fissures and the vermis portions of lobules I–X. Designation of these lobules follows the method developed by Larsell.

Lobules I–V are the vermis parts of the anterior lobe; lobules VI–IX are the vermis parts of the posterior lobe; and lobule X (the nodulus) is the vermis part of the flocculonodular lobe. Note the striking similarities between the gross specimen (**A**) and a median sagittal view of the cerebellum in a T1- (**B**) and T2-weighted MRI (**C**).

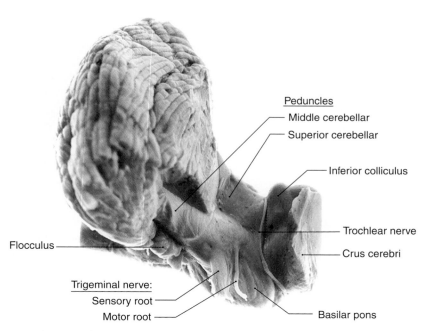

2-38 Lateral and slightly rostral view of the cerebellum and brainstem with the middle and superior cerebellar peduncles exposed. Note the relationship of the trochlear nerve to the inferior colliculus and the relative positions of, and distinction between, motor and sensory roots of the trigeminal nerve.

2-39 Lateral view of the left cerebral hemisphere with the frontal and parietal opercula removed and the temporal operculum retracted downward exposing the insula. Structures characteristic of the insular cortex (including the long and short gyri and the central sulcus of the insula), and immediately adjacent areas, are clearly seen in the two MRIs in the sagittal plane through lateral portions of the hemisphere (inversion recovery—upper; T1-weighted image—lower).

Prerolandic branches of MCA (M₄)

Temporal and parietal opercula removed

Orbitofrontal branches of MCA

M₂ segments of MCA on insula cortex

Rolandic branches of MCA (M₄)

Anterior and posterior parietal branches of MCA (M₄)

Deep middle cerebral vein

Bifurcation of M₁ into superior and inferior trunks (M₂–M₄)

Anterior temporal branches of MCA (M₄)

Angular branches of MCA (M₄)

Deep middle cerebral vein

Posterior temporal branches of MCA (M₄)

Temporal operculum retracted

2-40 Lateral view of the left cerebral hemisphere showing the pattern of the middle cerebral artery (MCA) as it branches from M₁ into M₂ segments that pass over the insular cortex. Also shown are the M₄ branches on the surface of the cortex (having exited from the lateral sulcus) and the deep middle cerebral vein on the surface of the insula. Compare this view of the vasculature of the insula with the anatomy from the same perspective in Figure 2-39 on the facing page.

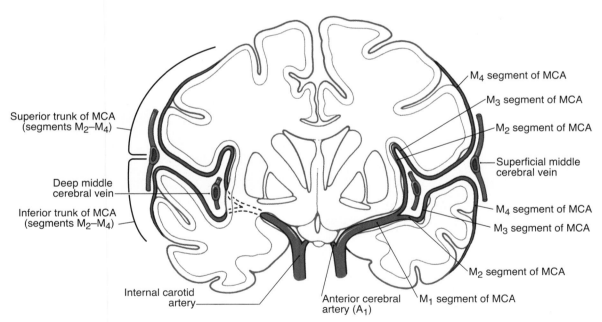

M₄ segment of MCA

M₃ segment of MCA

M₂ segment of MCA

Superficial middle cerebral vein

Superior trunk of MCA (segments M₂–M₄)

Deep middle cerebral vein

Inferior trunk of MCA (segments M₂–M₄)

M₄ segment of MCA

M₃ segment of MCA

M₂ segment of MCA

Internal carotid artery

Anterior cerebral artery (A₁)

M₁ segment of MCA

2-41 Semi-diagrammatic cross-sectional representation of the cerebral hemispheres showing the main arteries and veins related to the insular cortex. The internal carotid artery branches into the anterior and middle cerebral (MCA) arteries. The first segment of the MCA (M₁) passes laterally and diverges into superior and inferior trunks at the limen insulae (entrance to the insular cortex). In general, distal branches of the superior trunk course upward and eventually serve the cortex above the lateral sulcus, and distal branches of the inferior trunk course downward to serve the cortex below the lateral sulcus. En route, these respective branches form the M₂ (insular part of MCA), M₃ (opercular part of MCA), and M₄ (cortical part of MCA) segments, as shown here.

The deep middle cerebral vein receives small branches from the area of the insula and joins with the anterior cerebral vein to form the basal vein (see Figures 2-16 and 2-19 on pp. 21 and 23). The superficial middle cerebral vein collects blood from the lateral aspect of the hemisphere and drains into the cavernous sinus (see also Figures 2-13, 2-16, and 2-19 on pp. 19, 21, and 23).

2-42 Early in development, the posterior cerebral artery (PCA) originates from the internal carotid artery (**A**). At this stage, the cerebral arterial circle (circle of Willis) is not complete. Vascular sprouts from the basilar artery are growing to meet the PCAs and from the anterior cerebral arteries (ACA) to meet on the midline where they will form the *anterior communicating artery* (*ACom*). The initial connection between the basilar artery and the PCA is small (**B**); this will become the adult P_1 segment. As development progresses, the initially small P_1 segment enlarges in diameter (to form the major connection between the basilar and the distal PCA, the adult P_1) and the initially large portion of the PCA between the internal carotid artery and the PCA–P_1 junction becomes smaller in diameter (to form the *posterior communicating artery* [*PCom*] of the adult, **C**).

In 22%–25% of adult individuals, the territory served by the PCA is perfused mainly from the internal carotid artery. This is due to the fact that the fetal pattern of the PCA arising from the internal carotid persists into the adult. This is called a *fetal PCA*, or a *persistent fetal PCA*. Examples of a *fetal PCA* are shown here in a specimen (**D**, fetal PCA is on the patient's right, normal pattern on patient's left) and in MRI (**E**, arrows) and CT angiogram (**F**, arrows). Note that in the MRI-T2 (**E**, axial), the PCA can be easily followed from the internal carotid into the occipital lobe (arrows) with no evidence of any substantive connection to a P_1. A fetal PCA in the adult may co-exist with other vascular patterns that deviate from normal. For example, in the axial images in **F** and **G** (CTA), a fetal PCA is present on the patient's left (**F**, arrows) and in the same patient, at a slightly different axial plane, a single trunk from the left internal carotid artery (**G**) gives origin to both the right and left *anterior cerebral arteries* (ACA$_1$ becomes the right ACA; ACA$_2$ becomes the left ACA).

3

Cranial Nerves

■ Cranial Nerve Deficits in Representative Brainstem Lesions (Figures 3-1 to 3-8) ■

Table 3-1

Synopsis of Cranial Nerves*

Cranial Nerve	Component(s)	Function	Attachment to Brain	Associated Foramen/Foramina	Deficits
Olfactory (CN I)	Special sense (SVA/VA)	Sense of smell	Olfactory bulb, olfactory trigone	Ethmoid foramina of cribriform plate	Anosmia, hyposmia, hyperosmia, and olfactory hypesthesia/hyperesthesia
Visual (CN II)	Special sense (SSA/SA)	Vision	Optic chiasm (optic nerve to chiasm to tract)	Optic canal	Blindness, hemianopia, quadrantanopia, and loss of afferent limb corneal reflex (see Figs. on pp. 258–260, 262–263)
Oculomotor (CN III)	Somatic motor (GSE/SE)	Eye movement	Oculomotor sulcus, medial part of cerebral peduncle	Superior orbital fissure	Paralysis of most eye movement and diplopia (see Figs. on pp. 222–225)
	Visceral motor (SVE/VE)	Pupil constriction	With root of CN III	Superior orbital fissure	Pupillary dilation and loss of efferent limb corneal reflex (see Figs. on pp. 222–225)
Trochlear (CN IV)	Somatic motor (GSE/SE)	Eye movement	Midbrain, caudal to inferior colliculus	Superior orbital fissure	Inability to look down-and-out and diplopia (see Figs. on pp. 222–225)
Trigeminal (CN V)	Somatic sense (GSA/SA)	Sensation in face, sinuses, oral cavity, teeth, cornea, tongue, forehead, TMJ, and palate (see Figs. on pp. 198–201)	Lateral aspect of pons	Superior orbital fissure (V_1); Foramen rotundum (V_2); Foramen ovale (V_3)	Loss of sensation on areas of face and in oral cavity served by each division; loss of afferent limb corneal and jaw-jerk reflexes (see Figs. on pp. 198–201)
	Pharyngeal motor (SVE/SE)	Motor to masticatory muscles plus others (see Figs. on pp. 226–229)	Lateral aspect of pons	Foramen ovale	Masticatory muscle weakness/paralysis and loss of efferent limb jaw-jerk reflex (see Figs. on pp. 226–229)
Abducens (CN VI)	Somatic motor (GSE/SE)	Eye movement	Pons–medulla junction (medial location)	Superior orbital fissure	Lateral gaze palsy and diplopia (see Figs. on pp. 222–225)
Facial (CN VII)	Pharyngeal motor (SVE/SE)	Motor to muscles of facial expression plus others (see Figs. on pp. 226–229)	Pons–medulla junction (intermediate location)	Internal acoustic meatus and stylomastoid foramen	Weakness/paralysis of facial muscles and loss of efferent limb corneal reflex (see Figs. on pp. 226–229)
	Visceral motor (GVE/VE)	To parasympathetic ganglia (see Figs. on pp. 226–229)		Internal acoustic meatus	Decrease in secretions
	Special sense (SVA/VA)	Taste from anterior two-thirds of tongue (see Figs. on pp. 198–199, 202–203)		Internal acoustic meatus and stylomastoid foramen	Loss of taste on anterior two-thirds of tongue (see Figs. on pp. 202–203, 228–229)
	Somatic sense (GSA/SA)	Sensation on pinna (see Figs. on pp. 198–199)		Internal acoustic meatus and stylomastoid foramen	Loss of ear sensation (see Figs. on pp. 228–229)
	Visceral sense (GVA/VA)	Visceral sense from salivary glands		Internal acoustic meatus and stylomastoid foramen	
Vestibulocochlear (CN VIII)	Special sense (SSA/SA)	Hearing, balance, and equilibrium (see Figs. on pp. 266–269)	Pons–medulla junction (lateral location)	Internal acoustic meatus	Deafness, tinnitus, vertigo, unsteady gait, and nystagmus (see Figs. on pp. 266–269)

Cranial Nerve	Component(s)	Function	Attachment to Brain	Associated Foramen/Foramina	Deficits
Glosso-pharyngeal (CN IX)	Pharyngeal motor (SVE/SE)	Motor to stylopharyngeus muscle (see Figs. on pp. 226–229)	Postolivary sulcus	Jugular foramen	Difficulty swallowing and loss of gag reflex (see Figs. on pp. 228–229)
	Visceral motor (GVE/VE)	To otic ganglion then parotid (see Figs. on pp. 226–229)			Decrease of secretory function
	Special sense (SVA/VA)	Taste from posterior third of tongue (see Figs. on pp. 202–203, 228–229)	Postolivary sulcus	Jugular foramen	Loss of taste on posterior third of tongue; not tested (see Figs. on pp. 228–229)
	Somatic sense (GSA/SA)	Sensation in external auditory meatus (see Figs. on pp. 198–199, 228–229)			Loss of sensation in external auditory meatus (see Figs. on pp. 228–229)
	Visceral sense (GVA/VA)	From carotid body/sinus, parotid, and pharynx			Possible bradycardia or tachycardia
Vagus (CN X)	Pharyngeal motor (SVE/SE)	Motor to constrictors of pharynx, intrinsic laryngeal muscles, much of palate, upper esophagus, and vocalis (see Figs. on pp. 226–227)	Postolivary sulcus	Jugular foramen	Dysphagia, dysarthria, loss of vocalis function (hoarseness), and loss of gag reflex (see Figs. on pp. 212–213, 228–229)
	Visceral motor (GVE/VE)	To ganglia in/on trachea, bronchi, gut, and heart (see Figs. on pp. 226–227)			Decrease in secretory action and effect on intestinal motility and heart rate (see Figs. on pp. 226–229)
	Special sense (SVA/VA)	From taste buds on epiglottis, base of tongue, and palate (see Figs. on pp. 202–203)			Loss of taste; not tested
	Somatic sense (GSA/SA)	Sensation on eardrum, external auditory meatus, and dura of posterior fossa (see Figs. on pp. 198–199)			Loss of sensation in external auditory meatus and on eardrum (see Figs. on pp. 226–229)
	Visceral sense (GVA/VA)	From larynx, pharynx, heart, trachea and bronchi, esophagus, and gut (see Figs. on pp. 202–203)			Decrease/loss of sensations from viscera; may affect gag reflex
Accessory (CN XI)	Somatic motor (GSE/SE)	Motor to sternocleidomastoid and trapezius muscles (see Figs. on pp. 222–223)	Lateral aspect of spinal cord C1–C4/C5	Enters foramen magnum; exits jugular foramen	Weakness of trapezius and sternocleidomastoid muscles (see Figs. on pp. 212–213)
Hypoglossal (CN XII)	Somatic motor (GSE/SE)	Motor to extrinsic and intrinsic tongue muscles (see Figs. on pp. 222–223)	Preolivary sulcus	Hypoglossal canal	Deviation of the tongue on protrusion (see Figs. on pp. 212–213, 224–225)

* This table is not intended to be all inclusive, but to serve as a brief overview. Details of structures innervated and their functions and of the various deficits seen following root lesions of cranial nerves (or central lesions that influence cranial nerve function) are available in the respective figures indicated in this table and in other portions of this chapter and Chapter 8. The functional component designations used on this table integrate the traditional and contemporary versions that are explained in Figure 8-1 on p. 184.
CN, cranial nerve; TMJ, temporomandibular joint; V$_1$, ophthalmic nerve; V$_2$, maxillary nerve; V$_3$, mandibular nerve.

3-1 Inferior view of the hemisphere showing the optic nerve (II), chiasm, tract, and related structures (**A**). The MRIs of cranial nerve (CN) II are shown in axial (**B**, T1-weighted; **D**, T2-weighted) and in oblique sagittal (**C**, T1-weighted) planes. Note the similarity between the axial planes, especially (**B**), and the gross anatomical specimen. In addition, note the relationship between the anterior cerebral artery, anterior communicating artery, and the structures around the optic chiasm (**D**).

The anterior communicating artery or its junction with the anterior cerebral artery (**D**) is the most common site of supratentorial (carotid system) *aneurysms*. Rupture of aneurysms at this location is one of the more common causes of *spontaneous* (also called *non-traumatic) subarachnoid hemorrhage*. The proximity of these vessels to optic structures and the hypothalamus (**D**) explains the variety of visual and hypothalamic disorders experienced by these patients. A lesion of the optic nerve results in *blindness* in that eye and loss of the afferent limb of the *pupillary light reflex*. Lesions caudal to the optic chiasm result in deficits in the visual fields of both eyes (*contralateral [right or left] homonymous hemianopia*).

The anterior choroidal artery serves the optic tract and portions of the internal capsule immediately internal to this structure. This explains the unusual combination of a *homonymous hemianopia* coupled with a contralateral *hemiplegia* and *hemianesthesia* (to all somatosensory modalities) in the *anterior choroidal artery syndrome*.

A

Optic chiasm

Posterior cerebral artery

Basilar artery

Basilar pons

Internal carotid artery

Middle cerebral artery

Posterior communicating artery

Oculomotor nerve

Superior cerebellar artery

B

Bulb of the eye

Optic tract

Posterior cerebral artery

Superior cerebellar artery

Oculomotor nerve

C

Internal carotid artery

Oculomotor nerve

Basilar pons (rostral portion)

Fourth ventricle (rostral portion)

Oculomotor nerve

Temporal lobe

Uncus

D

Frontal lobe

Interpeduncular fossa

Optic chiasm

Oculomotor nerve

Corpus callosum

Dorsal thalamus

Superior colliculus

Inferior colliculus

Cerebellum

Basilar pons

3-2 Inferior view of the hemisphere showing the exiting fibers of the oculomotor nerve (III), and their relationship to the posterior cerebral and superior cerebellar arteries (**A**). The MRIs of cranial nerve III are shown in sagittal (**B**, T2-weighted; **D**, T1-weighted) and in axial (**C**, T1-weighted) planes. Note the relationship of the exiting fibers of the oculomotor nerve to the posterior cerebral and superior cerebellar arteries (**A, B**) and the characteristic appearance of CN III as it passes through the subarachnoid space toward the superior orbital fissure (**C**). The sagittal section (**D**) is just off the midline and shows the position of the oculomotor nerve in the interpeduncular fossa rostral to the basilar pons and caudal to optic structures.

That portion of the posterior cerebral artery located between the basilar artery and posterior communicating artery (**A**) is the P_1 segment. The most common site of *aneurysms* in the infratentorial area (vertebrobasilar system) is at the bifurcation of the basilar artery, also called the basilar tip. Patients with aneurysms at this location may present with *eye movement disorders*, *pupillary dilation* caused by damage to the root of the third nerve, and *diplopia*.

Rupture of a *basilar tip aneurysm* may result in the cardinal signs (sudden *severe headache, nausea, vomiting*, and possibly *syncope*) that signal a stroke as broadly defined. In addition, the extravasated blood may dissect its way into the ventricular system through the floor of the third ventricle.

A
Lamina terminalis
Supraoptic recess
Optic chiasm
Infundibular recess
Mammillary body
Interpeduncular fossa
Cerebral aqueduct
Oculomotor nerve
Basilar pons

B
Optic tract
Optic nerve
Posterior cerebral artery
Superior cerebellar artery
Oculomotor nerve
Basilar pons

C
Oculomotor nerve
Posterior cerebral artery
Interpeduncular fossa
Midbrain
Posterior cerebral artery
Superior cerebellar artery
Crus cerebri
Anterior lobe of cerebellum

D
Middle cerebral artery
Hypothalamus
Interpeduncular fossa
Crus cerebri
Midbrain tegmentum
Fourth ventricle (rostral portion)
Anterior cerebral artery
Optic tract
Mammillary body
Posterior cerebral artery
Trochlear nerve (in ambient cistern)

3-3 A median sagittal view of the brainstem and diencephalon (**A**) reveals the position of the oculomotor nerve (III) in relation to adjacent structures. The MRI in **B** and **C** show the position of the oculomotor nerve in sagittal (**B**, T1-weighted) and in axial (**C**, T2-weighted) planes. Note the relationship of the oculomotor nerve to the adjacent posterior cerebral and superior cerebellar arteries (**B**, **C**). Also compare these images with that of Figure 3-2B on p. 45. In **D** (T2-weighted), the trochlear nerve is seen passing through the ambient cistern around the lateral aspect of the midbrain (compare with Figure 2-38 on p.37).

The oculomotor (III) and trochlear (IV) nerves are the cranial nerves of the midbrain. The third nerve exits via the interpeduncular fossa to innervate four major extraocular muscles (see Figure 8-21 on p. 223), and through the ciliary ganglion, the sphincter pupillae muscles. Damage to the oculomotor nerve may result in *paralysis of most eye movement*, a *dilated pupil*, and loss of the efferent limb of the *pupillary light reflex*, all in the ipsilateral eye. The fourth nerve is unique in that it is the only cranial nerve to exit the posterior (dorsal) aspect of the brainstem and is the only cranial nerve motor nucleus to innervate, exclusively, a muscle on the contralateral side of the midline. Damage to the third and fourth nerves also results in *diplopia*.

A
Basilar pons
Trigeminal nerve
Facial nerve
Abducens nerve
Flocculus
Pyramid
Vestibulocochlear nerve

B
Internal carotid artery
Temporal lobe
Trigeminal nerve
Basilar artery
Middle cerebellar peduncle
Trigeminal nerve
Fourth ventricle
Basilar pons
Pontine tegmentum
Cerebellum

C
Temporal lobe
Trigeminal ganglion
Trigeminal ganglion
Basilar artery
Superior cerebellar artery
Trigeminal nerve
Tegmentum of pons
Fourth ventricle
Basilar pons
Anterior lobe of cerebellum

D
Midbrain tegmentum
Root of trigeminal nerve
Basilar pons
Pyramid

E
Third ventricle
Crus cerebri
Interpeduncular fossa
Sensory root of the trigeminal nerve
Basilar pons

3-4 The trigeminal nerve (V) is the largest of the cranial nerve roots of the brainstem (**A**). It exits at an intermediate position on the lateral aspect of the pons roughly in line with CNs VII, IX, and X. The fifth nerve and these latter three are mixed nerves in that they have motor and sensory components. The trigeminal nerve is shown in axial MRI (**B**, T1-weighted; **C**, T2-weighted) and coronal planes (**D**, **E**, both T1-weighted images). Note the characteristic appearance of the root of the trigeminal nerve as it traverses the subarachnoid space (**B**, **C**), origin of the trigeminal nerve, and position of the sensory root of the nerve at the lateral aspect of the pons in the coronal plane (**D**, **E**). In addition, the MRI in **C** clearly illustrates the position of the trigeminal ganglion in the middle cranial fossa.

Trigeminal neuralgia (*tic douloureux*) is a lancinating paroxysmal pain within the V_2–V_3 territories frequently triggered by stimuli around the corner of the mouth. The causes probably are multiple and may include neurovascular compression by aberrant branches of the superior cerebellar artery (see the apposition of this vessel to the nerve root in **C**), *multiple sclerosis*, *tumors*, and ephaptic transmission within the nerve or ganglion.

There are multiple medical treatments for *trigeminal neuralgia*; when these fail, surgical therapy may include *peripheral nerve section* or *neurectomy*, *microvascular decompression*, or *percutaneous trigeminal rhizotomy*.

A

Vestibulocochlear nerve

Facial nerve

Pyramid

Olivary eminence

Abducens nerve

Facial nerve

Vestibulocochlear nerve

Glossopharyngeal nerve

Vagus nerve

Hypoglossal nerve

B

Cochlea

Semicircular canals

Vestibulocochlear nerve

Facial nerve

Basilar artery

Abducens nerve

Pons-medulla junction

Lateral recess of fourth ventricle

Fourth ventricle

Tonsil of cerebellum

1-27 180   SP SL FoV 150

C

Cochlea

Semicircular canals

VPVIII

CPVIII

Fourth ventricle

Cerebellum

Abducens nerve

Cochlea

Cochlear portion of eighth nerve (CPVIII)

Semicircular canals

Vestibular portion of eighth nerve (VPVIII)

Basilar pons

Pontine tegmentum

D

Anterior inferior cerebellar artery

Cochlea

Semicircular canals

Cerebellar vermis

Cerebellar hemisphere

Cochlear portion of eighth nerve

Cochlea

Semicircular canals

Vestibular portion of eighth nerve

Cerebellar tonsil

3-5 The cranial nerves at the pons–medulla junction are the abducens (VI), the facial (VII), and the vestibulocochlear (VIII) (**A**). The facial and vestibulocochlear nerves both enter the internal acoustic meatus, the facial nerve distributing eventually to the face through the stylomastoid foramen, and the vestibulocochlear nerve to structures of the inner ear. MRIs in the axial plane, **B, C, D** (all T2-weighted images) show the relationships of the vestibulocochlear root and the facial nerve to the internal acoustic meatus. Also notice the characteristic appearance of the cochlea (**B, C**) and the semicircular canals (**B, C**). In addition to these two cranial nerves, the labyrinthine branch of the anterior inferior cerebellar artery also enters the internal acoustic meatus and sends branches to serve the cochlea and semicircular canals and their respective ganglia.

The so-called acoustic neuroma, a tumor associated with the eighth nerve, is actually a *vestibular schwannoma* because it arises from the neurilemma sheath of the vestibular root. Most patients with this tumor have *hearing loss, tinnitus,* and *equilibrium problems,* or *vertigo.* As the tumor enlarges (to more than about 2 cm) it may cause *facial weakness* (seventh root), numbness (fifth root), or abnormal *corneal reflex* (fifth or seventh root). Treatment is usually by surgery, radiation therapy, or a combination thereof.

A
Abducens nerve
Olivary eminence
Postolivary sulcus
Preolivary sulcus
Facial nerve
Vestibulocochlear nerve
Glossopharyngeal nerve
Vagus nerve
Hypoglossal nerve

B
Preolivary sulcus
Retroolivary sulcus (postolivary sulcus)
Glossopharyngeal nerve
Flocculus
Fourth ventricle
Cerebellum
Pyramid
Olive (inferior)
Glossopharyngeal nerve
Restiform body
Tonsil of cerebellum

C
Retroolivary sulcus
Tonsil of cerebellum
Cerebellum
Pyramid
Olive (inferior)
Vagus nerve
Fourth ventricle

D
Vagus nerve
Restiform body
Fourth ventricle
Pyramid
Olivary eminence
Postolivary sulcus
Vagus nerve
Tonsil of cerebellum

3-6 The glossopharyngeal (IX) and vagus (X) nerves (**A**) exit the lateral aspect of the medulla via the postolivary sulcus; the ninth nerve exits rostral to the row of rootlets comprising the tenth nerve (**A**). These nerves are generally in line with the exits of the facial and trigeminal nerves; all of these are mixed nerves. The exit of the glossopharyngeal nerve (**A, B**) is close to the pons–medulla junction and correlates with the corresponding shape (more rectangular) of the medulla. The vagus nerve exits at a slightly more caudal position (**A, C, D**); the shape of the medulla is more square and the fourth ventricle is smaller. The ninth and tenth cranial nerves and the spinal portion of the accessory nerve (XI) exit the skull via the jugular foramen.

Glossopharyngeal neuralgia is a lancinating pain originating from the territories served by the ninth and tenth nerves at the base of the tongue and throat. Trigger events may include chewing and swallowing. Lesions of nerves passing through the jugular foramen (IX, X, XI) may result in loss of the *gag reflex* (motor limb via ninth nerve), and drooping of the ipsilateral shoulder accompanied by an inability to turn the head to the opposite side against resistance (eleventh nerve). There are a number of syndromes associated with lesions of the contents of the jugular foramen or with lesions immediately internal or external to this foramen (e.g., the *Avellis, Villaret, Vernet*, and *Collet-Sicard syndromes*).

A
Abducens nerve
Olivary eminence
Postolivary sulcus
Preolivary sulcus
Facial nerve
Vestibulocochlear nerve
Glossopharyngeal nerve
Vagus nerve
Hypoglossal nerve

B
Olivary eminence
Restiform body
Tonsil of cerebellum
Pyramid
Preolivary sulcus
Hypoglossal nerve
Postolivary sulcus
Vagus nerve

C
Tonsil of cerebellum
Cerebellum
Hypoglossal nerve
Medulla

3-7 The hypoglossal nerve (XII) (**A**) exits the inferolateral aspect of the medulla via the preolivary sulcus. This cranial nerve exits in line with the abducens nerve found at the pons–medulla junction and in line with the exits of the third and fourth nerves of the midbrain. The twelfth nerve exit is characteristically located laterally adjacent to the pyramid, which contains corticospinal fibers.

In axial MRI (**B**, T2-weighted; **C**, T1-weighted), note the characteristic position of the hypoglossal nerve in the subarachnoid space and its relation to the overall shape of the medulla. This shape is indicative of a cranial nerve exiting at more mid-to-caudal medullary levels. In **B**, note its relationship to the preolivary sulcus and olivary eminence. The hypoglossal exits the base of the skull by traversing the hypoglossal canal. A lesion of the hypoglossal root, or in its peripheral distribution, will result in a deviation of the tongue to the side of the root damage on attempted protrusion; the

genioglossus muscle on that side is paralyzed. A lesion in the medulla, such as a *medial medullary syndrome (Déjèrine syndrome)*, can result in the same deviation of the tongue (to the side of the lesion on protrusion) plus additional motor (corticospinal) and sensory (medial lemniscus) deficits on the opposite side of the body.

The total picture of deficits seen in medullary lesions that involve the hypoglossal nucleus, or nerve, or in posterior fossa lesions that involve the hypoglossal root and other roots, will depend on what additional structures are recruited into the lesion or are damaged. For example, the *Collet-Sicard syndrome* involves the roots of CNs IX, X, XI (with the corresponding deficits) and the root of XII (with the appropriate deficit). Recall that the jugular foramen (CNs IX, X, XI) and the hypoglossal canal (CN XII) are closely adjacent to each other, separated only by a small bar of bone. These roots may be collectively damaged in a basal skull fracture involving both foramina or by a tumor involving these roots in a confined area.

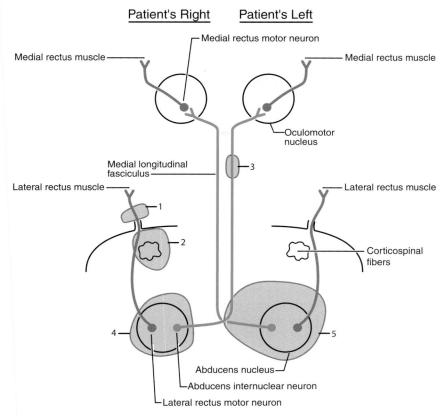

Patient's Right   Patient's Left

Medial rectus motor neuron

Medial rectus muscle

Medial rectus muscle

Oculomotor nucleus

Medial longitudinal fasciculus — 3

Lateral rectus muscle

Lateral rectus muscle

1

Corticospinal fibers

2

4   5

Abducens nucleus

Abducens internuclear neuron

Lateral rectus motor neuron

3-8 Lesions (#1 to #5) of the abducens nerve and/or nucleus and of the medial longitudinal fasciculus that result in deficits of eye movements in the horizontal plane.

Lesion of the abducens root (#1): Motor neurons in the abducens nucleus innervate the ipsilateral lateral rectus muscle. Consequently, a patient with a lesion of the abducens root external to the pons (see Figure 3-5 for the position of the sixth root) experiences a loss of voluntary lateral gaze in the eye on the side of the lesion, indicating a paralysis of the lateral rectus muscle. Other movements in the affected eye, and all movements in the contralateral eye, are normal. This patient will experience *diplopia*. When looking straight ahead, the eye on the lesioned side will deviate slightly toward the midline (unopposed action of the medial rectus in the same eye) and the diplopia is made worse when attempting to look toward the lesioned side in a horizontal plane.

Caudal basilar pontine lesion (#2): As axons arising from abducens motor neurons pass through the basilar pons, they are located laterally adjacent to corticospinal fibers (see Figure 6-17 on pp. 126–127). A lesion in this portion of the pons may simultaneously damage the exiting abducens fibers and corticospinal axons. A patient with this lesion experiences an *alternating* (or *crossed*) *hemiplegia*, a paralysis of the lateral rectus muscle on the side of the lesion (loss of voluntary lateral gaze to that side, and *diplopia*), and a paralysis of the upper and lower extremities on the opposite side of the body. Alternating, or crossed, deficits are characteristic of brainstem lesions.

Internuclear ophthalmoplegia (INO) (#3): In addition to abducens motor neurons that innervate the ipsilateral lateral rectus muscle, the abducens nucleus also contains interneurons. The axons of these interneurons cross the midline, enter the medial longitudinal fasciculus (MLF), and ascend to terminate on motor neurons in the oculomotor nucleus that innervate the medial rectus muscle on that

side. A lesion in the MLF interrupts these axons and results in a loss of medial gaze (medial rectus paralysis) in the eye on the side of the lesion during attempted conjugate eye movements. Other movements in the affected eye and all movements in the contralateral eye are normal. The laterality of the deficit reflects the side of the lesion and of the deficit. For example, a *right internuclear ophthalmoplegia* specifies a lesion in the right MLF and paralysis of the right medial rectus muscle; a *left internuclear ophthalmoplegia* indicates a lesion in the left MLF and left medial rectus weakness.

Lesion of the abducens nucleus (#4): A lesion of the abducens nucleus damages alpha motor neurons innervating the ipsilateral lateral rectus muscle and the interneurons that terminate on medial rectus alpha motor neurons residing in the contralateral oculomotor nucleus. A patient with this lesion experiences a loss of horizontal gaze in both eyes during attempted voluntary eye movement toward the side of the lesion; horizontal gaze toward the contralateral side is normal. This is basically an abducens root lesion plus an INO.

The one-and-a-half syndrome (#5): This syndrome is so named because a unilateral pontine lesion may result in a loss of medial and lateral voluntary eye movement on the side of the lesion (the "one") and a loss of medial horizontal eye movement on the contralateral side (the "one-half"). The lesion resulting in this pattern of deficits involves the abducens nucleus on one side (deficits = lateral rectus paralysis on the side of the lesion, medial rectus paralysis on the contralateral side) and the immediately adjacent MLF conveying the axons of abducens interneurons originating in the opposite abducens nucleus (deficit = medial rectus paralysis on the side of the lesion). These lesions are usually large and involve portions of the paramedian pontine reticular formation, commonly called the horizontal gaze center.

Table 3-2 Summary of Brainstem Lesions that Involve Cranial Nerve Nuclei and/or the Roots of Cranial Nerves and the Correlated Deficits of Cranial Nerve Function

LESION(S)/SYNDROME	STRUCTURES DAMAGED	DEFICITS
Medulla Medial medullary (Déjérine) syndrome Lateral medullary (PICA or Wallenberg) syndrome	—Hypoglossal nerve/nucleus —Corticospinal fibers —Medial lemniscus —Spinal trigeminal tract nucleus ——Nucleus ambiguus —Vestibular nuclei —Anterolateral system	—Ipsilateral paralysis of tongue —Contralateral hemiplegia —Contralateral loss of discriminative touch, vibratory and position sense on UE, trunk, and LE —Ipsilateral loss of pain and thermal sense on face —Dysphagia, hoarseness, deviation of uvula to contralateral side —Nystagmus, vertigo, nausea —Contralateral loss of pain and thermal sense on UE, trunk, and LE
Pons Raymond syndrome* (Foville syndrome) Gubler syndrome	—Corticospinal fibers —Abducens fibers in pons —Corticospinal fibers —Facial nucleus or fibers —(Anterolateral system) —(Trigeminal nerve) —Corticospinal fibers —Trigeminal nerve	—Contralateral hemiplegia —Ipsilateral abducens palsy, diplopia —Contralateral hemiplegia —Ipsilateral paralysis of facial muscles —(Contralateral loss of pain and thermal sensation on UE, trunk, and LE) —(Ipsilateral paralysis of masticatory muscles, ipsilateral loss of pain and thermal sensation on face) —Contralateral hemiplegia —Ipsilateral paralysis of masticatory muscles, ipsilateral loss of pain and thermal sensation on face
Midbrain Weber (cerebral peduncle) syndrome Claude (red nucleus) syndrome	—Corticospinal fibers —Oculomotor fibers —Corticonuclear fibers —Oculomotor nerve —Cerebellothalamic fibers	—Contralateral hemiplegia —Ipsilateral oculomotor paralysis, diplopia, dilated pupil —Contralateral weakness of facial muscles on lower face; deviation of tongue to contralateral side on protrusion; ipsilateral trapezius + sternocleidomastoid weakness —Ipsilateral oculomotor palsy, diplopia, dilated pupil —Contralateral ataxia, tremor, + red nucleus hyperkinesias

Benedikt syndrome = Deficits of Weber syndrome + deficits of Claude syndrome

*According to Wolf (1971) in his excellent book describing brainstem syndromes from their original sources, Fulgence Raymond described a female patient, with several medical complications, with right hemiparesis and left abducens palsy. Raymond localized the probable lesion (he acknowledged more than one potential cause) to the basilar pons involving corticospinal fibers and the abducens root. This is also commonly called the Foville syndrome, although Foville is also described as recruiting adjacent structures with their corresponding deficits. Both eponyms are acceptable.

LE = lower extremity; UE = upper extremity.

■ Cranial Nerves in Their Larger Functional/Clinical Context (Figures 3-9 to 3-15) ■

Cranial nerves are usually an integral part of any neurological examination; this is certainly the case in injuries and/or diseases that involve the head and neck. This chapter details their exit points (or, one could argue, the entrance points in the case of sensory nerves), their corresponding appearance in MRI, and examples of lesions causing deficits of eye movements in the horizontal plane and of brainstem lesions that include cranial nerve deficits.

This is, however, only part of a much larger picture that places cranial nerves in a functional context and views their connections in the periphery as well as within the central nervous system. Although these more comprehensive cranial nerve connections, and their corresponding functions, are illustrated in Chapter 8 in their appropriate *systems context*, they are briefly listed here to facilitate cross reference for those users wishing to consider cranial nerves in a more integrated format at this point.

Functional Components of Spinal and Cranial Nerves (See Figures 8-1 and 8-2 on pp. 184–185.)

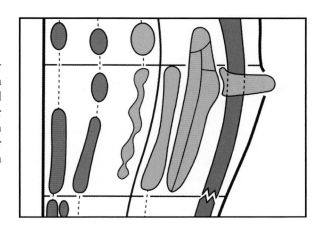

3-9 The columns of cells within the spinal cord are rostrally continuous with comparable cell columns in the brainstem that have similar functions. For example, general motor cell columns of the spinal cord are continuous with the groups of motor nuclei that innervate the tongue and the extraocular muscles; both cell columns innervate skeletal muscles. The same is the case for general sensation. Nuclei conveying special senses are found only in the brainstem and are associated with only certain cranial nerves.

Trigeminal Pathways and Deficits (See Figures 8-9 and 8-10A,B on pp. 198–201.)

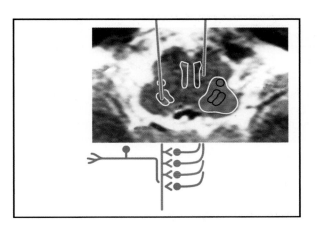

3-10 The trigeminal nerve conveys sensory input from the face and oral cavity and provides motor innervation to the muscles of mastication. The spinal trigeminal tract and nucleus also receive general sensation via CNs VII, IX, and X. In this respect, the *spinal trigeminal tract is the center for all general sensory sensations entering the brainstem on all cranial nerves.* In the same sense, the solitary tract and nucleus (Figure 8-11 on pp. 202–203) is *the brainstem center for all visceral sensation that enters the brainstem on CNs VII, IX, and X.* Both of these cranial nerve brainstem nuclei convey information to the thalamus and eventually to the cerebral cortex.

Corticonuclear Pathways and Deficits (See Figures 8-15 and 8-16A,B on pp. 210–213.)

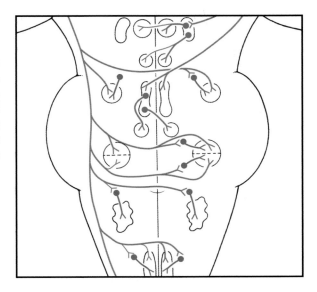

3-11 The cerebral cortex influences cranial nerve nuclei via corticonuclear fibers. In the neurological examination, this is most evident when testing motor functions of CNs VII, IX, X, XI and XII. In many situations, the deficit is seen by the inability of the patient to perform a movement "against resistance." Comparing the deficit(s) of a lesion of these fibers to damage of cranial nerves within the brainstem, or the periphery, is essential to localizing the lesion within the central nervous system.

Cranial Nerve Efferents (III–VII and IX–XII) and Deficits (See Figures 8-21 to 8-24B on pp. 222–229.)

3-12 Cranial nerve nuclei are either motor to skeletal muscle or visceromotor to ganglia in the periphery. Lesions involving the nuclei, or roots, of motor nuclei result in paralysis of the muscles served, with the predictable deficits, such as weakness of the facial muscles or deviation of the tongue on protrusion. Lesions that damage the visceromotor fibers of a cranial nerve result in an expected visceromotor response, such as dilation of the pupil, or a decrease in secretory function or smooth muscle motility.

Cranial Nerve Reflex Pathways and Deficits (See Figures 8-29 to 8-34 on pp. 232–235.)

3-13 Testing cranial nerve reflexes is a routine part of any complete neurological examination. This part of the neurological exam tests the integrity of the afferent and efferent limbs of the reflex. Sometimes both of these are on the same cranial nerve; sometimes they are on different cranial nerves. In addition, deficits may be seen that reflect damage *affecting* cranial nerve function, but this damage is not in the afferent or efferent limbs of the reflex; this suggests a broader problem within the central nervous system.

Pupillary and Visual Pathways and Deficits (See Figures 8-46 to 8-49B on pp. 258–263.)

3-14 The pupillary reflex (commonly called the *pupillary light reflex*) has its afferent limb via the second cranial nerve and its efferent limb via the third cranial nerve. The reaction of the pupil when light is shined in one eye is a clear hint as to the location of the lesion. The optic nerve, chiasm, tract, and radiations and the visual cortex have a retinotopic representation throughout. Lesions of any of these structures result in visual deficits, such as a *hemianopia* or *quadrantanopia*, that reflect the particular portion of the visual system that is damaged. Because visual pathways are widespread within the brain, lesions at various different locations may result in visual deficits.

Auditory and Vestibular Pathways and Deficits (See Figures 8-51 and 8-52 on pp. 266–269.)

3-15 The auditory portion of the eighth cranial nerve is concerned with the perception of sound. Damage to the cochlea itself, or the cochlear root, may profoundly alter one's perception of sound or may result in deafness. The vestibular portion of the eighth cranial nerve functions in the arena of balance, equilibrium, and maintenance of posture. Damage to the semicircular canals, to the vestibular root, or to central structures that receive vestibular input, may result in *vertigo, ataxia*, difficulty walking or maintaining balance, and/or a variety of eye movement problems.

4

Meninges, Cisterns, Ventricles, and Related Hemorrhages

Table 4-1 Comparison of Cerebral Versus Spinal Meninges

CEREBRAL	SPINAL
Dura	**Dura**
• Adherent to inner table of skull (no epidural space)	• Separated from vertebrae by epidural space
• Composed of two fused layers (periosteal and meningeal), which split to form sinuses	• Composed of one layer (spinal dura only; vertebrae have their own periosteum)
Arachnoid (outer part of leptomeninges)	**Arachnoid (outer part of leptomeninges)**
• Attached to dura in living condition (no subdural space)	• Attached to dura in living condition (no subdural space)
• Arachnoid villi (in superior sagittal sinus)	• No arachnoid villi
• Arachnoid trabeculae	• Few or no arachnoid trabeculae but larger arachnoid septae
• Subarachnoid space with many cisterns	• Subarachnoid space with one cistern
Pia (inner part of leptomeninges)	**Pia (inner part of leptomeninges)**
• Intimately adherent to surface of brain	• Intimately adherent to surface of cord
• No pial specializations	• Specializations in the form of denticulate ligaments, filum terminale, and linea splendens
• Follows vessels as they pierce the cerebral cortex	• Follows vessels as they pierce the cord

■ Meningitis, Meningeal Hemorrhages, and Meningioma ■

A wide variety of disease processes and lesions may involve the meninges; only a few examples are mentioned here.

Infections of the meninges (**bacterial meningitis**) may be called **leptomeningitis** because the causative organisms localize to the subarachnoid space and involve the pia and arachnoid. Extension into the dura is called **pachymeningitis**. A variety of organisms cause *bacterial meningitis*, those most commonly associated with certain groups are as follows: neonate = *Streptococcus agalactiae, Escherichia coli, Listeria monocytogenes;* neonate to about 24 months = *S. agalactiae, E. coli, Haemophilus influenza;* about 2–50 years = *S. pneumonia, Neisseria meningitides;* about 50 years+ = *S. pneumonia, N. meningitides, L. monocytogenes;* basal skull fracture = *S. pneumonia, H. influenza;* head trauma = *Staphylococcus.* The patient becomes acutely ill (i.e., headache, confusion, fever, stiff neck (*meningismus*), stupor), may have generalized or focal signs/symptoms, and, if not rapidly treated (with appropriate antibiotics), will likely die. Patients with **viral meningitis** may become ill over a period of several days, experience headache, confusion, and fever, but, with supportive care, will recover after an acute phase of approximately 1 to 2 weeks. These patients usually recover with no permanent deficits.

The most common cause of an **epidural (extradural) hematoma** is a skull fracture that results in a laceration of a major dural vessel, such as the middle meningeal artery. In approximately 15% of cases, bleeding may come from a venous sinus. The extravasated blood dissects the dura mater off the inner table of the skull; there is no pre-existing (extradural) space for the blood to enter. These lesions are frequently large, lens (lenticular) shaped, may appear loculated, and are "short and thick" compared with subdural hematomas (see Figure 4-2 on p. 59). The fact that epidural hematomas do not cross suture lines correlates with their characteristic shape. The patient may lapse into a coma and, if the lesion is left untreated, death may result. In some cases, the patient may be unconscious initially, followed by a lucid interval (the patient is wide awake), then subsequently deteriorate rapidly and die; this is called "talk and die." Treatment of choice for large lesions is surgical removal of the clot and coagulation of the damaged vessel.

Tearing of bridging veins (veins passing from the brain outward through the arachnoid and dura), usually the result of trauma, is a common cause of **subdural hematoma**. This designation is somewhat a misnomer because the extravasated blood actually dissects through a specialized, yet structurally weak, cell layer at the dura–arachnoid interface; this is the dural border cell layer. There is no pre-existing "subdural space" in the normal brain. Acute subdural hematomas, more commonly seen in younger patients, usually are detected immediately or within a few hours after the precipitating incident. Chronic subdural hematomas, usually seen in the elderly, are frequently of unknown origin; may take days or weeks to become symptomatic; and cause a progressive change in the mental status of the patient. This lesion appears "long and thin" compared with an epidural hematoma, follows the surface of the brain, and may extend for considerable distances (see Figure 4-2 on p. 58 and Figure 4-5 on p. 61). Treatment is surgical evacuation (for larger or acute lesions) or close monitoring for small, asymptomatic, or chronic lesions.

The most common cause of **subarachnoid hemorrhage** is trauma. In approximately 75%–80% of patients with **spontaneous (nontraumatic) subarachnoid hemorrhage,** the precipitating event is rupture of an intracranial aneurysm. Symptomatic bleeding from an arteriovenous malformation occurs in approximately 5% of cases. Blood collects in and percolates through the subarachnoid space and cisterns (see Figure 4-5 on p. 61). Sometimes, the deficits seen (assuming the patient is not in a coma) may be a clue as to location, especially if cranial nerves are nearby. Onset is sudden; the patient complains of a sudden and excruciatingly painful headache ("the worst of my life," "thunderclap," "felt like my head exploded") and may remain conscious, become lethargic and disoriented, or may be comatose. Treatment of an aneurysm is to surgically separate the sac of the aneurysm from the parent vessel (by clip or coil), if possible, and protect against the development of vasospasm. During surgery, some blood in the subarachnoid space and cisterns may be removed.

Tumors of the meninges (**meningiomas**) are classified in different ways, but usually they arise from arachnoid cap(stem cells (a small number are dural in origin) around the villi or at places where vessels or cranial nerves penetrate the dura-arachnoid. These tumors grow slowly (symptoms may develop almost imperceptibly over years), are histologically benign, may result in hyperostosis of the overlying skull, and frequently contain calcifications. In decreasing order, meningiomas are found in the following locations: parasagittal area + falx cerebri (together 29%), convexity 15%, sella 13%, sphenoid ridge 12%, and olfactory groove 10%. Treatment is primarily by surgical removal, although some meningiomas are treated by radiotherapy.

4-1 Semi-diagrammatic representation of the central nervous system and its associated meninges. The details show the relationships of the meninges in the area of the superior sagittal sinus, on the lateral aspect of the cerebral hemisphere, and around the spinal cord. Cerebrospinal fluid is produced by the choroid plexuses of the lateral, third, and fourth ventricles. It circulates through the ventricular system (small arrows) and enters the subarachnoid space via the medial foramen of Magendie and the two lateral foramina of Luschka. In the living situation, the arachnoid is attached to the inner surface of the dura. There is no *actual* or *potential* subdural space.

4-2 Examples of *meningitis* (**A–D**, all axial) in the adult. Meningitis is a disease that generally involves the subarachnoid space (SAS) and the membranes bordering on this space, namely the *arachnoid mater* and the *pia mater*. Consequently, it is commonly called *leptomeningitis* (or *arachnoiditis*, or *pia-arachnitis*). Meningitis may preferentially affect one side more that the other in some cases.

Source of infections that may lead to meningitis are those involving the paranasal sinuses or the mastoid air cells (*mastoiditis*, **A**). Once this infection accesses the central nervous system, it may involve the venous sinuses (**A**), which appear bright when enhanced. The infection will layer out over the surface of brain within the SAS, enter the sulci, and occupy the SAS immediately above and below the tentorium cerebelli (see arrows in **A, B, C**). The SAS and the sulci enhance when the patient is treated with IV gadolinium (**C, D**) and appear bright in the image. In addition to these features, small enhancements may appear within the SAS (**D**, arrows) that indicate the formation of small abscesses. This inflammation may also extend to involve the dura mater in which case it is called *pachymeningitis*.

4-3 Examples of *meningitis (leptomeningitis)* that extensively involves both sides of the central nervous system (**A–D**, all axial) in the adult. In **A**, note the enhancement of the meninges over the temporal lobe, at the location of the tentorium cerebelli, and of the venous sinuses (SSS = superior sagittal; S = sigmoid; TS = transverse). At different axial levels, enhancement is clearly visible on the brain surface (**B, C**, arrows), along the dural reflections (tentorium cerebelli and falx cerebri, **B–D**), and within the sulci (**C**). In addition, enhancements over the curvature of the hemisphere are suggestive of focal collections of inflammation.

As seen in these samples, meningitis can be imaged using gadolinium and to a reasonable level its degree and extent visualized. However, it is also apparent that the lesion, the inflamed meninges, and SAS, are more subtle than lesions such as meningioma, hemorrhage, or brain tumor. Vessels located within the subarachnoid space may also enhance as they most likely contain infectious material and the organisms may infiltrate the vessel walls. As noted in Figure 4-2, the inflammation may also extend to involve the dura mater (*pachymeningitis*).

Hemorrhage in brain

4-4 Examples of *epidural (extradural) hemorrhage/hematoma* (A, B) and of acute (C, D) and subacute (E) subdural *hematoma/hemorrhage*. Note the lenticular shape of the epidural lesions (they do not cross suture lines—A, B), their loculated appearance, and their location external to the substance of the brain. In contrast, the acute subdural lesions (C, D, arrows) are quite thin and extend over a longer distance on the cortex; they are not constrained by suture lines. Note the midline shift in patients A and D.

In E, the subdural hematoma has both chronic and subacute phases. The chronic phase is indicated by the upper two and lower two arrows where the blood is replaced by fluid, and the subacute phase by the middle arrow, where fresher blood has entered the lesion. Note the extent of this lesion on the surface of the cortex and its narrowness compared with epidural lesions. The patient in E also has small hemorrhages into the substance of the brain in the region of the genu of the internal capsule. Images A–E are CT. For additional comments on epidural and subdural hemorrhages, see p. 56.

The treatment of choice for *epidural hematoma*, especially if the patient is symptomatic, or if the patient is asymptomatic but the acute lesion is greater than 1 cm thick at its widest point, is surgical removal and hemostasis of bleeders. In *subdural hematoma*, surgical evacuation is the preferred treatment in symptomatic patients with acute lesions that are 1 cm thick (0.5 in pediatric patients). On the other hand, asymptomatic patients with thin subdural lesions may be followed medically and may not require surgery.

4-5 Examples of *epidural* (extradural) *hemorrhage/hematoma* (**A, B**) and *subdural hematoma/hemorrhage* (**C, D**) resultant to trauma to the head; all are CT and all are in the axial plane.

Epidural hematoma may occur in cases of skull fracture (**A**, on the right side) in which the middle meningeal artery (or its larger branches) is lacerated. The resulting hematoma is formed between the inner table of the skull and the outer aspect of the dura (*epidural*, **B**, on the right). In this significant trauma, there is a large epidural, a small lesion, probably also an epidural (small arrows), and small amounts or air within the cranial cavity (**B**, black dots). The mechanism of epidural hematoma formation is most likely twofold. First, the dura is stripped from the inner table of the skull during the traumatic event creating an artifactual space. Second, the sharp edges of bone lacerate arteries, which bleed into this space,

and, it is believed, may further dissect the dura from the skull. Epidural hematomas do not cross suture lines.

Trauma to the head, without skull fracture, may result in subdural hemorrhage/hematoma; in such cases, it is called *acute subdural hematoma* (**C, D**). Subdural hematomas may also be *subacute* or *chronic* and do occur in cases where trauma is not involved. In these examples, trauma on the right side of the head (**C**, soft tissue damage at arrows) resulted in a large *acute subdural hematoma* on the patient's right side, and trauma on the left side of the head (**D**, soft tissue damage at arrows) resulted in a subdural lesion on the patient's right. This latter lesion is a type of *contrecoup injury* in which the lesion is on the side opposite the initial impact. Note that the larger subdural lesion (**C**) has caused considerable midline shift. Subdural hematomas are not restrained by suture lines.

A

Lamina terminalis cistern

Chiasmatic cistern

Interpeduncular cistern

Prepontine cistern

Premedullary cistern

Paracallosal cistern

Quadrigeminal cistern

B

Fourth ventricle

C

D

Cisterna magna

B

Sylvian cistern
Crural cistern

Midbrain

Quadrigeminal cistern

Lamina terminalis cistern
Optic tract

Interpeduncular cistern

Ambient cistern

Inferior colliculus

C

Trigeminal nerve

Superior cerebellopontine cistern

Prepontine cistern

Basilar artery

Basilar pons

Fourth ventricle

D

Medulla

Cisterna magna

Premedullary cistern

Inferior cerebellopontine cistern

4-6 A median sagittal MRI (**A**—T2-weighted) of the brain showing the positions of the major cisterns associated with midline structures. Axial views of the midbrain (**B**—T1-weighted), pons (**C**—T2-weighted), and medulla (**D**—T2-weighted) represent the corresponding planes indicated in the sagittal view (**A**).

Cisterns are the enlarged portions of the subarachnoid space that contain arteries and veins, roots of cranial nerves, and, of course, cerebrospinal fluid. Consequently, the subarachnoid space and cisterns are continuous one with the other. In addition, the subarachnoid space around the brain is continuous with that around the spinal cord. Compare these cisterns with blood-filled parts of the subarachnoid space and cisterns in Figure 4-5 on the facing page.

A

Lamina terminalis cistern

Supraoptic recess

Interpeduncular cistern

Temporal horn

Midbrain

Quadrigeminal cistern

Sylvian cistern

Crural cistern

Ambient cistern

B

Subdural hemorrhage

Blood on insular cortex

C

Lamina terminalis cistern

Blood on insula

Interpeduncular cistern

Cerebellum

Blood on tentorium cerebelli

Third ventricle

Sylvian cistern

Crural cistern

Ambient cistern

D

Rostral part of fourth ventricle

4-7 Blood in the *subarachnoid space* and *cisterns (subarachnoid hemorrhage)*. In these CT examples, blood occupies the subarachnoid space and cisterns, outlining these areas in white. Consequently, the shape of the cisterns is indicated by the configuration of the white area, the white area representing blood.

Around the base of the brain (**A**), it is easy to identify the cisterns related to the midbrain, the supraoptic recess, which is devoid of blood, and blood extending laterally into the Sylvian cistern. In some cases (**B**), subdural hemorrhage may penetrate the arachnoid membrane and result in blood infiltrating between gyri, such as this example with blood on the cortex of the insula. In **C**, the blood is located around the midbrain (crural and ambient cisterns), extends into the Sylvian cistern, and into the cistern of the lamina terminalis. The sharp interface between the lamina terminalis cistern (containing blood) and the third ventricle (devoid of blood) repre-

sents the position of the lamina terminalis. In **D**, blood is located in cisterns around the pons, but avoids the rostral part of the fourth ventricle. Also note the clearly enlarged temporal horn of the lateral ventricle in **D**; enlargement of this particular part of the ventricle is indicative of increased pressure within the ventricular system.

Subarachnoid hemorrhage (SAH) is always a serious medical event. In the case of SAH resulting from aneurysm rupture (about 75%–80% of all spontaneous cases), 10%–15% die prior to reaching medical attention, 40%–50% die within about 2–4 weeks of the precipitating event, and about 30% of those who survive have moderate to severe deficits. About 65% of patients who have the aneurysms successfully clipped have a diminished quality of life.

Compare these images with the locations of some of the comparable cisterns as seen in Figure 4-6 on the facing page. Images **A–D** are CT.

4-8 Examples of a right-sided convexity meningioma (**A, B**) and a meningioma of the tentorium cerebelli (**C, D**). Meningiomas are slow-growing, usually benign extra-axial tumors that are curable assuming they can be completely removed (91%+, 5-year survival). They may present with headache or seizure, but many are asymptomatic and some are discovered as an incidental finding. The *convexity meningoma* (**A**—sagittal, **B**—coronal) is located in the medial aspect of the superior frontal gyrus rostral to the paracentral gyri. It is slightly off the midline; meningiomas that are directly adjacent to the midline and involve the superior sagittal sinus are called *parasagittal meningiomas*. Note its attachment to the dura (**A**,

arrow); this attachment, seen in many meningiomas, is commonly called the *dural tail*. Convexity meningiomas are seen in about 15% of cases.

The *tentorial meningioma* (**C**—sagittal, **D**—coronal) is located on the midline, close to the rostral edge of the tentorium, and on its inferior surface. The tumor significantly impinges on the cerebellum (**C, D**), but does not involve the occipital lobes. This patient has motor deficits of the cerebellar type due to the involvement of the cerebellum. Due to its location, this tumor presents a greater surgical challenge than does the convexity meningioma. Tentorial meningiomas are seen in 3%–4% of cases.

4-9 Examples of meningiomas that are located on the midline. The *sellar meningioma* (**A**—sagittal, **B**—coronal, also called *tuberculum sellae meningioma*), arises from the sella turcica and, due to its position, may impinge on optic structures and/or cause deficits indicative of involvement of the hypothalamus. Note that, although the tumor has reached significant size, major structures in the central region of the hemisphere, such as large veins and the corpus callosum (G = genu, B = body, S = splenium), are in their normal positions. Tumors are seen in this area in about 8%–12% of cases and may require special surgical approaches.

The large meningioma in **C** and **D** was diagnosed as a *falcine meningioma*, a tumor that arises from the falx cerebri. Such tumors may arise at any point along the course of the falx cerebri, are frequently bilateral, and may impinge on the medial aspects of both hemispheres. Note that the central portions of the hemisphere have been pushed caudally as seen by the foreshortened internal cerebral vein and the change in shape and position of the corpus callosum (G = genu, S = splenium). At the same time, *olfactory groove meningiomas* are also seen in this location and have a very similar appearance. These arise from the area of the cribriform plate and enlarge upward to impinge on the frontal lobes. Falcine meningiomas constitute about 8% and olfactory groove meningiomas about 10% of all tumors of this type.

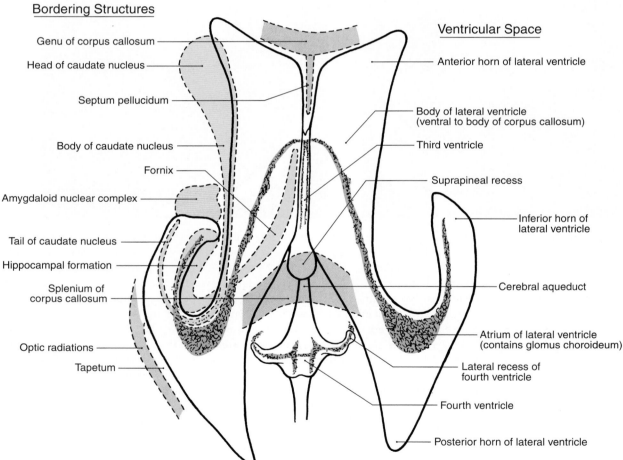

4-10 Lateral (above) and dorsal (below) views of the ventricles and the choroid plexus. The dashed lines show the approximate positions of some of the important structures that border on the ventricular space. The choroid plexus is shown in red, and structures bordering on the various portions of the ventricular spaces are color-coded; these colors are continued in Figure 4-11 on the facing page. Note the relationships between the choroid plexus and various parts of the ventricular system. The large expanded portion of the choroid plexus found in the area of the atrium is the glomus (*glomus choroideum*).

A
- Corpus callosum (body)
- Anterior horn of lateral ventricle
- Septum pellucidum
- Caudate nucleus (head)
- Corpus callosum (rostrum)
- Gyrus rectus

B
- Caudate nucleus
- Corpus callosum (body)
- Septum pellucidum
- Fornix (F)
- Body of lateral ventricle
- Interventricular foramen
- Anterior commissure
- Third ventricle
- Hypothalamus
- Optic chiasm
- F

C
- Caudate nucleus (body)
- Stria terminalis
- Corpus callosum (body)
- Body of lateral ventricle
- Choroid plexus (CP)
- Fornix
- CP
- Third ventricle
- Dorsal thalamus
- Massa intermedia
- Mammillary body
- Hypothalamus

D
- Caudate nucleus
- Fornix
- Dorsal thalamus
- Third ventricle
- Amygdaloid nuclear complex
- Optic tract
- Inferior horn of lateral ventricle

E
- Body of lateral ventricle
- Corpus callosum
- Pulvinar
- Pineal
- Cerebral aqueduct
- Inferior horn of lateral ventricle
- Hippocampal formation
- Caudate nucleus (tail)

F
- Optic radiations
- Tapetum
- Corpus callosum (splenium)
- Atrium of lateral ventricle
- Hippocampal formation

G
- Optic radiations
- Tapetum
- Calcarine sulcus
- Calcar avis
- Posterior horn of lateral ventricle

(Lateral view labels: A, B, C, D, E, F, G)

4-11 Lateral view of the ventricular system and corresponding semi-diagrammatic cross-sectional representations from rostral (**A**) to caudal (**G**) identifying specific structures that border on the ventricular space. In the cross-sections, the ventricle is outlined by a heavy line, and the majority of structures labeled have some direct relevance to the ventricular space at that particular level. The color coding corresponds to that shown in Figure 4-10 on the facing page.

4-12 Examples of hemorrhage occupying portions of the ventricular system (*intraventricular hemorrhage*). In these CT images, blood appears white within the ventricles. Consequently, the shape of the ventricular system is outlined by the white area, and the specific portion of the ventricular system is correspondingly labeled.

Note blood in the anterior horn, atrium, and posterior horn of the lateral ventricles (**A, B**), and blood clearly outlining the shape of the third ventricle (**B**). Blood also clearly outlines central portions of the fourth ventricle (**C**) and caudal portions of the fourth ventricle (**D**), including an extension of blood into the left lateral recess of the fourth ventricle. In addition to these images, Figure 4-13C on p. 69 shows blood in the cerebral aqueduct and the most inferior portions of the third ventricle. Images **A—D** are CT.

A

B

Epidural
hematoma

Blood in
brain

Blood in lateral
ventricle

Blood in third
ventricle

C

Blood in third
ventricle

Blood in atrium of
lateral ventricle

Subarachnoid blood on
tentorium cerebelli

4-13 Examples of blood in the ventricles resulting from head trauma and traumatic brain injuries. Note the soft tissue damage and skull fractures (especially in patients **A** and **B**). In patient **A**, there is blood in the right anterior horn of the lateral ventricle. Patient **B** has blood in the right anterior horn, in the third ventricle, in the substance of the brain in the right frontal lobe as well as a small epidural at the right frontal pole. Patient C has blood in the third ventricle and in the atrium of the lateral ventricle on the right side. In addition to trauma, as illustrated here, *intraventricular hemorrhage* (also called *intraventricular blood*) may occur in a variety of situations. *Intracerebral hemorrhage*, a bleed into the substance of the brain (also called *parenchymatous hemorrhage*), may extend into a ventricular space, bleeding from a brain tumor, arteri-

ovenous malformation, or from a tumor of the choroid plexus. In addition, blood from a ruptured aneurysm may preferentially dissect into adjacent ventricular spaces. For example, a ruptured basilar tip aneurysm may result in blood in the third ventricle; a ruptured aneurysm of the anterior communicating artery may result in blood in the third ventricle or in the anterior horn of the lateral ventricle; and rupture of a PICA aneurysm may result in blood in the fourth ventricle.

These images illustrate the important fact that, especially in patients with head trauma, blood may be found at different locations (meningeal, intraventricular, within the substance of the brain [*parenchymatous*]) in the same patient. All images are axial CTs.

A

Choroid plexus (CP) in body of lateral ventricle

CP in atrium of lateral ventricle

CP in roof of third ventricle

CP in temporal horn of lateral ventricle

CP in fourth ventricle

Anterior choroidal artery

AICA

PICA

Posterior communicating artery

Lateral posterior choroidal artery

BA

Medial posterior choroidal artery

VA

B

Medial striate artery

Internal carotid artery

A_1 P_1

Middle cerebral artery (M_1)

Anterior choroidal artery

Anterior choroidal artery

Posterior communicating artery

Posterior cerebral artery (P_2)

Lateral posterior choroidal artery

Superior cerebellar artery

Medial posterior choroidal artery

Basilar artery (BA)

Anterior inferior cerebellar artery (AICA)

AICA branch to choroid plexus at the foramen of Luschka

Vertebral artery (VA)

Posterior inferior cerebellar artery (PICA)

PICA branch to choroid plexus in the fourth ventricle

4-14 Blood supply to the choroid plexus of the lateral, third, and fourth ventricles. Those branches of the vertebrobasilar system and of the internal carotid artery and P_2 segment of the posterior cerebral artery that supply the choroid plexus are accentuated by appearing in a darker red shade. In **A,** a representation of these vessels (origin, course, termination) is shown from the lateral aspect. Anterior, medial posterior, and lateral posterior choroidal arteries serve the plexuses of the lateral and third ventricles. The choroid plexus in the fourth ventricle and the clump of choroid plexus protruding out of the foramen of Luschka are served by posterior inferior and anterior inferior cerebellar arteries, respectively. In **B,** the origins of these branches from their main arterial trunks are shown. See also Figures 2-24 (p. 27), 2-32 (p. 33), and 2-35 (p. 35).

4-15 Tumors of the choroid plexus (CP) constitute about 1% of all intracranial tumors and are generally classified as *choroid plexus papilloma* (benign, most common of CP tumors) or *choroid plexus carcinoma* (malignant, rare). These tumors are most commonly seen in children under 2 years of age and may present with *symptoms/signs of increased intracranial pressure (nausea/ vomiting, lethargy, headache, enlarged ventricles, craniomegaly).* The CP is highly vascularized; consequently, tumors of this structure may bleed into the ventricular space and create a cast outlining its shape.

Examples of tumors of the choroid plexus in axial (A–D), coronal (E), and sagittal (F) planes. The tumor in A–C is from the same patient and shows the lesion in the area of the atrium of the lateral ventricle on the left (A) with bleeding from the tumor into the posterior and temporal horns of the lateral ventricle on the same side (B, C). Note the enlarged ventricles (A–C). The image in D shows a large tumor originating from the choroid plexus in the roof of the third ventricle. This tumor has partially obstructed the interventricular foramina, with consequent enlargement of the lateral ventricles. Images E and F are of patients with tumors in the glomus choroideum of the choroid plexus of the lateral ventricle. Images A–C are CT, and D–F are MRI with enhancement of the tumor.

Blood in frontal lobe

Temporal horn

Blood in third ventricle

Blood in cerebral aqueduct

4-16 Examples of *hemorrhages* into the substance of the brain that, in some cases, have also resulted in blood in the ventricular system. The large hemorrhages into the hemisphere (**A, B**) have resulted in enlargement of the ventricles, a *midline shift*, and, in the case of **A,** a small amount of blood in the posterior horn of the lateral ventricle. In these examples, the lesion is most likely a result of hemorrhage from lenticulostriate branches of the M$_1$ segment.

Blood in the substance of the brain and in the ventricular system may also result from trauma (**C**). In this example (**C**), blood is seen in the frontal lobe and in the third ventricle and cerebral aqueduct. The enlarged temporal horns (**C**) of the lateral ventricles are consistent with the interruption of CSF flow through the cerebral aqueduct (noncommunicating *hydrocephalus*). Images **A–C** are CT.

5

Internal Morphology of the Brain in Unstained Slices and MRI

Part I

Brain Slices in the Coronal Plane Correlated with MRI

Orientation to Coronal MRIs: When looking at a coronal MRI image, you are viewing the image as if you are looking at the face of the patient. Consequently, the observer's right is the left side of the brain in the MRI and the left side of the patient's brain. Conversely, the observer's left is the right side of the brain in the MRI and the right side of the patient's brain. Obviously, the concept of what is the left side versus what is the right side of the patient's brain is enormously important when using MRI (or CT) to diagnose a neurologically impaired individual.

To reinforce this concept, the rostral surface of each coronal brain slice appears in each photograph. So, when looking at the slice, the observer's right field of view is the left side of the brain slice, and the observer's left field of view is the right side of the brain slice. This view of the slice correlates exactly with the orientation of the brain as seen in the accompanying coronal MRIs.

Orientation to Axial MRIs: When looking at an axial MRI image, you are viewing the image as if standing at the patient's feet and looking toward his or her head while the patient is lying on his or her back. Consequently, and as is the case in coronal images, the observer's right is the left side of the brain in the MRI and the left side of the patient's brain. It is absolutely essential to have a clear understanding of this right-versus-left concept when using MRI (or CT) in the diagnosis of the neurologically impaired patient.

To reinforce this concept, the ventral surface of each axial slice was photographed. So, when looking at the slice, the observer's right is the left side of the brain slice. This view of the slice correlates exactly with the orientation of the brain as seen in the accompanying axial MRIs.

Cingulate gyrus (CinGy)

Cingulum (Cin)

Body of corpus callosum (BCorCl)

Head of caudate nucleus (HCaNu)

Anterior horn of lateral ventricle (AH of LVen)

Septum pellucidum

Anterior limb of internal capsule (ALIntCap)

Rostrum of corpus callosum (RCorCl)

Putamen (Put)

External capsule (ExtCap)

Subcallosal gyrus

Claustrum (Cl)

Insula (In)

Extreme capsule (ExtrmCap)

Middle cerebral artery

Temporal lobe (TemLb)

Nucleus accumbens (NuAcc)

Optic nerve (OpNr)

BCorCl

AH of LVen

In

ExtrmCap

NuAcc

OpNr

HCaNu

ALIntCap

Put

ExtCap

Cl

ExtrmCap

CinGy

Cin

BCorCl

AH of LVen

RCorCl

TemLb

Olfactory tract

5-1 The rostral surface of a coronal section of brain through the *anterior limb of the internal capsule* and the *head of the caudate nucleus.* The head of the *caudate nucleus* is especially prominent at this coronal plane. In patients with *Huntington disease* (an inherited neurodegenerative disease), the head of the cau-

date has largely, or completely, disappeared, and the anterior horn of the lateral ventricle would be noticeably large at this level. The two MRI images (both are inversion recovery) are at the same plane and show many of the structures identified in the brain slice.

Body of corpus callosum (BCorCl)

Septum (Sep)

Corona radiata (CorRad)

Column of fornix (ColFor)

Insula (In)

Anterior commissure (AC)

Claustrum

Ventral striatum

Ventral pallidum

Supraoptic recess

Optic chiasm (OpCh)

Infundibulum (Inf)

Uncus

Head of caudate nucleus (HCaNu)

Anterior limb of internal capsule (ALIntCap)

Putamen (Put)

External Capsule (ExtCap)

Claustrum (Cl)

Extreme capsule (ExtCap)

Globus pallidus (GP)

Middle cerebral artery

Sep

CorRad

ColFor

In

GP
AC

Optic tract

BCorCl

HCaNu

ALIntCap

Put

Cl

AC

Third ventricle

Inf

ExtrmCap

Sep

CorRad

GP

AC

OpCh

5-2 The rostral surface of a coronal section of brain through the level of the *anterior commissure* and the *column of the fornix*. The *caudate nucleus* is smaller in size (when compared to the more rostral plane in Figure 5-1) and the *globus pallidus* is obvi- ous in its position medially adjacent to the *putamen*. The two MRI images (both are inversion recovery) are at the same plane and show many of the structures identified in the brain slice.

Body of corpus callosum (BCorCl)

Anterior tubercle of
thalamus (AntTub)

Head of caudate nucleus
(HCaNu)

Body of lateral
ventricle (BLatVen)

Corona radiata (CorRad)

Internal capsule (IntCap,
level of Genu)

Stria terminalis and
terminal vein

Insula (In)

Putamen (Put)

External capsule
(ExtCap)

Globus pallidus (GP)

Claustrum (Cl)

Insula (In)

Extreme capsule
(ExtrmCap)

Column of fornix
(ColFor)

Column of fornix
(ColFor)

Third ventricle (ThrVen)

Amygdaloid nuclear
complex (AmyNu)

Amygdaloid nuclear
complex (AmyNu)

Hypothalamus (Hyth)

Optic Tract (OpTr)

BLatVen

BCorCl

HCaNu

IntCap

CorRad

Anterior
nucleus

Put

Body of
fornix

AntTub

ExtCap

In

ThrVen

Ventral
anterior
nucleus

GP

OpTr

Hippo-
campus

Hyth

ThrVen

OpTr

AmyNu

5-3 The rostral surface of a coronal section of brain through the level of the *anterior tubercle of the thalamus* and the *column of the fornix* just caudal to the anterior commissure. A level that includes these structures also passes through the *genu of the internal capsule*. Portions of the columns of the fornix and the septum (drawn in as black lines) were removed to more adequately expose the anterior tubercles of the thalamus. This section also includes the two portions of the globus pallidus: a *medial* or *internal segment* and a *lateral* or *external segment*. The terminal vein is also called the superior thalamostriate vein. The two MRI images (both are inversion recovery) are at the same plane and show many of the structures identified in the brain slice.

The hippocampus is located in the ventromedial aspect of the temporal horn of the lateral ventricle and appears to have texture in MRI representing its alternating layers of cell bodies and fibers. The amygdaloid nucleus is located in the rostral end of the temporal horn and appears very homogenous in MRI. An easy way to recall these relationships is: ventricular space + texture = hippocampus, whereas no ventricular space + homogenous appearance = amygdala. Based on the coronal plane, the transition from one to the other may take place quickly.

Septum

Body of corpus callosum (BCorCl)

Body of fornix (BFor)

Body of lateral ventricle (BLatVen)

Anterior nucleus of thalamus (AntNu)

Body of caudate nucleus (BCaNu)

Stria terminalis and terminal vein

Ventral anterior nucleus of thalamus (VA)

Corona radiata (CorRad)

Posterior limb of internal capsule (PLIntCap)

Ventral anterior nucleus of thalamus (VA)

Putamen (Put)

Mammillothalamic tract

Insula (In)

External capsule (ExtCap)

Globus pallidus (GP)

Claustrum

Extreme capsule (ExtrmCap)

Third ventricle (ThrVen)

Dorsomedial nucleus of thalamus

Amygdaloid nuclear complex (AmyNu)

Optic Tract

Mammillary body (MB)

Hippocampal formation

Inferior horn of lateral ventricle (IHLatVen)

Oculomotor nerve

Hippocampal formation (Hip)

Interpeduncular fossa

Posterior cerebral artery

Basilar pons (BP)

BCorCl

BLatVen

BFor

Thalamus

Put

GP

IHLatVen

BP

BLatVen
BCaNu

AntNu
VA

PLIntCap

Put

IHLatVen
Hip

BLatVen
BCaNu

BCorCl

BFor
AntNu

VA
PLIntCap

In

Hip

MB

5-4 The rostral surface of a section of brain through the *anterior nucleus of the thalamus, mammillothalamic tract,* and *mammillary bodies.* This plane also includes the basilar pons (seen in the slice and MRI) and structures associated with the interpeduncular fossa (seen in the slice). The two MRI images (both are inversion recovery) are at the same plane and show many of the structures identified in the brain slice. The globus pallidus is clearly divided into its lateral and medial segments in the brain slice. Additionally, the terminal vein is also called the superior thalamostriate vein.

Body of fornix (BFor)

Stria terminalis and terminal vein

Corona radiata (CorRad)

Third ventricle and massa intermedia

Posterior limb of internal capsule (PLIntCap)

External capsule

Claustrum

Extreme capsule

Subthalamic nucleus

Red nucleus

Substantia nigra (SN)

Interpeduncular fossa (IPF)

Basilar pons (BP)

Body of corpus callosum (BCorCl)

Body of lateral ventricle (BLatVen)

Body of caudate nucleus (BCaNu)

Dorsomedial nucleus of thalamus (DMNu)

Ventral lateral nucleus of thalamus (VL)

Putamen (Put)

Insula (In)

Internal medullary lamina (IML)

Globus pallidus (GP)

Third ventricle (ThrVen)

Tail of caudate nucleus

Inferior horn of lateral ventricle

Hippocampal formation (Hip)

Optic tract

Crus cerebri (CC)

Corticospinal fibers

BFor

ThrVen

PLIntCap
Put
GP

Hip

IPF

BCorCl
BCaNu
DMNu
VL

In

Put

CC

SN

BP

BFor

IML
ThrVen

SN

IPF

5-5 The rostral surface of a coronal section of brain through caudal parts of the *ventral lateral nucleus, massa intermedia, subthalamic nucleus,* and *basilar pons.* This slice beautifully illustrates that fibers within the internal capsule (posterior limb in this slice) traverse the crus cerebri and enter the basilar pons (MRI and brain slice); these within the crus are the *corticospinal, cortico-* *pontine (parieto-, occipito-, tempro-, and frontopontine),* and the *corticonuclear fibers.* The two MRI images (both are inversion recovery) are at the same plane and show many of the structures identified in the brain slice. The terminal vein is also called the superior thalamostriate vein.

Body of fornix (BFor)

Body of corpus callosum (BCorCl)

Body of lateral ventricle (BLatVen)

Body of caudate nucleus (BCaNu)

Stria terminalis and terminal vein

Corona radiata

Lateral dorsal nucleus of thalamus

Dorsomedial nucleus of thalamus (DMNu)

Ventral posterolateral nucleus of thalamus (VPL)

Internal medullary lamina (IML)

Centromedian nucleus of thalamus

External capsule

Claustrum

Insula

Putamen (Put)

Ventral posteromedial nucleus of thalamus

Posterior limb of internal capsule (PLIntCap)

Tail caudate nucleus

Optic tract

Inferior horn of lateral ventricle (IHLatVen)

Hippocampal formation (Hip)

Third ventricle

Red nucleus (RNu)

Interpeduncular fossa (IPF)

Crus Cerebri (CC)

Trigeminal nerve (TriNr)

Substantia nigra

Basilar pons

BFor

BCorCl

BLatVen

IML

BCaNu

PLIntCap

DMNu

VPL

RNu

Put

Hip

CC

TriNr

TriNr

IPF

BP

5-6 The rostral surface of a coronal section of brain through the *lateral dorsal* and *centromedian nuclei*, rostral midbrain (*red nucleus*), *crus cerebri*, and corticospinal fibers in the *basilar pons*. The trajectory of *corticospinal (and related) fibers* through the posterior limb, crus cerebri, and basilar pons is also seen in this slice (also compare with Figure 5-5). The MRI image (inversion recovery) is at the same plane and shows many of the structures identified in the brain slice. The terminal vein is also called the superior thalamostriate vein.

Body of fornix (BFor)

Fimbria of fornix (FFor)

Stria terminalis and terminal vein

Pulvinar (Pul)

Medial geniculate nucleus (MGNu)

Lateral geniculate nucleus (LGNu)

Inferior horn of lateral ventricle (IHLatVen)

Hippocampal formation (Hip)

Cerebral aqueduct (CA)

Decussation of superior cerebellar peduncle

Pyramid

Body of corpus callosum (BCorCl)

Body of lateral ventricle (BLatVen)

Body of caudate nucleus (BCaNu)

Pulvinar (Pul)

Retrolenticular limb of internal capsule

Posterior commissure

Tail of caudate nucleus

Lateral geniculate nucleus (LGNu)

Pretectal area (PrTecAr)

Periaqueductal gray

Middle cerebellar peduncle (MCP)

BCorCl

BLatVen

BCaNu

Pul

MGNu

LGNu

Basilar pons

BFor

Pul

LGNu

MGNu

CA

FFor

Pul

PrTecAr

IHLatVen

Hip

Basilar pons

Trigeminal nerve

5-7 The rostral surface of a coronal section of brain through the *pulvinar, medial, and lateral geniculate nuclei; the basilar pons; and middle cerebellar peduncle.* Note that in this coronal plane the geniculate bodies are characteristically located inferior to the overlying pulvinar nucleus in both the brain slice and MRI. The two MRI images (both are inversion recovery) are at the same plane and show many of the structures in the brain slices. The terminal vein is also called the superior thalamostriate vein. For details of the cerebellum see Figures 2-36 and 2-37 (pp. 36–37).

Crus of fornix (CrF)

Body of corpus callosum (BCorCl)

Body of lateral ventricle (BLatVen)

Fimbria of fornix (FFor)

Body of caudate nucleus (BCaNu)

Pulvinar (Pul)

Retrolenticular limb of internal capsule

Stria terminalis and terminal vein

Fimbria of hippocampus

Pineal

Tail caudate nucleus

Hippocampal formation (Hip)

Inferior horn of lateral ventricle (IHLatVen)

Superior colliculus (SC)

Cerebral aqueduct (CA)

Periaqueductal gray (Pag)

Flocculus

Medulla (Med)

Middle cerebellar peduncle (MCP)

BCorCl

BLatVen

SC

Hip

Pag

Med

FFor

Pul

SC

CA

MCP

Splenium of corpus callosum

BLatVen

IHLatVen

Hip

Pag

MCP

Pyramid

5-8   The rostral surface of a coronal section of brain through the *pulvinar nucleus, superior colliculus, middle cerebellar peduncle,* and rostral portion of the *medulla oblongata.* The two MRI images (both are inversion recovery) are at the same plane and show many of the structures identified in the brain slice. The terminal vein is also called the superior thalamostriate vein. For details of the cerebellum, see Figures 2-36 and 2-37 (pp. 36–37).

5-9 The rostral surface of a coronal section of brain through the *splenium of the corpus callosum,* the *inferior colliculus,* the middle cerebellar peduncle in the base of the cerebellum, and the rostral portion of the medulla oblongata. The plane of the section is also through the atrium of the lateral ventricles. The two MRI images (both are inversion recovery) are at the same plane and show many of the structures identified in the brain slice. For details of the cerebellum, see Figures 2-36 and 2-37 (pp. 36–37).

Internal Morphology of the Brain in Unstained Slices and MRI

Part II

Brain Slices in the Axial Plane Correlated with MRI

Orientation to Axial MRIs: When looking at an axial MRI image, you are viewing the image as if standing at the patient's feet and looking toward his or her head while the patient is lying on his or her back. Consequently, and as is the case in coronal images, the observer's right is the left side of the brain in the MRI and the left side of the patient's brain, and the observer's left is the right side of the brain in MRI and the right side of the patient's brain. It is absolutely essential to have a clear understanding of this right-versus-left concept when using MRI or CT in the diagnosis of the neurologically impaired patient.

To reinforce this concept, the ventral surface of each axial slice was photographed. So, when looking at the slice, the observer's right is the left side of the brain slice, and the observer's left is the right side of the brain slice. This view of the slice correlates exactly with the orientation of the brain as seen in the accompanying axial MRIs.

5-10 Ventral surface of an axial section of brain through dorsal portions of the *corpus callosum*. The plane of the section just touches the upper portion of *the body of the caudate nucleus*.

The two MRI images (both are inversion recovery) are at a similar plane and show some of the structures identified in the brain slice. The terminal vein is also called the superior thalamostriate vein.

Cingulate gyrus

Anterior cerebral arteries

Genu of corpus callosum

Head of caudate nucleus (HCaNu)

Anterior horn of lateral ventricle (AHLatVen)

Stria terminalis and terminal vein

Body of fornix

Anterior nucleus of thalamus

Anterior tubercle

Ventral anterior nucleus of thalamus

Corona radiata (CorRad)

Lateral thalamic nuclei

Tail of caudate nucleus

Dorsomedial nucleus of thalamus

Lateral ventricle (LatVen)

Tail of caudate nucleus

Crus of fornix

Splenium of corpus callosum

LatVen

Caudate nucleus

AHLatVen

Putamen

HCaNu

CorRad

Internal capsule

Septum pellucidum

Dorsal thalamus

Atrium of lateral ventricle

5-11 Ventral surface of an axial section of brain through the *splenium of the corpus callosum* and the *head of the caudate nucleus.* This plane includes only a small portion of the *dorsal thalamus.* The two MRI images (inversion recovery—left; T2-weighted—right) are at a comparable plane and show some of the structures identified in the brain slice. The terminal vein is also called the superior thalamostriate vein.

5-12 Ventral surface of an axial section of brain through the *genu of the corpus callosum, head of the caudate nucleus, centromedian nucleus,* and dorsal portions of the *pulvinar.* The two MRI images (inversion recovery—left; T2-weighted—right) are at the same plane and show many of the structures identified in the brain slice. The arrowheads in the brain slice and MRIs are pointing to the mammillothalamic tract. The terminal vein is also called the superior thalamostriate vein.

Genu of corpus callosum

Subcallosal gyri

Anterior limb of internal capsule (ALIntCap)

Putamen (Put)

Globus pallidus (GP)

Insula (In)

Posterior limb of internal capsule (PLIntCap)

Subthalamic nucleus

Red nucleus (RNu)

Lateral geniculate nucleus (LGNu)

Retrolenticular limb of internal capsule

Fimbria of hippocampus

Hippocampal formation (Hip)

Medial geniculate nucleus (MGNu)

Pineal

Splenium of corpus callosum (SpCorCl)

Anterior commissure (AC)

Head of caudate nucleus (HCaNu)

Column of fornix (ColFor)

Third ventricle

Mammillothalamic tract (MtTr)

External capsule

Claustrum

Extreme capsule

Ventral posterior thalamic nuclei

Brachium of superior colliculus

Pulvinar

Tail of caudate nucleus

Tapetum (Tap)

Optic radiation (OpRad)

Atrium of lateral ventricle (ALatVen)

Posterior horn of lateral ventricle (PHLatVen)

Superior colliculus (SC)

ALIntCap

Put

GP

PLIntCap

Lateral thalamic nuclei

Dorsomedial nucleus

Crus of fornix

SpCorCl

AC

HCaNu

ColFor

MtTr

Massa intermed.

Pul

ALatVen

OpRad

ColFor

In

AC

MtTr

RNu

LGNu

MGNu

Tap

SC

PHLatVen

Hip

5-13 Ventral surface of an axial section of brain through the *anterior commissure, column of the fornix, medial and lateral geniculate nuclei,* and *superior colliculus*. The *medial* and *lateral segments* of the globus pallidus are visible on the slice. The lateral and medial segments of the globus pallidus can be discerned on the right side of the brain. The MRI images (both T2-weighted) are at approximately the same plane and show many of the structures identified in the brain slice.

Hypothalamus (HyTh)

Head of
caudate nucleus

Nucleus accumbens

Anterior perforated
substance

Crus cerebri (CC)

Inferior horn of
lateral ventricle
(IHLatVen)

Hippocampal
formation

Substantia
nigra (SN)

Decussation of superior
cerebellar peduncle

Inferior colliculus (IC)

Cerebellum (Cbl)

Anterior cerebral arteries (ACA)

Lamina terminalis

Third ventricle (ThrVen)

Optic tract (OpTr)

Uncus

Amygdaloid
nuclear complex

Mammillary body (MB)

Interpeduncular
fossa (IPF)

Lateral geniculate
nucleus

Tail of caudate nucleus

Hippocampal formation (Hip)

Choroid plexus in
inferior horn

Periaqueductal gray

Cerebral Aqueduct (CA)

ThrVen

Un

SN

IC

Cbl

OpTr

HyTh

MB

CC

IPF

CA

Posterior
cerebral
artery

ACA

ThrVen

IHLatVen

Hip

Posterior horn
lateral ventricle

5-14 Ventral surface of an axial section of brain through the *hypothalamus, mammillary body, crus cerebri,* and *inferior colliculus.* The two MRI images (inversion recovery—left; T2-weighted—right) are at similar planes and show many of the structures identified in the brain slice. For details of the cerebellum, see Figures 2-36 and 2-37 (pp. 36–37).

Corticospinal fibers

Basilar artery (BA)

Medial lemniscus (ML)

Basilar pons (BP)

Tegmentum of pons (TegP)

Fourth ventricle (ForVen)

Nucleus coeruleus

Superior cerebellar peduncle (SCP)

Vermis of anterior lobe of cerebellum (VCbl)

Hemisphere of anterior lobe of cerebellum (HCbl)

Hemisphere of posterior lobe of cerebellum

BA

BP

ML

TegP

SCP

ForVen

HCbl

VCbl

Occipital lobe

Temporal lobe

HCbl

VCbl

Occipital lobe

5-15 Ventral surface of an axial section of brain through rostral parts of the *basilar pons* and the *anterior lobe of the cerebellum*. The two MRI images (T2-weighted—left; inversion recovery— right) are at the same plane and show many of the structures identified in the brain slice. For details of the cerebellum, see Figures 2-36 and 2-37 (pp. 36–37).

Basilar artery (BA)

Basilar pons (BP)

Trigeminal nerve (TriNr)

Medial lemniscus

Tegmentum of pons (TegP)

Middle cerebellar peduncle (MCP)

Fourth ventricle (ForVen)

Dentate nucleus (DNu)

Hemisphere of posterior lobe of cerebellum (HCbl)

Vermis of posterior lobe of cerebellum (VCbl)

BP

TriNr

MCP

ForVen

HCbl

Temporal lobe

Trigeminal ganglion

TriNr

TegP

BA

Temporal lobe

Lesion in BP

BP

TegP

ForVen

BP

MCP

DNu

BA

TegP

ForVen

VCbl

5-16   Ventral surface of an axial section of brain through the middle regions of the *basilar pons, exit of the trigeminal nerve, fourth ventricle,* cerebellar nuclei. The three MRI images (inverted inversion recovery—upper left; T2-weighted—upper right; T1-weighted—lower) are at the same plane and show many of the structures identified in the brain slice. Note the lesion in the basilar pons (upper right). For details of the cerebellum, see Figures 2-36 and 2-37 (pp. 36–37).

5-17 Ventral surface of an axial section of brain through portions of the *medulla oblongata,* just caudal to the pons–medulla junction and the *posterior lobe* of the cerebellum. The three MRI images (T1-weighted—upper left and right; T2-weighted—lower) are at the same plane and show many of the structures identified in the brain slice. Note the lateral medullary lesion (lower), also known as the *posterior inferior cerebellar artery syndrome* or the *lateral medullary syndrome (PICA or Wallenberg syndrome).* For details of the cerebellum, see Figures 2-36 and 2-37 (pp. 36–37).

NOTES

6

Internal Morphology of the Spinal Cord and Brain in Stained Sections

Basic concepts that are essential when one is *initially* learning how to diagnose the neurologically impaired patient include 1) an understanding of cranial nerve nuclei and 2) how these structures relate to long tracts. The importance of these relationships is clearly seen in the combinations of deficits that generally characterize lesions at different levels of the neuraxis. First, deficits of the body only, excluding the head, that may present as motor or sensory losses (long tracts) on the same side, or opposite sides, are indicative of spinal cord lesions (e.g., Brown-Séquard syndrome). Spinal cord injuries characteristically have *motor and sensory levels;* these are the *lowest functional levels* remaining in the compromised patient. Second, cranial nerve deficits (on one side of the head) in combination with long tract signs (on the opposite side of the body) characterize lesions in the brainstem (e.g., lateral medullary and Weber syndromes). These patterns of loss are frequently called *alternating* or *crossed deficits*. In these examples cranial nerve signs are better *localizing signs* than are long tract signs. A *localizing sign* can be defined as an objective neurologic abnormality that correlates with a lesion (or lesions) at a specific neuroanatomical location (or locations). Third, motor and sensory deficits on the same side of the head and body are usually indicative of a lesion in the forebrain.

■ Color-Coded Cranial Nerve Nuclei and Long Tracts ■

Cranial nerve nuclei are coded by their function: pink, sensory; red, motor. These structures are colored bilaterally to make it easy to correlate cranial nerve and long tract function on both sides of the midline. For example, one can easily correlate damage to the hypoglossal nerve root and the adjacent corticospinal fibers on one side, while comparing this pattern with the clinical picture of a lateral medullary syndrome on the other side.

Long tracts are color-coded beginning at the most caudal spinal cord levels (e.g., see Figures 6-1 and 6-2), with these colors extending into the dorsal thalamus (see Figure 6-30) and the posterior limb of the internal capsule (see Figures 6-31 and 6-32). The colorized spinal tracts are the fasciculus gracilis (dark blue), the fasciculus cuneatus (light blue),* the anterolateral system (dark green), and the lateral corticospinal tract (grey). In the brainstem, these spinal tracts are

joined by the spinal trigeminal tract and ventral trigeminothalamic fibers (both are light green). The long tracts are color-coded on one side only, to emphasize: 1) laterality of function and dysfunction; 2) points at which fibers in these tracts may decussate; and 3) the relationship of these tracts to cranial nerves.

A color key appears on each page. This key identifies the various tracts and nuclei by their color and specifies the function of each structure on each page.

■ Correlation of MRI and CT with Internal Spinal Cord and Brainstem Anatomy ■

As one is learning basic anatomical concepts, it is absolutely essential to understand how this information is used in the clinical environment. To show the relationship between basic anatomy and how MRI (T1- and T2-weighted) and CT (myelogram/cisternogram) are viewed, a series of self-explanatory illustrations is provided on each set of facing pages in the spinal cord and brainstem sections of this chapter. This continuum of visual information consists of: 1) a small version of the colorized line drawing in an *Anatomical Orientation*; 2) a top-to-bottom flip of this illustration that brings it into a *Clinical Orientation*; and 3) a CT (spinal cord) or MRI and CT (brainstem) that follows this clinically oriented image. To further enhance the seamless application of basic neuroscience to clinical images (and to do so in their proper context), especially important anatomical structures are outlined, in white, on CT (spinal cord) and on the T1-weighted MRI (brainstem) images. This allows the user to understand where these anatomical structures are located in clinical images as viewed in the *Clinical Orientation*. One essential aspect of diagnosis is developing the ability to visualize what structures are involved in brainstem lesions and how the patient's deficits correlate with the location and extent of the lesion.

Every effort is made to identify and use MRI and CT that correlate, as closely as possible, with their corresponding line drawing and stained section. This approach recognizes and retains the strength of the anatomical approach and introduces essential clinical concepts while at the same time allowing the user to customize the material to suit a range of educational applications.

---

*The dark and light blue colors represent information originating from lower and upper portions of the body, respectively.

6-1A   Transverse section of the spinal cord showing the characteristics of a sacral level. The gray matter occupies most of the cross-section; its H-shaped appearance is not especially obvious at sacral–coccygeal levels. The white matter is a comparatively thin mantle. The sacral cord, although small, appears round in the CT myelogram. Note the appearance of the sacral spinal cord surrounded by the upper portion of the cauda equina (left) and the cauda equina as it appears caudal to the conus medullaris in the lumbar cistern (right). Compare with Figure 2-4 on p. 12.

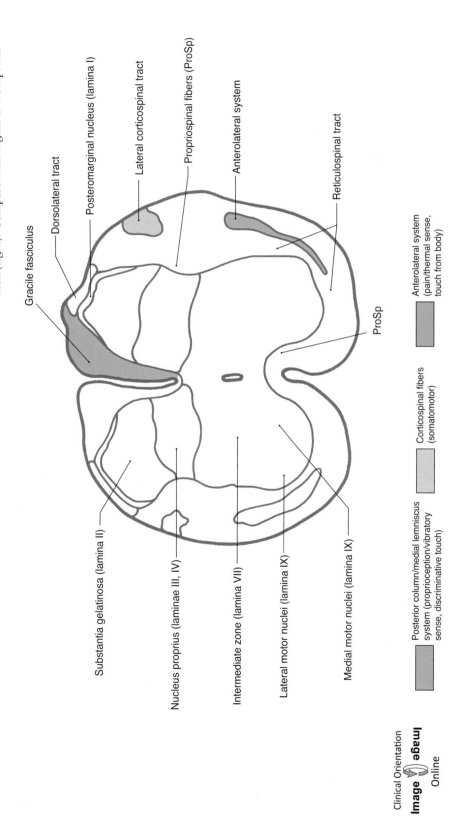

Gracile fasciculus

Dorsolateral tract

Posteromarginal nucleus (lamina I)

Lateral corticospinal tract

Propriospinal fibers (ProSp)

Anterolateral system

Reticulospinal tract

ProSp

Substantia gelatinosa (lamina II)

Nucleus proprius (laminae III, IV)

Intermediate zone (lamina VII)

Lateral motor nuclei (lamina IX)

Medial motor nuclei (lamina IX)

Posterior column/medial lemniscus system (proprioception/vibratory sense, discriminative touch)

Corticospinal fibers (somatomotor)

Anterolateral system (pain/thermal sense, touch from body)

Clinical Orientation

Image Online

Lumbar cistern
Anterior horn
Cauda equina
Posterior horn
Filum terminale internum

CT myelogram

CT myelogram

Clinical orientation

Anatomical orientation

Clinical Orientation
Image
Online

6-1B

6-2A   Transverse section of the spinal cord showing its characteristic appearance at lumbar levels (L4). Posterior and anterior horns are large in relation to a modest amount of white matter, and the general shape of the cord is round. Fibers of the medial division of the posterior root directly enter the gracile fasciculus. The lumbar spinal cord appears round in the CT myelogram. The roots of upper portions of the cauda equina surround the lower levels of the lumbar spinal cord (right).

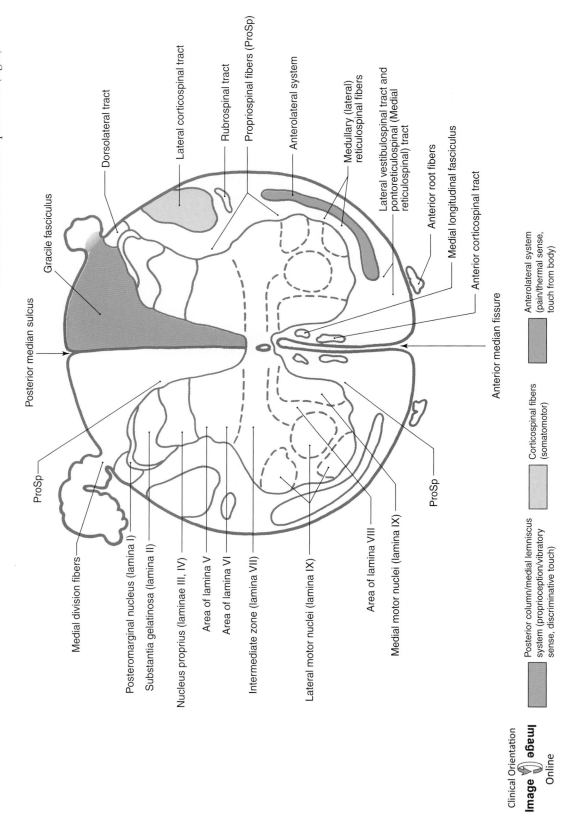

Posterior median sulcus

Gracile fasciculus

Dorsolateral tract

Lateral corticospinal tract

Rubrospinal tract

Propriospinal fibers (ProSp)

Anterolateral system

Medullary (lateral) reticulospinal fibers

Lateral vestibulospinal tract and pontoreticulospinal (Medial reticulospinal) tract

Anterior root fibers

Medial longitudinal fasciculus

Anterior corticospinal tract

Anterior median fissure

ProSp

Medial division fibers

Posteromarginal nucleus (lamina I)

Substantia gelatinosa (lamina II)

Nucleus proprius (laminae III, IV)

Area of lamina V

Area of lamina VI

Intermediate zone (lamina VII)

Lateral motor nuclei (lamina IX)

Area of lamina VIII

Medial motor nuclei (lamina IX)

ProSp

Posterior column/medial lemniscus system (proprioception/vibratory sense, discriminative touch)

Corticospinal fibers (somatomotor)

Anterolateral system (pain/thermal sense, touch from body)

Clinical Orientation

Image Online

CT myelogram

CT myelogram

Anterior root

Anterior horn

Posterior root

Posterior horn

Clinical orientation

Anatomical orientation

Clinical Orientation
Image
Image
Online

6-2B

6-3A   Transverse section of the spinal cord showing its characteristic appearance at thoracic levels (T4). The white matter appears large in relation to the rather diminutive amount of gray matter. Posterior and anterior horns are small, especially when compared to low cervical levels and to lumbar levels. The overall shape of the cord is round. The thoracic spinal cord appears round in CT myelogram.

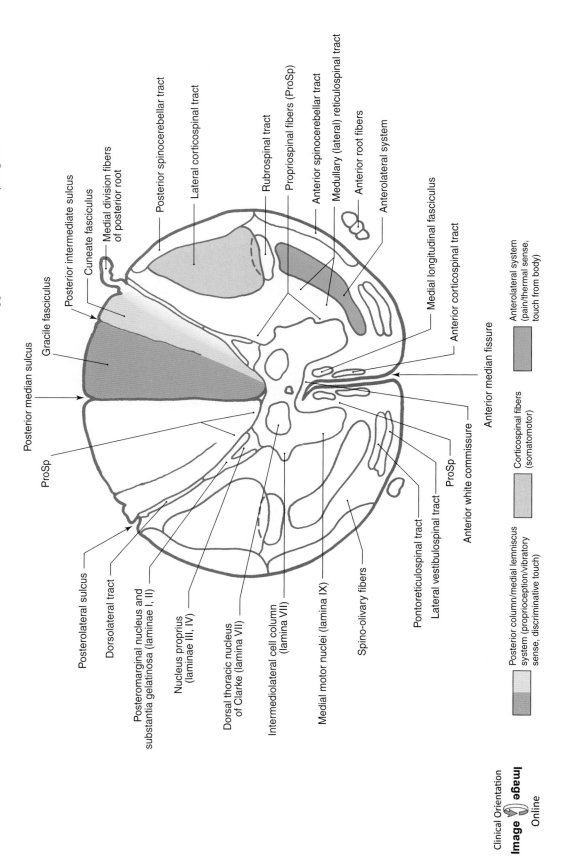

Posterior intermediate sulcus
Cuneate fasciculus
Medial division fibers of posterior root
Posterior spinocerebellar tract
Lateral corticospinal tract
Rubrospinal tract
Propriospinal fibers (ProSp)
Anterior spinocerebellar tract
Medullary (lateral) reticulospinal tract
Anterior root fibers
Anterolateral system

Posterior median sulcus
Gracile fasciculus
ProSp

Medial longitudinal fasciculus
Anterior corticospinal tract
Anterior median fissure
ProSp
Anterior white commissure

Posterolateral sulcus
Dorsolateral tract
Posteromarginal nucleus and substantia gelatinosa (laminae I, II)
Nucleus proprius (laminae III, IV)
Dorsal thoracic nucleus of Clarke (lamina VII)
Intermediolateral cell column (lamina VII)
Medial motor nuclei (lamina IX)
Spino-olivary fibers
Pontoreticulospinal tract
Lateral vestibulospinal tract

Posterior column/medial lemniscus system (proprioception/vibratory sense, discriminative touch)
Corticospinal fibers (somatomotor)
Anterolateral system (pain/thermal sense, touch from body)

Clinical Orientation
Image Online

CT myelogram

Anterior horn
Anterior root
Lateral horn
Posterior root
Posterior horn

CT myelogram

Clinical orientation

Anatomical orientation

Clinical Orientation
Image
Online

6-3B

6-4A Transverse section of the spinal cord showing its characteristic appearance at lower cervical levels (C7). The anterior horn is large, and there is—proportionally and absolutely—a large amount of white matter. The overall shape of the cord is oval. The lower portions of the cervical spinal cord (beginning at about C4 and extending through C8) appear oval in MRI (left) and in CT myelogram (center and right). Although frequently called lamina X, Rexed (1954) clearly describes nine laminae (I–IX) and an "area X, the central gray substance." This original designation is used here.

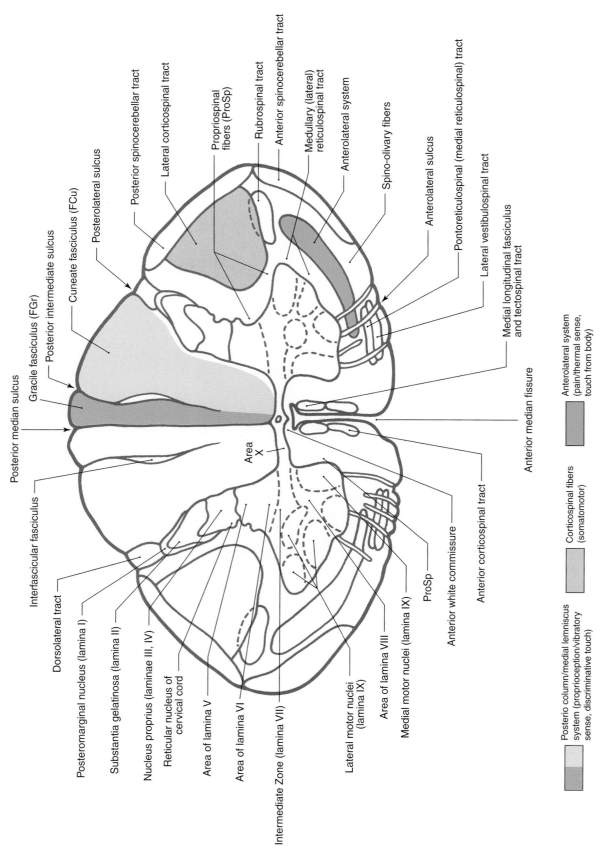

Posterior median sulcus

Gracile fasciculus (FGr)

Posterior intermediate sulcus

Cuneate fasciculus (FCu)

Posterolateral sulcus

Posterior spinocerebellar tract

Lateral corticospinal tract

Propriospinal fibers (ProSp)

Rubrospinal tract

Anterior spinocerebellar tract

Medullary (lateral) reticulospinal tract

Anterolateral system

Spino-olivary fibers

Anterolateral sulcus

Pontoreticulospinal (medial reticulospinal) tract

Lateral vestibulospinal tract

Medial longitudinal fasciculus and tectospinal tract

Anterior median fissure

Area X

Interfascicular fasciculus

Dorsolateral tract

Posteromarginal nucleus (lamina I)

Substantia gelatinosa (lamina II)

Nucleus proprius (laminae III, IV)

Reticular nucleus of cervical cord

Area of lamina V

Area of lamina VI

Intermediate Zone (lamina VII)

Lateral motor nuclei (lamina IX)

Area of lamina VIII

Medial motor nuclei (lamina IX)

ProSp

Anterior white commissure

Anterior corticospinal tract

Posterio column/medial lemniscus system (proprioception/vibratory sense, discriminative touch)

Anterolateral system (pain/thermal sense, touch from body)

Corticospinal fibers (somatomotor)

CT myelogram

CT myelogram

Anterior horn
Anterior root
Posterior root
Posterior horn
FGr + FCu

MRI, T2 weighted image

Clinical orientation

Anatomical orientation

Clinical Orientation
Image
Online

6-4B

6-5A Transverse section of the spinal cord at the C1 level. Lateral corticospinal fibers are now located medially toward the decussation of the corticospinal fibers, also called the motor decussation or pyramidal decussation (see also Figure 6-8, p. 108). At this level, fibers of the spinal trigeminal tract are interdigitated with those of the dorsolateral tract. The spinal cord at C1 and C2 levels appears round in CT myelogram when compared to low cervical levels (see Figure 6-4).

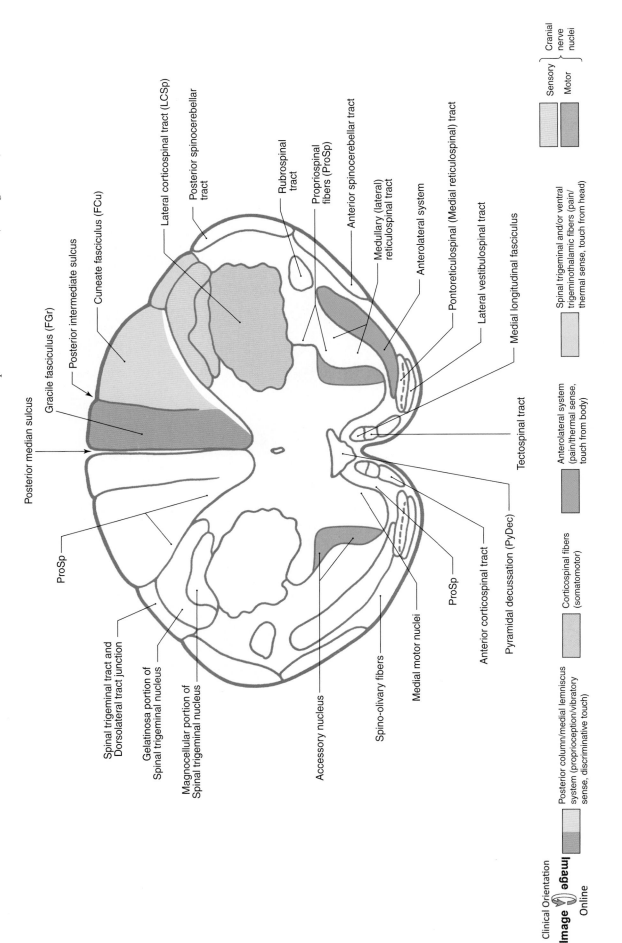

Posterior median sulcus

Gracile fasciculus (FGr)

Posterior intermediate sulcus

Cuneate fasciculus (FCu)

Lateral corticospinal tract (LCSp)

Posterior spinocerebellar tract

Rubrospinal tract

Propriospinal fibers (ProSp)

Anterior spinocerebellar tract

Medullary (lateral) reticulospinal tract

Anterolateral system

Pontoreticulospinal (Medial reticulospinal) tract

Lateral vestibulospinal tract

Medial longitudinal fasciculus

ProSp

Spinal trigeminal tract and Dorsolateral tract junction

Gelatinosa portion of Spinal trigeminal nucleus

Magnocellular portion of Spinal trigeminal nucleus

Accessory nucleus

Spino-olivary fibers

Medial motor nuclei

ProSp

Anterior corticospinal tract

Pyramidal decussation (PyDec)

Tectospinal tract

Anterolateral system (pain/thermal sense, touch from body)

Spinal trigeminal and/or ventral trigeminothalamic fibers (pain/thermal sense, touch from head)

Sensory
Motor } Cranial nerve nuclei

Posterior column/medial lemniscus system (proprioception/vibratory sense, discriminative touch)

Corticospinal fibers (somatomotor)

Clinical Orientation

Image ☉ Image
Online

CT myelogram

PyDec
C1 anterior horn
LCSp fibers
C1 posterior horn
FGr + FCu

CT myelogram

Clinical orientation

Anatomical orientation

Clinical Orientation

Image

Online

6-5B

■ Vascular Syndromes or Lesions of the Spinal Cord ■

Acute Central Cervical Spinal Cord Syndrome

This results from occlusion of the anterior spinal artery.

Deficit	Structure Damage
• Bilateral paresis or flaccid paralysis of upper extremities	• Medial portions of both lateral corticospinal tracts; ventral grey horns at cervical levels
• Irregular loss of pain and temperature sensations bilaterally over body below lesion	• Anterolateral system fibers (partial involvement bilaterally)

Hyperextension of the neck may cause damage to the vertebral arteries (which give rise to the anterior spinal artery), or it may directly damage the anterior spinal artery, causing a spasm. This vascular damage leads to a temporary or permanent interruption of blood supply. Deficits may resolve within a few hours or may be permanent, depending on the extent of vascular complication. Sparing of the posterior columns (proprioception, vibratory sense) is a hallmark; approximately the anterior two-thirds of the spinal cord is ischemic.

Thrombosis of Anterior Spinal Artery

This may occur in a hypotensive crisis, as a result of trauma resulting from a dissecting aortic aneurysm, or in patients with atherosclerosis. It may occur at all spinal levels, but is more frequently seen in thoracic and lumbosacral levels unless trauma is the primary cause. Results are *bilateral flaccid paraplegia* (if the lesion is below cervical levels) or *quadriplegia* (if the lesion is in cervical levels), *urinary retention*, and *loss of pain and temperature sensation*. Flaccid muscles may become spastic over a period of a day to weeks, with *hyperactive muscle stretch reflexes* and *extensor plantar (Babinski) reflexes*. In addition, lesions at high cervical levels may also result in paralysis of respiratory muscles. The artery of Adamkiewicz (an especially large spinal medullary artery) is usually located at spinal levels T12–L1 and more frequently arises on the left side. Occlusion of this vessel may infarct lumbosacral levels of the spinal cord.

Hemorrhage in the Spinal Cord

This is *rarely* seen, but may result from trauma or bleeding from congenital vascular lesions. Symptoms may develop rapidly or gradually in stepwise fashion, and blood is usually present in the cerebrospinal fluid.

Arteriovenous Malformation in Spinal Cord

More frequently found in lower cord levels. Symptoms of a spinal AVM (*micturition problems* are seen early, *motor deficits*, *lower back pain*) may appear over time and may seem to resolve then recur (get better, then worse).These lesions are usually found external to the cord (extramedullary) and can be surgically treated, especially when the major feeding vessels are few in number and easily identified. *Foix-Alajouanine syndrome* is an inflammation of spinal veins, with subsequent occlusion that results in infarct of the spinal cord and a *necrotic myelitis*. The symptoms are *ascending pain* and a *flaccid paralysis*.

6-6 Semi-diagrammatic representation of the internal blood supply to the spinal cord. This is a tracing of a C4 level, with the positions of principal tracts superimposed on the left and the general pattern of blood vessels superimposed on the right.

ABBREVIATIONS

A	Representation of arm fibers	L	Representation of leg fibers
AH	Anterior (ventral) horn	N	Representation of neck fibers
AWCom	Anterior white commissure	PH	Posterior (dorsal) horn
CenC	Central canal	S	Representation of sacral fibers
IZ	Intermediate zone	T	Representation of truck fibers

Brown-Séquard Syndrome

This syndrome is a hemisection (functional hemisection) of the spinal cord that may result from trauma, compression of the spinal cord by tumors or hematomas, or significant protrusion of an intervertebral disc. The deficits depend on the level of the causative lesion. The classic signs are: 1) a loss of pain and thermal sensation on the contralateral side of the body beginning about one to two segments below the level of the lesion (*damage to anterolateral system fibers*); 2) a loss of discriminative touch and proprioception on the ipsilateral side of the body below the lesion (*interruption of posterior column fibers*); and 3) a paralysis on the ipsilateral side of the body below the lesion (*damage to lateral corticospinal fibers*). This syndrome is classified as an *incomplete spinal cord injury* (see below), and patients with this lesion may regain some degree of motor and sensory function. Compression of the spinal cord may result in some, but not all, of the signs and symptoms of the syndrome.

Syringomyelia

This condition is a cavitation within the central region of the spinal cord. A cavitation of the central canal with an *ependymal cell* lining is *hydromyelia*. A *syrinx* may originate in central portions of the spinal cord, may communicate with the central canal, and is most commonly seen in cervical levels of the spinal cord. The most common deficits are a *bilateral loss of pain and thermal sensation due to damage to the anterior white commissure*: the loss reflects the levels of the spinal cord damaged (e.g., a cape distribution over the shoulder and upper extremities). The other commonly seen deficit results from extension of the cavity into the anterior horn(s). The result is *unilateral or bilateral paralysis of the upper extremities* (cervical levels) or *lower extremities* (lumbosacral levels) due to damage to the anterior motor neuron cells. This paralysis is characteristically a *lower motor neuron deficit*. A syrinx in the spinal cord, particularly in cervical levels, may be associated with a variety of other developmental defects in the nervous system.

■ Spinal Cord Lesions ■

General Concepts

A *complete spinal cord lesion* is characterized by a bilateral and complete loss of motor and sensory function below the level of the lesion persisting for more than 24 hours. The vast majority of the patients with complete lesions (95%+) will suffer some permanent deficits. *Incomplete spinal cord lesions* are those with preservation of sacral cord function at presentation. The above described cases are examples of incomplete spinal cord lesions.

High Cervical

The *phrenic nucleus* is located in central areas of the anterior horn at levels C3–C7 and receives descending input from nuclei of the medulla (mainly in the reticular formation) that influence respiration, particularly inspiration. The *phrenic nerve* originates primarily from level C4 with some contributions from C3 and C5 and innervates the diaphragm. A *complete spinal cord lesion* between C1 and C3 interrupts medullary input to the phrenic nucleus and results in immediate respiratory (and cardiac) arrest. This constitutes a medical emergency necessitating intervention within minutes, or the patient will die.

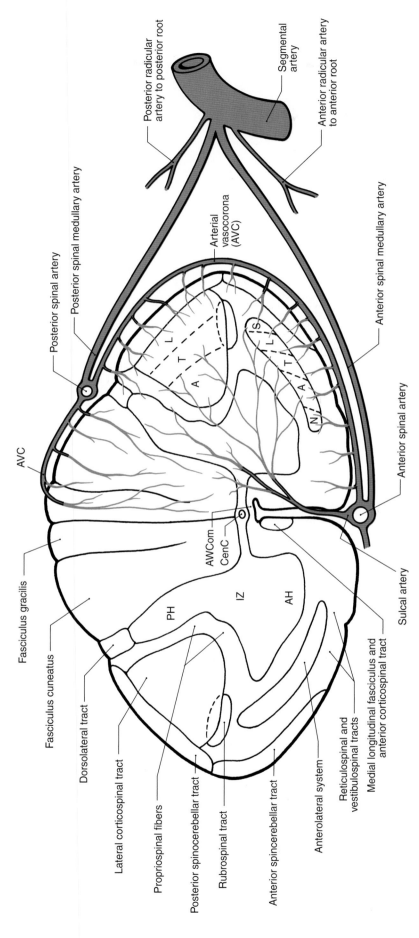

Posterior radicular artery to posterior root

Segmental artery

Anterior radicular artery to anterior root

Posterior spinal medullary artery

Anterior spinal medullary artery

Arterial vasocorona (AVC)

Posterior spinal artery

Anterior spinal artery

AVC

Anterior spinal artery

Fasciculus gracilis

AWCom
CenC

Sulcal artery

Fasciculus cuneatus

PH

IZ

AH

Dorsolateral tract

Lateral corticospinal tract

Propriospinal fibers

Posterior spinocerebellar tract

Rubrospinal tract

Anterior spincerebellar tract

Anterolateral system

Reticulospinal and vestibulospinal tracts

Medial longitudinal fasciculus and anterior corticospinal tract

6-6

6-7 All of the brainstem sections used in Figures 6-9 through 6-13 (medulla), 6-17 through 6-20 (pons), and 6-22 through 6-25 (midbrain) are from an individual who had an infarct (green in drawing) in the posterior limb of the internal capsule. This lesion damaged corticospinal fibers (grey in drawing), resulting in a contralateral hemiplegia of the arm and leg, and damaged sensory radiations that travel from thalamic nuclei to the somatosensory cortex through the posterior limb of the internal capsule. Although the patient survived the initial episode, corticospinal fibers (grey) distal to the lesion (green) underwent degenerative changes and largely disappeared. This Wallerian (anterograde) degeneration takes place because the capsular infarct effectively separates the descending corticospinal fibers from their cell bodies in the cerebral cortex. Consequently, the location of corticospinal fibers in the middle one-third of the crus cerebri of the midbrain, in the basilar pons, and in the pyramid of the medulla is characterized by the obvious lack of myelinated axons in these structures when compared to the opposite side. In the brainstem, these degenerated fibers are ipsilateral to their cells of origin, but are contralateral to their destination in the spinal cord—hence, the contralateral motor deficit. These photographs give the user the unique opportunity of seeing where corticospinal fibers are located at all levels of the human brainstem. Also, one is constantly reminded of: 1) the relationship of corticospinal fibers to other structures; 2) the deficits one can expect to see at representative levels due to this lesion; and 3) the general appearance of degenerated fibers in the human central nervous system. These images can be adapted to a wide range of instructional formats.

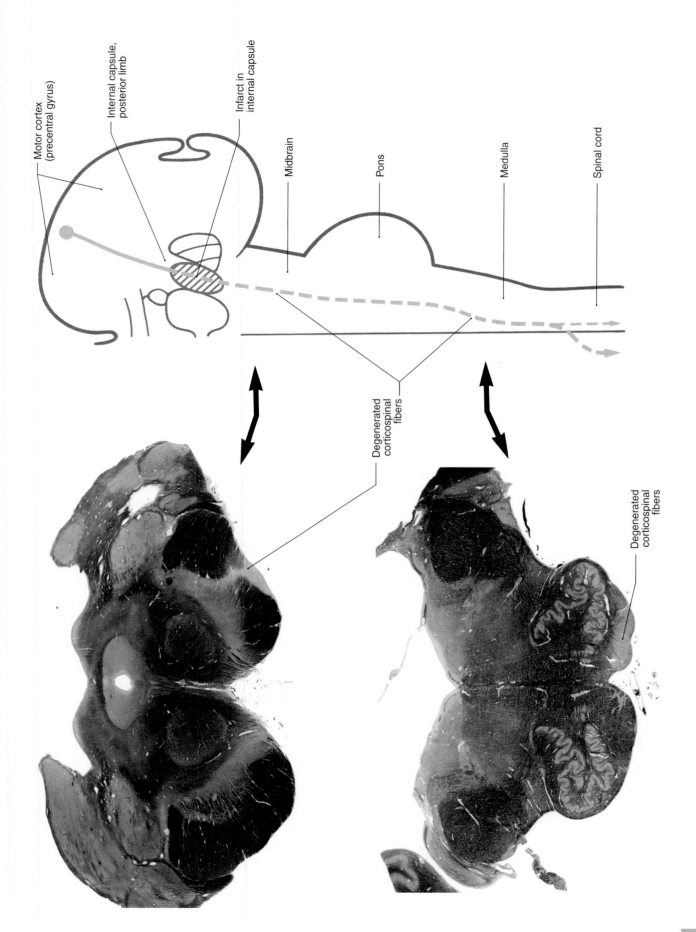

Motor cortex
(precentral gyrus)

Internal capsule,
posterior limb

Infarct in
internal capsule

Midbrain

Pons

Medulla

Spinal cord

Degenerated
corticospinal
fibers

Degenerated
corticospinal
fibers

6-8A Transverse section of the medulla through the *decussation of the pyramids* (motor decussation, pyramidal decussation, crossing of corticospinal fibers). This is the level of the spinal cord–medulla transition. The corticospinal fibers have moved from their location in the lateral funiculus to the motor decussation (compare this image with Figure 6-5A,B) and will cross to form the pyramid on the opposite side.

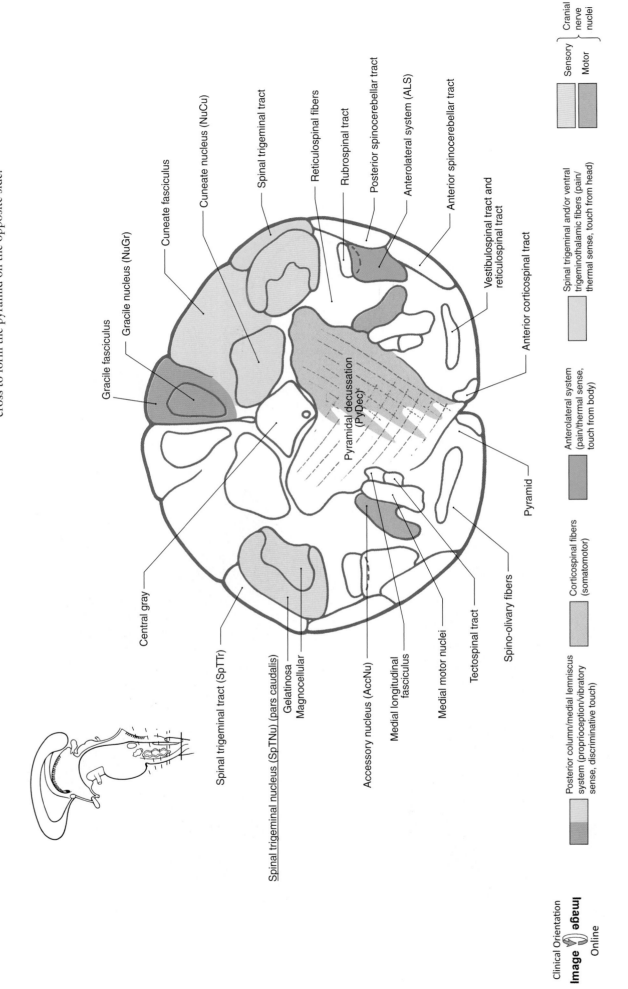

Gracile fasciculus

Gracile nucleus (NuGr)

Cuneate fasciculus

Cuneate nucleus (NuCu)

Spinal trigeminal tract

Reticulospinal fibers

Rubrospinal tract

Posterior spinocerebellar tract

Anterolateral system (ALS)

Anterior spinocerebellar tract

Vestibulospinal tract and reticulospinal tract

Anterior corticospinal tract

Pyramid

Pyramidal decussation (PyDec)

Central gray

Spinal trigeminal tract (SpTTr)

Spinal trigeminal nucleus (SpTNu) (pars caudalis)

Gelatinosa

Magnocellular

Accessory nucleus (AccNu)

Medial longitudinal fasciculus

Medial motor nuclei

Tectospinal tract

Spino-olivary fibers

Clinical Orientation

Image Online

Sensory ⎫
Motor ⎭ Cranial nerve nuclei

Posterior column/medial lemniscus system (proprioception/vibratory sense, discriminative touch)

Corticospinal fibers (somatomotor)

Anterolateral system (pain/thermal sense, touch from body)

Spinal trigeminal and/or ventral trigeminothalamic fibers (pain/thermal sense, touch from head)

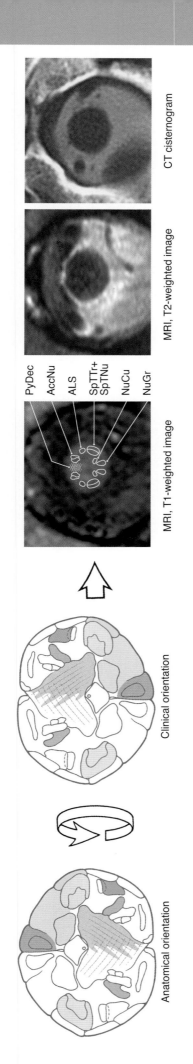

CT cisternogram

MRI, T2-weighted image

PyDec
AccNu
ALS
SpTTr+
SpTNu
NuCu
NuGr

MRI, T1-weighted image

Clinical orientation

Anatomical orientation

Clinical Orientation
Image
Online

6-8B

6-9A Transverse section of the medulla through the *posterior column nuclei* (nucleus gracilis and nucleus cuneatus), caudal portions of the *hypoglossal nucleus*, caudal end of the *principal olivary nucleus*, and middle portions of the *sensory decussation* (crossing of internal arcuate fibers).

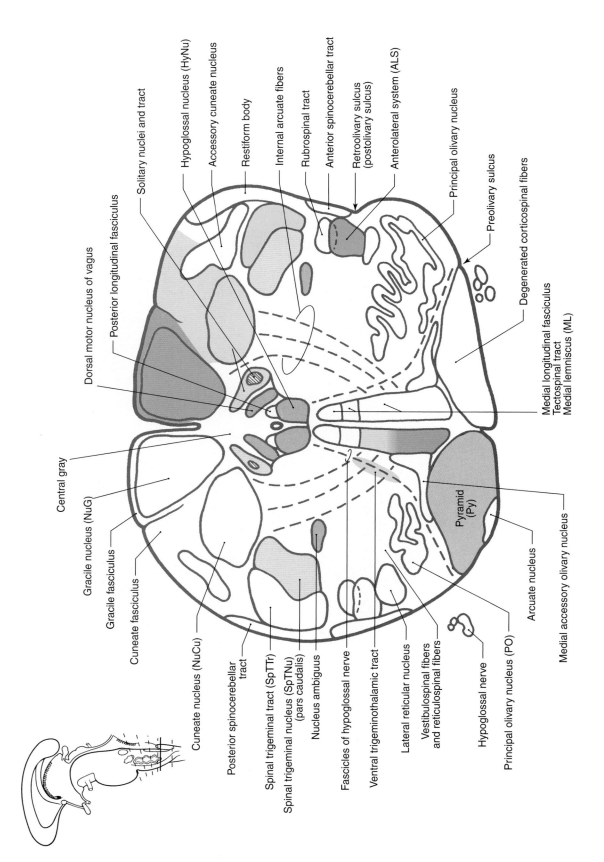

Solitary nuclei and tract

Hypoglossal nucleus (HyNu)

Accessory cuneate nucleus

Restiform body

Internal arcuate fibers

Rubrospinal tract

Anterior spinocerebellar tract

Retroolivary sulcus (postolivary sulcus)

Anterolateral system (ALS)

Principal olivary nucleus

Preolivary sulcus

Degenerated corticospinal fibers

Medial longitudinal fasciculus
Tectospinal tract
Medial lemniscus (ML)

Pyramid (Py)

Arcuate nucleus

Medial accessory olivary nucleus

Principal olivary nucleus (PO)

Hypoglossal nerve

Vestibulospinal fibers and reticulospinal fibers

Lateral reticular nucleus

Ventral trigeminothalamic tract

Fascicles of hypoglossal nerve

Nucleus ambiguus

Spinal trigeminal nucleus (SpTNu) (pars caudalis)

Spinal trigeminal tract (SpTTr)

Posterior spinocerebellar tract

Cuneate nucleus (NuCu)

Cuneate fasciculus

Gracile fasciculus

Gracile nucleus (NuG)

Central gray

Dorsal motor nucleus of vagus

Posterior longitudinal fasciculus

Sensory ⎫ Cranial
Motor ⎬ nerve
        ⎭ nuclei

Posterior column/medial lemniscus system (proprioception/vibratory sense, discriminative touch)

Corticospinal fibers (somatomotor)

Anterolateral system (pain/thermal sense, touch from body)

Spinal trigeminal and/or ventral trigeminothalamic fibers (pain/ thermal sense, touch from head)

CT cisternogram

MRI, T2-weighted image

Py
ML
PO
ALS
SpTTr+
SpTNu
NuCu
NuGr
HyNu

MRI, T1-weighted image

Clinical orientation

Anatomical orientation

Clinical Orientation

Image

Image

Online

6-9B

6-10A Transverse section of the medulla through rostral portions of the sensory decussation (*crossing of internal arcuate fibers*), *obex*, and the caudal one-third of the *hypoglossal* and *principal olivary nuclei*.

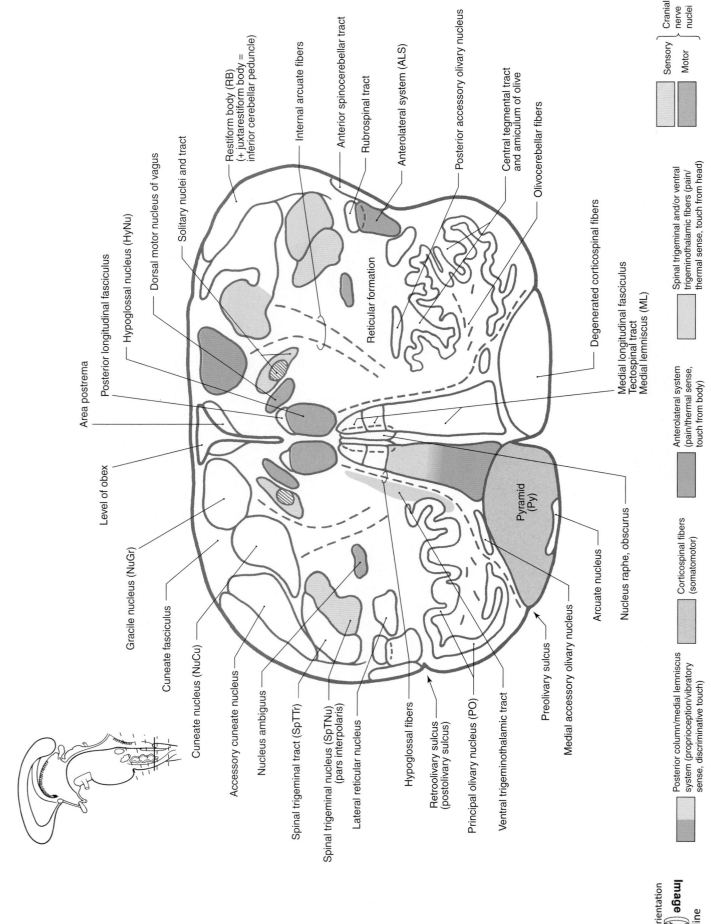

Restiform body (RB)
(+ juxtarestiform body =
inferior cerebellar peduncle)

Internal arcuate fibers

Anterior spinocerebellar tract

Rubrospinal tract

Anterolateral system (ALS)

Posterior accessory olivary nucleus

Central tegmental tract
and amiculum of olive

Olivocerebellar fibers

Degenerated corticospinal fibers

Medial longitudinal fasciculus
Tectospinal tract
Medial lemniscus (ML)

Solitary nuclei and tract

Dorsal motor nucleus of vagus

Hypoglossal nucleus (HyNu)

Posterior longitudinal fasciculus

Area postrema

Level of obex

Reticular formation

Pyramid
(Py)

Nucleus raphe, obscurus

Arcuate nucleus

Medial accessory olivary nucleus

Ventral trigeminothalamic tract

Principal olivary nucleus (PO)

Retroolivary sulcus
(postolivary sulcus)

Preolivary sulcus

Hypoglossal fibers

Lateral reticular nucleus

Spinal trigeminal nucleus (SpTNu)
(pars interpolaris)

Spinal trigeminal tract (SpTTr)

Nucleus ambiguus

Accessory cuneate nucleus

Cuneate nucleus (NuCu)

Cuneate fasciculus

Gracile nucleus (NuGr)

Clinical Orientation

Image

Online

Sensory ⎤ Cranial
        ⎥ nerve
Motor ⎦ nuclei

Spinal trigeminal and/or ventral
trigeminothalamic fibers (pain/
thermal sense, touch from head)

Anterolateral system
(pain/thermal sense,
touch from body)

Corticospinal fibers
(somatomotor)

Posterior column/medial lemniscus
system (proprioception/vibratory
sense, discriminative touch)

CT cisternogram

MRI, T2-weighted image

Py
ML
PO
ALS
SpTTr+
SpTNu
RB
NuCu+NuGr
HyNu

MRI, T1-weighted image

Clinical orientation

Anatomical orientation

Clinical Orientation
Image
Online

6-10B

6-11A Transverse section of the medulla through rostral portions of the *hypoglossal nucleus* and the middle portions of the *principal olivary nucleus*. The fourth ventricle has flared open at this level, and the restiform body is enlarging to become a prominent structure on the dorsolateral aspect of the medulla.

Solitary nuclei and tract
Spinal trigeminal nucleus (SpTNu) (pars interpolaris)
Spinal trigeminal tract (SpTTr)
Rubrospinal tract
Anterior spinocerebellar tract
Anterolateral system (ALS)
Central tegmental tract and amiculum of olive
Olivocerebellar fibers
Degenerated corticospinal fibers
Medial longitudinal fasciculus (MLF)
Tectospinal tract
Medial lemniscus (ML)
Pyramid (Py)
Nucleus raphe, pallidus
Arcuate nucleus
Medial accessory olivary nucleus
Ventral trigeminothalamic tract
Hypoglossal nerve
Principal olivary nucleus (PO)
Posterior accessory olivary nucleus
Lateral reticular nucleus
Vagus nerve
Nucleus ambiguus
Restiform body (RB) (+ juxtarestiform body = Inferior cerebellar peduncle)
Accessory cuneate nucleus
Inferior (spinal) vestibular nucleus (InfVNu)
Medial vestibular nucleus (MVNu)
Dorsal motor nucleus of the vagus
Nucleus raphe, obscurus
Posterior longitudinal fasciculus
Hypoglossal nucleus (HyNu)
Sulcus limitans
Reticular formation

Clinical Orientation

Image **Online**

Sensory } Cranial nerve nuclei
Motor

Posterior column/medial lemniscus system (proprioception/vibratory sense, discriminative touch)

Corticospinal fibers (somatomotor)

Anterolateral system (pain/thermal sense, touch from body)

Spinal trigeminal and/or ventral trigeminothalamic fibers (pain/ thermal sense, touch from head)

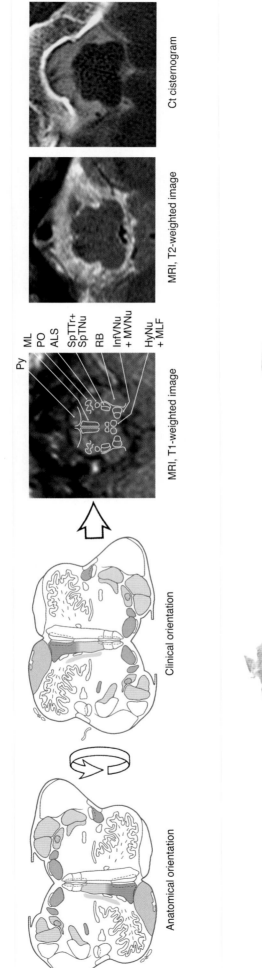

Ct cisternogram

MRI, T2-weighted image

Py ML
PO
ALS
SpTTr+
SpTNu
RB
InfVNu
+ MVNu
HyNu
+ MLF

MRI, T1-weighted image

Clinical orientation

Anatomical orientation

Clinical Orientation

Image
Image
Online

6-11B

6-12A Transverse section of the medulla through the *posterior (dorsal)* and *anterior (ventral) cochlear nuclei* and root of the *glossopharyngeal nerve.* This corresponds to approximately the rostral third to fourth of the *principal olivary nucleus,* to the location of the *lateral recess of the fourth ventricle,* and to the general area of the *medulla–pons junction.*

Posterior (dorsal) cochlear nucleus

Anterior (ventral) cochlear nucleus

Inferior (or spinal) vestibular nucleus (InfVNu)

Medial vestibular nucleus (MVNu)

Striae medullares of fourth ventricle

Nucleus prepositus (NuPre)

Posterior longitudinal fasciculus

Pontobulbar nucleus

Spinal trigeminal tract (SpTTr)

Spinal trigeminal nucleus (SpTNu) (pars oralis)

Rubrospinal tract

Nucleus ambiguus

Anterolateral system (ALS)

Central tegmental tract and amiculum of olive

Olivocerebellar fibers

Degenerated corticospinal fibers

Reticular formation

Nucleus raphe, pallidus

Medial longitudinal fasciculus (MLF)
Tectospinal tract
Medial lemniscus (ML)

Anterolateral system (pain/thermal sense, touch from body)

Pyramid (Py)

Nucleus raphe, obscurus

Inferior salivatory nucleus

Solitary nuclei

Solitary tract

Restiform body (RB)

Cerebellum

Posterior (dorsal) cochlear nucleus

Anterior (ventral) cochlear nucleus

Cochlear nerve

Glossopharyngeal nerve

Anterior spinocerebellar tract

Reticulospinal fibers

Posterior accessory olivary nucleus

Principal olivary nucleus

Ventral trigeminothalamic tract

Medial accessory olivary nucleus

Arcuate nucleus

Sensory
Motor } Cranial nerve nuclei

Spinal trigeminal and/or ventral trigeminothalamic fibers (pain/thermal sense, touch from head)

Corticospinal fibers (somatomotor)

Posterior column/medial lemniscus system (proprioception/vibratory sense, discriminative touch)

Clinical Orientation
Image Online

CT cisternogram

MRI, T2-weighted image

Py
ML
ALS
SpTTr+
SpTNu
RB
InfVNu
+ MVNu
NuPre
+MLF

MRI, T1-weighted image

Clinical orientation

Anatomical orientation

6-13A Transverse section of the medulla–pons junction through the rostral pole of the *principal olivary nucleus* and through the *facial motor nucleus*. This plane is just caudal to the main portions of the abducens nucleus. Pontine nuclei at this level may also be called arcuate nuclei. CochNu = posterior and anterior cochlear nuclei.

Juxtarestiform body
Restiform body (RB)
Inferior cerebellar peduncle

Abducens nucleus
Solitary tract
Facial nerve
Facial nucleus (FacNu)
Rubrospinal tract
Anterior spinocerebellar tract
Anterolateral system (ALS)
Superior olive
Secondary cochlear fibers
Central tegmental tract
Degenerated corticospinal fibers

Superior cerebellar peduncle
Superior medullary velum
Medial longitudinal fasciculus
Nucleus raphe, obscurus
Medial lemniscus (ML)
Posterior longitudinal fasciculus
Reticular formation
Pyramid (Py)
Pontine nuclei

Superior vestibular nucleus
Medial vestibular nucleus (MVNu)
Lateral vestibular nucleus (LVNu)
Solitary nuclei and tract
Spinal trigeminal nucleus (SpTNu) (pars oralis)
Anterior (ventral) cochlear nucleus
Vestibular root of eighth nerve
Pontobulbar nucleus (or body)
Spinal trigeminal tract (SpTTr)
Secondary cochlear fibers
Superior olive
Tectospinal tract
Ventral trigeminothalamic tract
Principal olivary nucleus
Nucleus raphe, magnus
Nucleus raphe, pallidus
Corticospinal fibers (CSp)

Sensory | Cranial nerve nuclei
Motor

Posterior column/medial lemniscus system (proprioception/vibratory sense, discriminative touch)

Anterolateral system (pain/thermal sense, touch from body)

Corticospinal fibers (somatomotor)

Spinal trigeminal and/or ventral trigeminothalamic fibers (pain/thermal sense, touch from head)

Clinical Orientation
Image
Online

CT cisternogram

MRI, T2-weighted image

Py/CSp
ML
ALS
FacNu
SpTTr+
SpTNu
RB
CochNu
MVNu
+LVNu

MRI, T1-weighted image

Clinical orientation

Anatomical orientation

6-14 Semi-diagrammatic representation of the internal distribution of arteries in the medulla oblongata. Selected main structures are labeled primarily on the left side of each section, and the general pattern of arterial distribution overlies these structures on the right side. The general distribution patterns of arteries in the medulla, as illustrated here, may vary from patient to patient. For example, the territories served by adjacent vessels may overlap to differing degrees at their margins, or the territory of a particular vessel may be smaller or larger than seen in the typical pattern.

ABBREVIATIONS

FCu	Cuneate fasciculus	Py	Pyramid
FGr	Gracile fasciculus	RB	Restiform body (+ juxtarestiform body = inferior cerebellar peduncle)
ML	Medial lemniscus	RetF	Reticular formation
NuCu	Cuneate nucleus		
NuGr	Gracile nucleus		

Vascular Syndromes or Lesions of the Medulla Oblongata

Medial Medullary Syndrome

This results from occlusion of branches of the anterior spinal artery.

Deficit	Structure Damage
• Contralateral hemiplegia of upper extremity (UE), trunk, and lower extremity (LE)	• Pyramid (corticospinal fibers)
• Contralateral loss of position sense, vibratory sense, and discriminative touch (UE, trunk, LE)	• Medial lemniscus
• Deviation of tongue to ipsilateral side when protruded; muscle atrophy and fasciculations	• Hypoglossal nerve in medulla or hypoglossal nucleus

The *medial medullary syndrome* (*Déjèrine syndrome*) is rare compared to the more common occurrence of the lateral medullary syndrome. *Nystagmus* may result if the lesion involves the medial longitudinal fasciculus or the nucleus prepositus hypoglossi. The lesion may involve ventral trigeminothalamic fibers, but diminished pain and thermal sense from the contralateral side of the face is rarely seen. The combination of a contralateral hemiplegia and ipsilateral deviation of the tongue is called an *inferior alternating hemiplegia* when the lesion is at this level.

Lateral Medullary Syndrome

Results from occlusion of posterior inferior cerebellar artery or branches of PICA to dorsolateral medulla (*PICA syndrome, Wallenberg syndrome*). In some cases, the lateral medullary syndrome may result from occlusion of the vertebral artery at the origin of the PICA with consequent loss of flow into PICA.

Deficit	Structure Damage
• Contralateral loss of pain and thermal sense on body	• Anterolateral system fibers
• Ipsilateral loss of pain and thermal sense on face	• Spinal trigeminal tract and nucleus
• Dysphagia, soft palate paralysis, hoarseness, diminished gag reflex	• Nucleus ambiguus, roots of 9th and 10th nerves
• Ipsilateral Horner syndrome (miosis, ptosis, anhidrosis, flushing of face)	• Descending hypothalamospinal fibers
• Nausea, diplopia, tendency to fall to ipsilateral side, nystagmus, vertigo	• Vestibular nuclei (mainly inferior and medial)
• Ataxia to the ipsilateral side	• Restiform body and spinocerebellar fibers

In addition to the preceding, involvement of the solitary tract and nucleus may (rarely) cause *dysgeusia*. *Dyspnea* and *tachycardia* may be seen in patients with damage to the dorsal motor nucleus of the vagus. It is also possible that damage to respiratory centers in the reticular formation or to the vagal motor nucleus may result in hiccup (*singultus*). Bilateral medullary damage may cause the syndrome of the "Ondine curse," an inability to breathe without willing it or "thinking about it."

Tonsillar Herniation

Although the cerebellar tonsil is not part of the medulla, the herniation of this structure (*tonsillar herniation*) down through the foramen magnum has serious consequences for function of the medulla. Although the causes vary, such as a sudden increase in pressure in the posterior cranial fossa, or a shift in pressure in the cranial cavity (such as during a lumbar puncture in a patient with a mass lesion) in cases of tonsillar herniation, the cerebellar tonsils "cone" downward into and through the foramen magnum. The result is a compression of the medulla (mechanical damage to the medulla plus occlusion of vessels), damage to respiratory and cardiac centers, and *sudden respiratory and cardiac arrest*. This constitutes a medical emergency, especially if the onset is sudden, and must be addressed *immediately* or the patient may die.

Syringobulbia

A cavitation within the brainstem (*syringobulbia*) may exist with syringomyelia, be independent of syringomyelia, or, in some cases, both may exist and communicate with each other. The cavity in syringobulbia is usually on one side of the midline of the medulla. Signs and symptoms of syringobulbia may include *weakness of tongue muscles* (hypoglossal nucleus or nerve), *weakness of pharyngeal, palatal, and vocal musculature* (ambiguus nucleus), *nystagmus* (vestibular nuclei), and *loss of pain and thermal sensation on the ipsilateral side of the face* (spinal trigeminal tract and nucleus, or crossing of trigeminothalamic fibers).

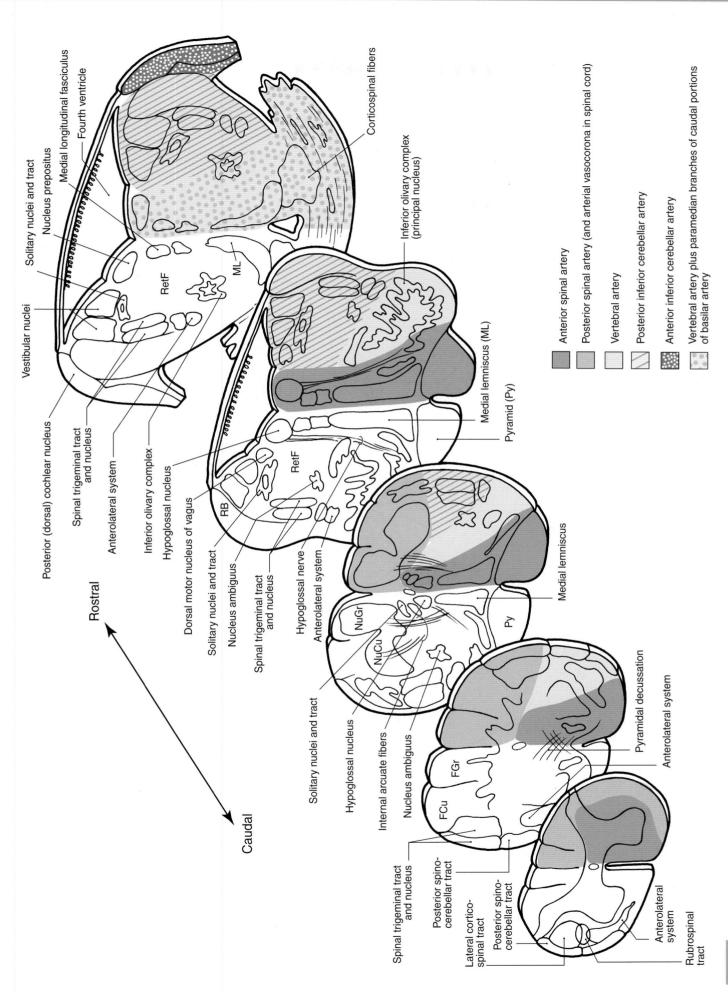

Medial longitudinal fasciculus

Fourth ventricle

Nucleus prepositus

Solitary nuclei and tract

Vestibular nuclei

Posterior (dorsal) cochlear nucleus

Spinal trigeminal tract and nucleus

Anterolateral system

Inferior olivary complex

Hypoglossal nucleus

Dorsal motor nucleus of vagus

Solitary nuclei and tract

Nucleus ambiguus

Spinal trigeminal tract and nucleus

Hypoglossal nerve

Anterolateral system

Solitary nuclei and tract

Hypoglossal nucleus

Internal arcuate fibers

Nucleus ambiguus

Spinal trigeminal tract and nucleus

Posterior spinocerebellar tract

Lateral corticospinal tract

Posterior spinocerebellar tract

Corticospinal fibers

Inferior olivary complex (principal nucleus)

Medial lemniscus (ML)

Pyramid (Py)

Medial lemniscus

Pyramidal decussation

Anterolateral system

Anterolateral system

Rubrospinal tract

RetF

ML

RetF

RB

NuGr

NuCu

Py

FGr

FCu

Rostral

Caudal

Anterior spinal artery

Posterior spinal artery (and arterial vasocorona in spinal cord)

Vertebral artery

Posterior inferior cerebellar artery

Anterior inferior cerebellar artery

Vertebral artery plus paramedian branches of caudal portions of basilar artery

6-14

6-15A   Transverse section through the dorsal aspects of the medulla at the level of the *cochlear nuclei* and the *cerebellar nuclei*. The plane corresponds to about the middle of *the dentate nucleus* and caudal portions of the *globose and emboliform nuclei*. For additional details of the medulla at this level, see Figure 6-12 on p. 116.

Dentate nucleus, DNu
(lateral cerebellar nucleus)

Globose nucleus, GNu
(posterior interposed cerebellar nucleus)

Fastigial nucleus, FNu
(medial cerebellar nucleus)

Tonsil of cerebellum
(Ton)

Posterior (dorsal)
cochlear nucleus

Lateral recess of
fourth ventricle

Restiform body
(RB)

Inferior (spinal)
vestibular nucleus

Solitary nuclei and tract

Medial vestibular nucleus

Medial longitudinal fasciculus (MLF)
Tectospinal tract

Anterolateral system
(pain/thermal sense,
touch from body)

Nucleus prepositus

Spinal trigeminal nucleus (pars oralis)

Spinal trigeminal tract

Choroid plexus

Tela choroidea

Nodulus

Uvula

DNu

GNu

DNu

FNu

Emboliform nucleus (ENu)
(anterior interposed
cerebellar nucleus)

Inferior medullary velum

Hilum of dentate nucleus

Anterior (ventral)
cochlear nucleus

Posterior column/medial lemniscus system
(proprioception/vibratory sense,
discriminative touch)

Corticospinal fibers
(somatomotor)

Anterolateral system
(pain/thermal sense,
touch from body)

Spinal trigeminal and/or ventral
trigeminothalamic fibers (pain/
thermal sense, touch from head)

Sensory   Cranial
          nerve
Motor   nuclei

Clinical Orientation
Image
Online

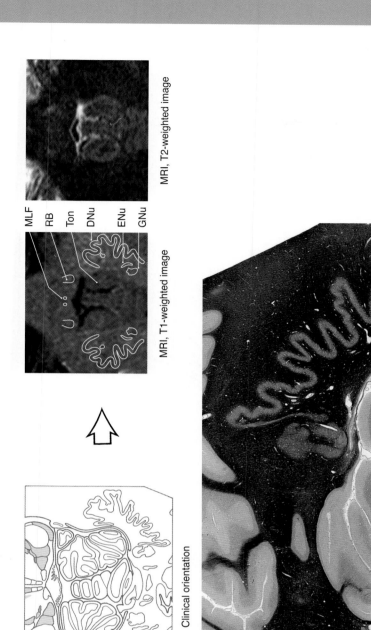

MLF
RB
Ton
DNu
ENu
GNu

MRI, T2-weighted image

MRI, T1-weighted image

Clinical orientation

Anatomical orientation

6-15B

6-16A Transverse section through dorsal portions of the pons at the level of the *abducens nucleus* (and *facial colliculus*) and through rostral portions of the *cerebellar nuclei*. For additional details of the pons at this level, see Figure 6-17 on p. 126.

Fastigial nucleus, FNu (medial cerebellar nucleus)

Globose nucleus, GNu (posterior interposed cerebellar nucleus)

Emboliform nucleus, ENu (anterior interposed cerebellar nucleus)

Dentate nucleus (DNu) (lateral cerebellar nucleus)

Juxtarestiform body (JRB)   Inferior cerebellar peduncle
Restiform body (RB)

Lateral vestibular nucleus (LVNu)

Facial nerve

Facial motor nucleus

Abducens nerve

Medial longitudinal fasciculus (MLF)
Tectospinal tract

Abducens nucleus

FNu

GNu

ENu

Facial nerve

Central tegmental tract

Superior cerebellar peduncle (SCP) (brachium conjunctivum)

Superior vestibular nucleus

Medial vestibular nucleus

Spinal trigeminal tract

Spinal trigeminal nucleus (pars oralis)

Sensory ⎱ Cranial
Motor ⎰ nerve nuclei

Spinal trigeminal and/or ventral trigeminothalamic fibers (pain/thermal sense, touch from head)

Anterolateral system (pain/thermal sense, touch from body)

Posterior column/medial lemniscus system (proprioception/vibratory sense, discriminative touch)

Corticospinal fibers (somatomotor)

Clinical Orientation
Image Online

MRI, T2-weighted image

MLF
LVNu
RB
JRB
SCP
DNu
ENu
GNu
FNu

MRI, T1-weighted image

Clinical orientation

Anatomical orientation

Clinical Orientation
Image
Image
Online

6-16B

6-17A Transverse section of the caudal pons through the *facial motor nucleus, abducens nucleus* (and *facial colliculus*), and the intramedullary course of fibers of *facial* and *abducens nerves.*

Superior vestibular nucleus

Restiform body (RB)

Facial nerve, internal genu

Mesencephalic tract and nucleus

Superior salivatory nucleus, SSNu

Principal sensory nucleus

Trigeminal motor nucleus

Trigeminal nerve

Anterior spinocerebellar tract

Rubrospinal tract

Anterolateral system (ALS)

Central tegmental tract

Trapezoid body and nuclei

Pontocerebellar fibers

Pontine nuclei

Degenerated corticospinal fibers

Superior vestibular nucleus

Medial longitudinal fasciculus (MLF)
Tectospinal tract

Superior cerebellar peduncle (SCP)

Superior medullary velum

Reticular formation

Medial lemniscus (ML)

Nucleus raphe, magnus

Posterior longitudinal fasciculus

Abducens nucleus (AbdNu)

SSNu

Superior vestibular nucleus

Medial vestibular nucleus (MVNu)

Juxtarestiform body

Lateral vestibular nucleus (LVNu)

Solitary nuclei and tract

Spinal trigeminal tract (SpTTr)

Spinal trigeminal nucleus (SpTNu)(pars oralis)

Facial nerve

Facial motor nucleus (FacNu)

Lateral lemniscus

Superior olive

Pontine nuclei

Abducens nerve

Corticospinal fibers (CSp)

Ventral trigeminothalamic tract

Clinical Orientation

Image Online

Posterior column—medial lemniscus system (proprioception/vibratory sense, discriminative touch)

Corticospinal fibers (somatomotor)

Anterolateral system (pain/thermal sense, touch from body)

Spinal trigeminal and/or ventral trigeminothalamic fibers (pain/thermal sense, touch from head)

Sensory ⎤ Cranial
Motor ⎦ nerve nuclei

CT cisternogram

MRI, T2-weighted image

CSp ML   ALS
           FacNu
           SpTTr+
           SpTNu
           RB
           LVNu+MVNu
           SCP
           AbdNu
      MLF
MRI, T1-weighted image

Clinical orientation

Anatomical orientation

Clinical Orientation
Image
Online

6-17B

6-18A Transverse section of the pons through the rostral pole of the *facial nucleus* and the internal *genu of the facial nerve* and rostral portions of the *abducens nucleus.*

Anterior spinocerebellar tract

Principal sensory nucleus (caudal part)

Trigeminal motor nucleus (caudal part)

Middle cerebellar peduncle

Trigeminal nerve

Anterolateral system (ALS)

Rubrospinal tract

Central tegmental tract

Mesencephalic nucleus and tract

Facial nerve, Internal genu (Fac,G)

Superior medullary velum

Superior cerebellar peduncle (SCP)

Reticular formation

Pontocerebellar fibers

Degenerated corticospinal fibers

Trapezoid body

Nucleus raphe, magnus

Medial longitudinal fasciculus
Tectospinal tract

Posterior longitudinal fasciculus

Fac,G

Medial lemniscus (ML)

Pontine nuclei

Pontine nuclei

Superior vestibular nucleus (SVNu)

Abducens nucleus (AbdNu)

Mesencephalic nucleus and tract

Superior salivatory nucleus

Spinal trigeminal nucleus and tract (SpTNu + Tr) (rostral end)

Facial nerve

Facial motor nucleus

Anterolateral system

Lateral lemniscus

Superior olive

Abducens nerve

Ventral trigeminothalamic tract

Corticospinal fibers (CSP)

Sensory ⎫ Cranial
Motor ⎬ nerve
       ⎭ nuclei

Spinal trigeminal and/or ventral trigeminothalamic fibers (pain/thermal sense, touch from head)

Anterolateral system (pain/thermal sense, touch from body)

Posterior column/medial lemniscus system (proprioception/vibratory sense, discriminative touch)

Corticospinal fibers (somatomotor)

Clinical Orientation
Image
Online

CSp
ML
ALS
SpTTr+
SpTNu
SVNu
SCP
AbdNu+
Fac,G

MRI, T1-weighted image

CT cisternogram

MRI, T2-weighted image

Clinical orientation

Anatomical orientation

Clinical Orientation

Image Online

6-18B

6-19A   Transverse section of the pons through the *principal sensory nucleus and motor nucleus of the trigeminal nerve.*

Central grey (periventricular grey)

Mesencephalic nucleus (MesNu + Tr)

Mesencephalic tract

Superior cerebellar peduncle (CP) (brachium conjunctivum)

Anterior spinocerebellar tract (ASCT)

Nucleus ceruleus

Trigeminal motor nucleus

Lateral lemniscus

Middle cerebellar peduncle (brachium pontis)

ASCT

Anterolateral system (ALS)

Rubrospinal tract

Central tegmental tract

Ventral trigeminothalamic tract

Pontocerebellar fibers

Degenerated corticospinal fibers

Pontine nuclei

Pontine nuclei

Nucleus raphe, pontis

Reticulotegmental nucleus

Medial lemniscus (ML)

Corticospinal fibers (CSP)

Lateral lemniscus, nucleus

Superior olive

Lateral lemniscus

Trigeminal nerve (TriNr)

Trigeminal motor nucleus (TriMotNu)

Principal sensory nucleus (PSNu)

Reticular formation

Tectospinal tract

Posterior longitudinal fasciculus

Medial longitudinal fasciculus (MLF)

Superior medullary velum

Clinical Orientation

Image Online

Posterior column/medial lemniscus system (proprioception/vibratory sense, discriminative touch)

Corticospinal fibers (somatomotor)

Anterolateral system (pain/thermal sense, touch from body)

Spinal trigeminal and/or ventral trigeminothalamic fibers (pain/thermal sense, touch from head)

Sensory ⎱ Cranial
Motor ⎰ nerve nuclei

CT cisternogram

MRI, T2-weighted image

CSp
ML
ALS
PSNu
TriMotNu
SCP
MesNu+Tr
MLF

TriNr

MRI, T1-weighted image

Clinical orientation

Anatomical orientation

Clinical Orientation
Image
Online

6-19B

6-20A   Transverse section of the rostral pons through the *exit of the trochlear nerve* and rostral portions of the *exit of the trigeminal nerve*. See also Figure 6-19 on p. 130.

Rubrospinal tract

Pontine nuclei

Pontocerebellar fibers

Medial longitudinal fasciculus (MLF)

Mesencephalic nucleus and tract (MesNu + Tr)

Reticular formation

Lateral lemniscus and nuclei of lateral lemniscus

Tectospinal tract

Degenerated corticospinal fibers

Locus ceruleus

Nucleus raphe, dorsalis

Frenulum

Cerebral aqueduct

Central gray (Periaqueductal gray)

Trochlear nerve, exit

Dorsal trigeminothalamic tract

Superior cerebellar peduncle (SCP) (brachium conjunctivum)

Central tegmental tract

Nucleus centralis, superior

Anterolateral system (ALS)

Medial lemniscus (ML)

Ventral trigeminothalamic tract

Middle Cerebellar peduncle (brachium pontis)

Trigeminal nerve

Basilar pons

Corticospinal fibers (CSP)

Clinical Orientation

Image Online

Sensory ⎤ Cranial
Motor ⎦ nerve nuclei

Posterior column/medial lemniscus system (proprioception/vibratory sense, discriminative touch)

Anterolateral system (pain/thermal sense, touch from body)

Spinal trigeminal and/or ventral trigeminothalamic fibers (pain/thermal sense, touch from head)

Corticospinal fibers (somatomotor)

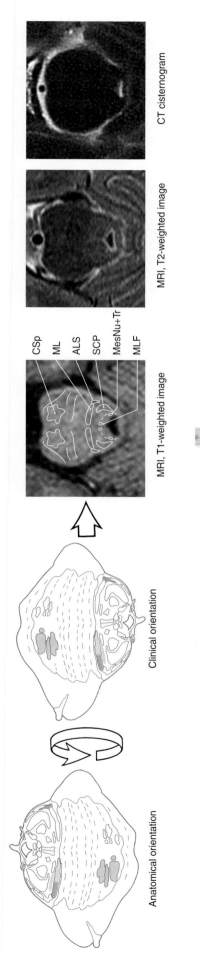

CSp
ML
ALS
SCP
MesNu+Tr
MLF

MRI, T1-weighted image

MRI, T2-weighted image

CT cisternogram

Clinical orientation

Anatomical orientation

Clinical Orientation

Image

Online

6-20B

6-21 Semi-diagrammatic representation of the internal distribution of arteries in the pons. Selected main structures are labeled on the left side of each section; the general pattern of arterial distribution overlies these structures on the right side. Some patients may have variations of the general distribution patterns of arteries to the pons as shown here. For example, the adjacent territories served by vessels may overlap to differing degrees at their margins, or the territory of a particular vessel may be smaller or larger than seen in the general pattern.

ABBREVIATIONS

BP	Basilar pons	**MLF**	Medial longitudinal fasciculus
CSp	Corticospinal fibers	**RB**	Restiform body (+ juxtarestiform body =
CTT	Central tegmental tract		inferior cerebellar peduncle)
MCP	Middle cerebellar peduncle	**RetF**	Reticular formation
	(brachium pontis)	**SCP**	Superior cerebellar peduncle (brachium
ML	Medial lemniscus		conjunctivum)

- Ipsilateral paralysis of masticatory muscles
- Ipsilateral Horner syndrome
- Ipsilateral loss of pain and thermal sense from face
- Contralateral loss of pain and thermal sense from UE, trunk, and LE
- Paralysis of conjugate horizontal gaze

- Trigeminal motor nucleus (midpontine levels)
- Descending hypothalamospinal fibers
- Spinal trigeminal tract and nucleus

- Anterolateral system

- Paramedian pontine reticular formation (at mid- to caudal levels)

The various combinations of these deficits may vary depending on whether the lesion is located in lateral pontine areas at caudal levels versus lateral pontine areas at rostral levels. As noted above, lesions located in lateral portions of the pontine tegmenti may also extend medial at either caudal or rostral levels and give rise to some of the deficits discussed above in the section on medial pontine syndrome.

Lesions that damage more lateral pontine areas generally are referred to as the *Gubler syndrome* (or the *Millard-Gubler syndrome*, although *Gubler* is preferred). In some instances, the term *midpontine base syndrome* is used to describe a basilar pontine lesion that involves the trigeminal root as well.

■ Vascular Syndromes or Lesions of the Pons ■

Medial Pontine Syndrome

This results from occlusion of paramedian branches of basilar artery.

Deficit	Structure Damage
• Contralateral hemiplegia of UE, trunk, and LE	• Corticospinal fibers in basilar pons
• Contralateral loss or decrease of position and vibratory sense and discriminative touch of UE, trunk, and LE	• Medial lemniscus
• Ipsilateral lateral rectus muscle paralysis	• Abducens nerve fibers or nucleus
• Paralysis of conjugate gaze toward side of lesion	• Paramedian pontine reticular formation (pontine gaze center)

The combination of corticospinal deficits on one side of the body coupled with a cranial nerve motor deficit on the opposite is called a *middle alternating hemiplegia* when the lesion is at this level. *Diplopia* will result (abducens nerve lesion) on gaze toward the side of the lesion. Involvement of the abducens nucleus may also result in an inability to adduct the contralateral medial rectus muscle (damage to abducens internuclear neurons).

At caudal levels, the lesion may extend lateral to involve the lateral lemniscus (*hypacusis*), parts of the middle cerebellar peduncle (some *ataxia*), the facial motor nucleus (*ipsilateral facial paralysis*), the spinal trigeminal tract and nucleus (*ipsilateral loss of pain and thermal sensation from the face*), and the anterolateral system (*contralateral loss of pain and thermal sensation from the body*).

At rostral pontine levels, the lesion may extend into the medial lemniscus or may involve only the arm fibers within this structure (*contralateral loss of vibratory sense, proprioception, and discriminative touch*), the motor nucleus of the trigeminal nerve (*ipsilateral paralysis of masticatory muscles*), or may damage the anterolateral system and rostral portions of the spinal trigeminal tract and *nucleus* (*loss of pain and thermal sensation from the body [contralateral] and from the face [ipsilateral]*).

Lesions in the medial pontine areas, especially at more caudal levels, may be known as the *Foville syndrome* or *Raymond syndrome*. The specifics of these syndromes are somewhat different but they may be used interchangeably. See Table 3-2 on p. 52 for more information on this point.

Lateral Pontine Syndrome

This results from occlusion of the long circumferential branches of the basilar artery.

Deficit	Structure Damage
• Ataxia, unsteady gait, fall toward side of lesion	• Middle and superior cerebellar peduncles (caudal and rostral levels)
• Vertigo, nausea, nystagmus, deafness, tinnitus, vomiting (at caudal levels)	• Vestibular and cochlear nerves and nuclei
• Ipsilateral paralysis of facial muscles	• Facial motor nucleus (caudal levels)

Rostral

Caudal

Trochlear nerve

Mesencephalic nucleus and tract

Medial longitudinal fasciculus (MLF)

Lateral lemniscus

Anterolateral system

Superior medullary velum

Fourth ventricle

Trigeminal nuclei:
Mesencephalic
Motor
Principal sensory

Trigeminal nerve

Anterolateral system

Abducens nucleus

MLF

Vestibular nuclei

Spinal trigeminal nucleus

Spinal trigeminal tract

Facial nerve

Facial motor nucleus

Anterolateral system

Abducens nerve

Basilar pons (BP)

SCP

ML

CSp

RetF

CTT

ML

SCP

MCP

BP

RB

MCP

ML

CSp

Ventral trigeminothalamic fibers

Paramedian branches of basilar artery

Long circumferential branches of basilar artery and branches of anterior inferior cerebellar artery

Short circumferential branches of basilar artery

Long circumferential branches of basilar artery and branches of superior cerebellar artery

6-21

6-22A   Transverse section of the brainstem at the pons–midbrain junction through the *inferior colliculus*, caudal portions of the decussation of the *superior cerebellar peduncle*, and rostral parts of the *basilar pons*. The plane of section is just caudal to the *trochlear nucleus*. IC = inferior colliculus on the cisternogram; the T1 and T2 are at a slightly different plane of section.

Sensory ⎤ Cranial
Motor ⎦ nerve nuclei

Spinal trigeminal and/or ventral trigeminothalamic fibers (pain/thermal sense, touch from head)

Anterolateral system (pain/thermal sense, touch from body)

Corticospinal fibers (somatomotor)

Posterior column/medial lemniscus system (proprioception/vibratory sense, discriminative touch)

Parietopontine fibers
Occipitopontine fibers
Temporopontine fibers

Pontocerebellar fibers

Pontine nuclei

Degenerated corticospinal fibers

Nucleus centralis, superior

Central tegmental tract

Tectospinal tract

Medial longitudinal fasciculus (MLF)

Nucleus ceruleus

Mesencephalic nucleus and tract (MesNu + Tr)

Nucleus raphe, dorsalis

Cerebral aqueduct

Central gray (periaqueductal gray)

Inferior colliculus, commissure

Inferior colliculus, pericentral nucleus

Inferior colliculus (IC), central nucleus

Posterior longitudinal fasciculus

Lateral lemniscus

Inferior colliculus, external nucleus

Reticular formation

Trochlear nerve

Dorsal trigeminothalamic tract

Anterolateral system (ALS)

Ventral trigeminothalamic tract

Medial lemniscus (ML)

Rubrospinal tract

Crus cerebri

Corticospinal fibers (CSp)

Superior cerebellar peduncle (SCP), decussation

Clinical Orientation
Image ⟳ Image
Online

IC

CT cisternogram

MRI, T2-weighted image

CSp
ML
ALS
SCP
MesNu+Tr
MLF

MRI, T1-weighted image

Clinical orientation

Anatomical orientation

Clinical Orientation
Image
Online

6-22B

6-23A Transverse section of the midbrain through the *trochlear nucleus* and *decussation of the superior cerebellar peduncle*. The section also includes caudal parts of the *superior colliculus* and the rostral tip of the *basilar pons*. IC = inferior colliculus on the T1-weighted MRI; at the plane of this section, the T2-weighted MRI and cisternogram are at a slightly more caudal plane compared to the line drawing.

Cerebral aqueduct

Central gray (periaqueductal gray)

Superior colliculus

Inferior colliculus, brachium

Mesencephalic nucleus and tract (MesNu + Tr)

Reticular formation

Dorsal trigeminothalamic tract

Medial longitudinal fasciculus (MLF)

Central tegmental tract

Ventral trigeminothalamic tract

Crus cerebri

PPon
OPon
TPon

Corticospinal fibers (CSp)

Corticonuclear fibers (corticobulbar fibers)

FPon

Pontine nuclei

Rubrospinal tract

Posterior longitudinal fasciculus

Nucleus raphe, dorsalis

Trochlear nucleus (TroNu)

Spinotectal fibers

Spinothalamic fibers

Anterolateral system (ALS)

Tectospinal tract

Medial lemniscus (ML)

Substantia nigra (SN), pars compacta

Parietopontine fibers (PPon)
Occipitopontine fibers (OPon)
Temporopontine fibers (TPon)

Degenerated corticospinal fibers

Frontopontine fibers (FPon)

Interpeduncular nucleus

Interpeduncular fossa

Superior cerebellar peduncle, decussation (SCPDec)

Sensory
Motor
Cranial nerve nuclei

Posterior column/medial lemniscus system (proprioception/vibratory sense, discriminative touch)

Corticospinal fibers (somatomotor)

Anterolateral system (pain/thermal sense, touch from body)

Spinal trigeminal and/or ventral trigeminothalamic fibers (pain/thermal sense, touch from head)

Clinical Orientation

Image Online

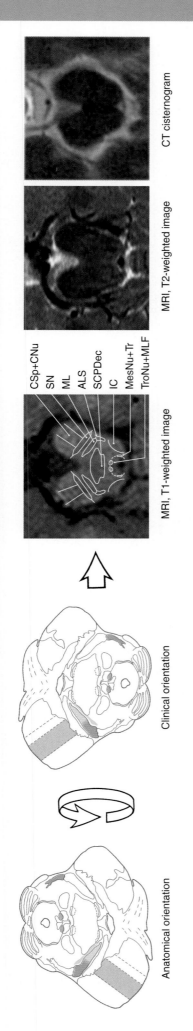

CT cisternogram

MRI, T2-weighted image

CSp+CNu
SN
ML
ALS
SCPDec
IC
MesNu+Tr
TroNu+MLF

MRI, T1-weighted image

Clinical orientation

Anatomical orientation

Clinical Orientation
Image
Online

6-23B

6-24A Transverse section of the midbrain through the *superior colliculus*, caudal parts of the *oculomotor nucleus*, and caudal parts of the *red nucleus*. The plane of section is caudal to the *Edinger-Westphal nucleus* but includes rostral portions of the *decussation of the superior cerebellar peduncle*, which, at this level, are intermingled with the caudal part of the red nucleus. Leg = lower extremity; Arm = upper extremity. At this level, spinothalamic fibers are the main constituents of the bundle indicated as the anterolateral system at lower levels.

Posterior longitudinal fasciculus

Oculomotor nucleus (OcNu)

Mesencephalic nucleus and tract (MesNu + Tr)

Spinotectal tract

Medial longitudinal fasciculus (MLF)

Spinothalamic fibers (SpThF)

Central tegmental tract

Posterior (dorsal) tegmental decussation

Red nucleus

Substantia nigra pars compacta (SNpc)

Substantia nigra pars reticulata (SNpr)

Parietopontine fibers (PPon)
Occipitopontine fibers (OPon)
Temporopontine fibers (TPon)

Degenerated corticospinal fibers

Superior cerebellar peduncle, decussation (SCPDec)

Frontopontine fibers (FPon)

Rubrospinal tract

Anterior (ventral) tegmental decussation

Interpeduncular nucleus

Oculomotor nerve

Cerebral aqueduct

Central gray (periaqueductal gray)

Superior colliculus

Dorsal trigeminothalamic tract

Reticular formation

Inferior colliculus, brachium

Ventral trigeminothalamic tract

Medial geniculate nucleus

Pallidonigral fibers
Nigrostriatal fibers
Corticonigral fibers

Crus cerebri

Medial lemniscus (ML)

SNpc

SNpr

Corticonuclear fibers (CNu) (corticobulbar fibers)

Leg
Trunk
Arm

Corticospinal fibers (CSp)

PPon
OPon
TPon

FPon

Red nucleus (RNu), caudal aspect

Clinical Orientation

Image Online

Posterior column/medial lemniscus system (proprioception/vibratory sense, discriminative touch)

Anterolateral system (pain/thermal sense, touch from body)

Corticospinal fibers (somatomotor)

Spinal trigeminal and/or ventral trigeminothalamic fibers (pain/thermal sense, touch from head)

Sensory
Motor
Cranial nerve nuclei

CT cisternogram

MRI, T2-weighted image

SCPDec
+RNu
CSp+CNu
SN
ML
SpThF
OcNu+MLF
MesNu+Tr

MRI, T1-weighted image

Clinical orientation

Anatomical orientation

Clinical Orientation
Image Online

6-24B

6-25A Transverse section of the midbrain through the *superior colliculus*, rostral portions of the *oculomotor nucleus*, including the *Edinger-Westphal nuclei*, and the exiting fibers of the *oculomotor nerve*. The plane of this section is also through caudal portions of the diencephalon including the *pulvinar nuclear complex* and the *medial* and *lateral geniculate nuclei*. Leg = lower extremity; Arm = upper extremity; CC = crus cerebri; OpTr = optic tract.

Parietopontine fibers (PPon)
Occipitopontine fibers (OPon)
Temporopontine fibers (TPon)

Inferior colliculus, brachium

Peripeduncular nucleus

Dorsal trigeminothalamic tract

Ventral trigeminothalamic tract

Cerebellorubral fibers and cerebellothalamic fibers

Degenerated corticospinal fibers

Central tegmental tract

Medial longitudinal fasciculus (MLF)

Frontopontine fibers (FPon)

Habenulopeduncular tract

Oculomotor nuclei (OcNu)

Oculomotor nerve

Posterior longitudinal fasciculus

Superior colliculus (SC)

Spinotectal tract

SNpr

SNpc

Cerebral aqueduct

Superior colliculus, commissure

Central grey (periaqueductal grey)

Edinger-Westphal preganglionic nucleus (EWpgNu)

Edinger-Westphal centrally projecting nucleus

Mesencephalic tract and nucleus (MesNu + Tr)

Superior colliculus, brachium

Pulvinar nuclear complex

Red nucleus (RNu)

Spinothalamic fibers (SpThF)

Medial geniculate nucleus (MGNu)

Lateral geniculate nucleus (LGNu)

Medial lemniscus (ML)

Optic tract

PPon

OPon

TPon

FPon

Leg
Trunk
Arm

Substantia nigra, pars compacta (SNpc)

Substantia nigra, pars reticulata (SNpr)

Corticonuclear fibers (CNu) (corticobulbar fibers)

Corticospinal fibers (CSp)

Corticonigral fibers
Pallidonigral fibers
Nigrostriatal fibers

Posterior column/medial lemniscus system (proprioception/vibratory sense, discriminative touch)

Anterolateral system (pain/thermal sense, touch from body)

Corticospinal fibers (somatomotor)

Spinal trigeminal and/or ventral trigeminothalamic fibers (pain/thermal sense, touch from head)

Sensory
Motor

Cranial nerve nuclei

Clinical Orientation
Image Online

OpTr

Crus
cerebri

SC

MRI, T2-weighted image

MRI, T2-weighted image

RNu
CSp+CNu
SN
ML
SpThF
OcNu+MLF
+EWpgNu
MesNu+Tr
SC

MRI, T1-weighted image

RNu
CC
ML
LGNu
MGNu

SpThF
SC

OcNu+MLF+EWpgNu

MRI, T1-weighted image

Clinical orientation

Anatomical orientation

6-26A Slightly oblique section through the midbrain–diencephalon junction. The section passes through the *posterior commissure*, the rostral end of the *red nucleus*, and ends just dorsal to the *mammillary body*. At this level, the structure labeled *mammillothalamic tract* probably also contains some *mammillotegmental fibers*. Structures at the midbrain–thalamus junction are best seen in an MRI angled to accommodate that specific plane. To make the transition from drawing to stained section to MRI easy, selected structures in the MRI are labeled.

Brachium of superior colliculus

Spinothalamic fibers

Lateral geniculate nucleus (LGNu)

Medial lemniscus

Cerebellorubral fibers and Cerebellothalamic fibers

Transition from crus cerebri (CC) to internal capsule

Cerebral aqueduct

Central grey (periaqueductal grey)

Nucleus of Darkschewitsch

Nucleus of Cajal

Medial longitudinal fasciculus

Medial geniculate nucleus (MGNu)

Optic tract (OpTr)

Subthalamic nucleus

Supraoptic nucleus

Fornix (F)

Red nucleus (RNu)

Mammillothalamic tract (MTTr)

Pineal

Posterior commissure

Superior colliculus

Pretectal nuclei

Hypothalamus

Third ventricle

Dorsal trigeminothalamic tract

Pulvinar nuclear complex (Pul)

Corticospinal fibers

Central tegmental tract

Ventral trigemino-thalamic tract

Peripeduncular nucleus

Parietopontine fibers
Occipitopontine fibers
Temporopontine fibers

Corticonuclear fibers (corticobulbar fibers)

Frontopontine fibers

Habenulopeduncular tract

Clinical Orientation

Image Online

Posterior column/medial lemniscus system (proprioception/vibratory sense, discriminative touch)

Corticospinal fibers (somatomotor)

Anterolateral system (pain/thermal sense, touch from body)

Spinal trigeminal and/or ventral trigeminothalamic fibers (pain/thermal sense, touch from head)

Sensory ⎫ Cranial
         ⎬ nerve
Motor   ⎭ nuclei

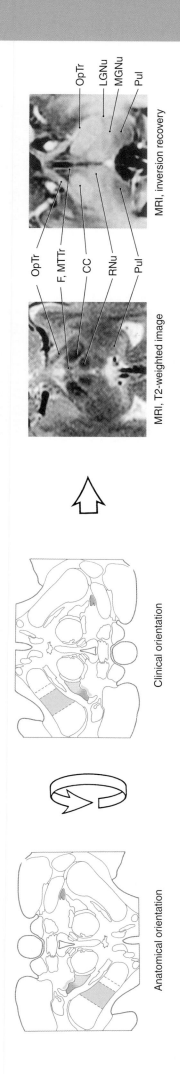

OpTr
LGNu
MGNu
Pul

MRI, inversion recovery

OpTr
F, MTTr
CC
RNu
Pul

MRI, T2-weighted image

Clinical orientation

Anatomical orientation

Clinical Orientation

Image

Online

6-26B

6-27 Semi-diagrammatic representation of the internal distribution of arteries in the midbrain. Selected main structures are labeled on the left side of each section; the typical pattern of arterial distribution overlies these structures on the right side. The general distribution patterns of the vessels to the midbrain, as shown here, may vary somewhat from patient to patient. For example, the adjacent territories served by neighboring vessels may overlap to differing degrees at their margins, or the territory of a particular vessel may be larger or smaller than seen in the general pattern.

ABBREVIATIONS

BP	Basilar pons	MGNu	Medial geniculate nucleus
CC	Crus cerebri	ML	Medial lemniscus
DecSCP	Decussation of the superior cerebellar peduncle	RNu	Red nucleus
		SC	Superior colliculus
IC	Inferior colliculus	SCP	Superior cerebellar peduncle
LGNu	Lateral geniculate nucleus	SN	Substantia nigra

Vascular Syndromes or Lesions of the Midbrain

Medial Midbrain (Weber) Syndrome

This may result from occlusion of the paramedian branches of the P_1 segment of the posterior cerebral artery (PCA).

Deficit	Structure Damage
• Contralateral hemiplegia of UE, trunk, and LE	• Corticospinal fibers in crus cerebri
• Ipsilateral paralysis of eye movement: eye oriented down and out and pupil dilated and fixed	• Oculomotor nerve

This combination of motor deficits at this level of the brainstem is called a *superior alternating hemiplegia*. This pattern consists of *ipsilateral paralysis of eye movement* and *contralateral hemiplegia* of the upper and lower extremities. Damage to the corticonuclear (corticobulbar) fibers in the crus cerebri may result in a partial deficit in tongue and facial movement on the contralateral side. These cranial nerve deficits are seen as a *deviation of the tongue* to the side opposite the lesion on attempted protrusion and a *paralysis of the lower half of the facial muscles* on the contralateral side. Although parts of the substantia nigra are frequently involved, *akinesia and dyskinesia* are not frequently seen.

Central Midbrain Lesion (Claude Syndrome)

Deficit	Structure Damage
• Ipsilateral paralysis of eye movement: eye oriented down and out and pupil dilated and fixed	• Oculomotor nerve
• Contralateral ataxia and tremor of cerebellar origin	• Red nucleus and cerebellothalamic fibers

The lesion in this syndrome may extend laterally into the medial lemniscus and the dorsally adjacent ventral trigeminothalamic fibers. If this was the case, there could conceivably be a loss or diminution of position and vibratory sense and of discriminative touch from the contralateral arm and partial loss of pain and thermal sensation from the contralateral face.

Benedikt Syndrome

This results from a larger lesion of the midbrain that essentially involves both of the separate areas of Weber and Claude. The main deficits are contralateral hemiplegia of the arm and leg (corticospinal fibers), ipsilateral paralysis of eye movement with dilated pupil (oculomotor nerve), and cerebellar tremor and ataxia (red nucleus and cerebellothalamic fibers). Slight variations may be present based on the extent of the lesion.

Parinaud Syndrome

This syndrome is usually caused by a tumor in the pineal region, such as germinoma, astrocytoma, pineocytoma/pineoblastoma, or any of a variety of other tumors that impinge on the superior colliculi. The potential for occlusion at the cerebral aqueduct in these cases also indicates that hydrocephalus may be a component of this syndrome. The deficits in these patients consist of a *paralysis of upward gaze* (superior colliculi), *hydrocephalus* (occlusion of the cerebral aqueduct), and eventually a *failure of eye movement* due to pressure on the oculomotor and trochlear nuclei. These patients also may exhibit *nystagmus* due to involvement of the medial longitudinal fasciculus.

Uncal Herniation

Herniation of the uncus occurs in response to large and/or rapidly expanding lesions in the cerebral hemisphere, this being a *supratentorial* location. *Uncal herniation* is an extrusion of the uncus through the tentorial notch (tentorial incisura) with resultant pressure on the oculomotor nerve and the crus cerebri of the midbrain. Initially, the pupils, unilaterally or bilaterally, may dilate or respond slowly to light, followed by weakness of oculomotor movement. As herniation progresses, the pupils become fully dilated, eye movements regulated by the oculomotor nerve may be slow or absent, and the eyes deviate slightly laterally because of the unopposed actions of the abducens nerves. There is usually weakness on the contralateral side of the body due to compression of corticospinal fibers in the crus cerebri. This combination of ipsilateral oculomotor palsy and a contralateral hemiplegia is also known as a *superior alternating hemiplegia*.

An alternative situation is when the pressure from the uncal herniation is sufficient to shift the entire midbrain to the opposite side. In this case, the oculomotor root may be stretched or *avulsed* on the side of the herniation (the ipsilateral side), and the crus cerebri on the contralateral side may be forced against the edge of the tentorium cerebelli with consequent damage to the corticospinal fibers located within the crus. In this case, the patient has an *oculomotor palsy and a hemiplegia of the UE and LE both on the same side of the body*. This combination of deficits is called the *Kernohan syndrome* (or *Kernohan phenomenon*).

Especially large, or bilateral, *supratentorial* lesions may also result in *decorticate rigidity* (in general, flexion of forearm, wrist, and fingers with adduction of UE; extension of LE with internal rotation and plantar flexion of foot). As the lesion descends into and through the tentorial notch into an *infratentorial* location, decorticate rigidity gives rise to *decerebrate rigidity* (UE and LE extended, toes pointed inward, forearm pronated, and head and neck extended—*opisthotonos*).

Rostral

Caudal

Edinger-Westphal preganglionic nucleus

Edinger-Westphal centrally projecting nucleus

Oculomotor nucleus

Anterolateral system

Ventral trigeminothalmic fibers

Oculomotor nerve

Mesencephalic nucleus

Trochlear nucleus

Medial longitudinal fasciculus

Anterolateral system

Ventral trigeminothalamic fibers

Cerebral aqueduct

Periaqueductal gray

Lateral lemniscus

Anterolateral system

Medial longitudinal fasciculus

Interpeduncular fossa

SC

RNu

ML

SN

CC

MGNu

LGNu

IC

DecSCP

ML

SN

CC

SCP

ML

CC

BP

Anteromedial (paramedian) branches of basilar bifurcation and P1 segment

Anterolateral (short circumferential) branches of the quadrigeminal and medial posterior choroidal arteries

Lateral branches of quadrigeminal (level of inferior colliculus), quadrigeminal and posterior medial choroidal arteries (level of superior colliculus)

Quadrigeminal and superior cerebellar arteries (level of inferior colliculus), quadrigeminal and posterior medial choroidal arteries (level of superior colliculus)

Thalamogeniculate artery

6-27

6-28A   Coronal section of forebrain through the *splenium of the corpus callosum* and the *crus of the fornix*, and extending into the *inferior colliculus* and exit of the *trochlear nerve*. Many of the structures labeled in this figure can be identified easily in the T1-weighted MRI adjacent to the photograph.

6-29A   Coronal section of the forebrain through the *pulvinar* and the *medial* and *lateral geniculate nuclei*. The section extends into upper portions of the *midbrain tegmentum*. Many of the structures labeled in this figure can be easily identified in the T1-weighted MRI adjacent to the photograph.

Cingulate gyrus

Cingulum

Lateral longitudinal stria of indusium griseum

Choroid plexus

External medullary lamina

Insula

Internal capsule

Retrolenticular limb
Sublenticular limb

Hippocampal formation

Lateral nucleus

Pulvinar nuclear complex

Medial nucleus

Hippocampus, fimbria of

Central grey (periaqueductal grey)

Trochlear nucleus

Superior cistern

Corpus callosum, body

Medial longitudinal stria

Fornix, body

Lateral ventricle, body

Caudate nucleus, body

Stria terminalis (StTer)

Superior colliculus, brachium

Inferior colliculus, brachium

Medial geniculate nucleus

Inferior pulvinar nucleus

Optic radiations

Lateral geniculate nucleus

StTer and bed nucleus

Caudate nucleus, tail

Alveus of hippocampus

Lateral ventricle, inferior horn

Sensory ⎤ Cranial
Motor ⎦ nerve nuclei

Spinal trigeminal and/or ventral trigeminothalamic fibers (pain/thermal sense, touch from head)

Anterolateral system (pain/thermal sense, touch from body)

Corticospinal fibers (somatomotor)

Posterior column/medial lemniscus system (proprioception/vibratory sense, discriminative touch)

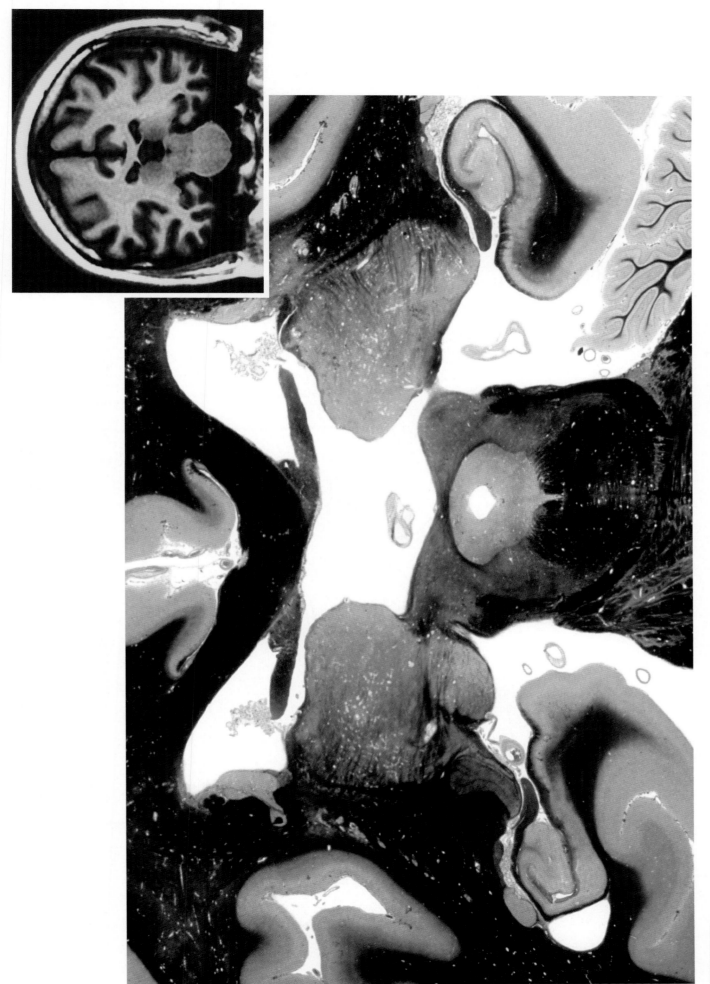

6-30A Slightly oblique section of the forebrain through the *pulvinar, ventral posteromedial,* and *ventral posterolateral nuclei.* The section extends rostrally through the *subthalamic nucleus* and ends in the *caudal hypothalamus,* just dorsal to the *mammillary bodies,* as seen by the position of the (postcommissural) fornix.

Centromedian nucleus of thalamus

Habenulopeduncular tract

Internal capsule, posterior limb

Ansa lenticularis

Anterior commissure

Dorsomedial nucleus of thalamus

Column of fornix

Pineal

Habenular commissure

Habenular nucleus

Third ventricle

Medial nucleus

Hypothalamus

Pulvinar nuclear complex

Mammillothalamic tract

Lateral nucleus

Zona incerta

Lenticular fasciculus

Thalamic fasciculus

Ventral posterolateral nucleus of thalamus

Ventral posteromedial nucleus of thalamus

Globus pallidus:
Lateral segment
Medial segment

Subthalamic nucleus

Clinical Orientation

Image Online

Sensory ⎱ Cranial
Motor ⎰ nerve nuclei

Spinal trigeminal and/or ventral trigeminothalamic fibers (pain/thermal sense, touch from head)

Anterolateral system (pain/thermal sense, touch from body)

Corticospinal fibers (somatomotor)

Posterior column/medial lemniscus system (proprioception/vibratory sense, discriminative touch)

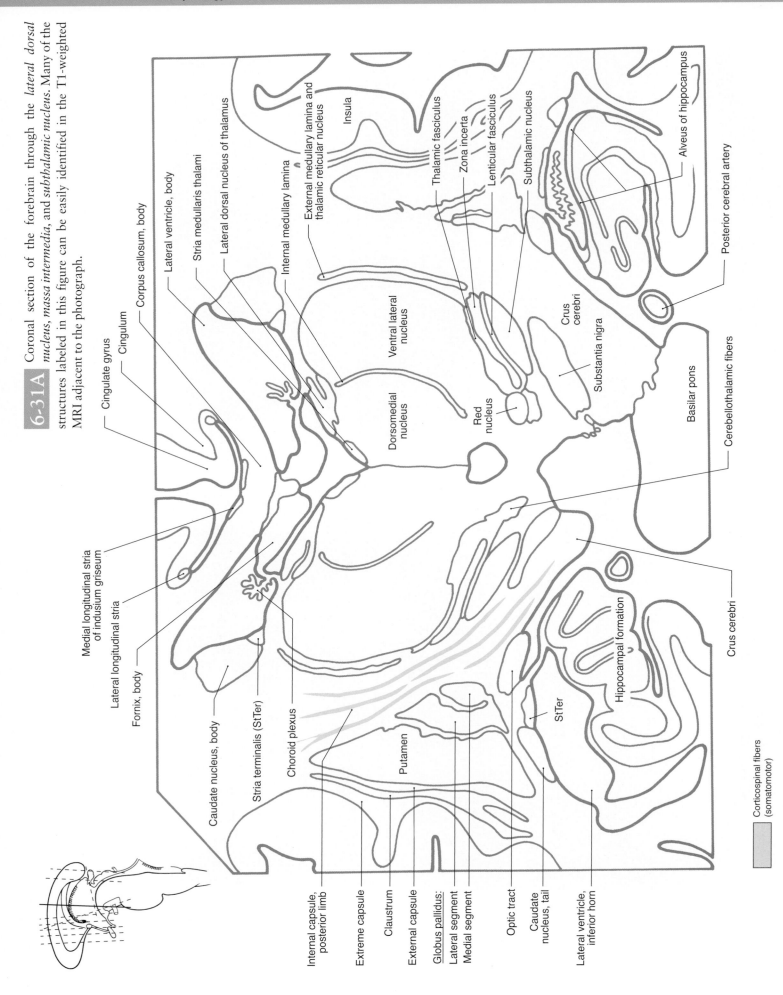

6-31A Coronal section of the forebrain through the *lateral dorsal nucleus, massa intermedia,* and *subthalamic nucleus.* Many of the structures labeled in this figure can be easily identified in the T1-weighted MRI adjacent to the photograph.

Cingulate gyrus

Cingulum

Corpus callosum, body

Lateral ventricle, body

Stria medullaris thalami

Lateral dorsal nucleus of thalamus

Internal medullary lamina

External medullary lamina and thalamic reticular nucleus

Insula

Thalamic fasciculus

Zona incerta

Lenticular fasciculus

Subthalamic nucleus

Alveus of hippocampus

Posterior cerebral artery

Crus cerebri

Substantia nigra

Basilar pons

Cerebellothalamic fibers

Crus cerebri

Hippocampal formation

StTer

Ventral lateral nucleus

Dorsomedial nucleus

Red nucleus

Medial longitudinal stria of indusium griseum

Lateral longitudinal stria

Fornix, body

Stria terminalis (StTer)

Choroid plexus

Caudate nucleus, body

Internal capsule, posterior limb

Extreme capsule

Claustrum

External capsule

Globus pallidus:
Lateral segment
Medial segment

Putamen

Optic tract

Caudate nucleus, tail

Lateral ventricle, inferior horn

Corticospinal fibers (somatomotor)

6-32A Coronal section of the forebrain through the *anterior nucleus of the thalamus* and *mammillary body*. Many of the structures labeled in this figure can be easily identified in the T1-weighted MRI. lat. = Lateral segment, med. = Medial segment.

Cingulum — Corpus callosum, body

Lateral ventricle, body

Choroid plexus

Stria medullaris thalami

Dorsomedial nucleus of thalamus

External medullary lamina and thalamic reticular nucleus

Internal medullary lamina

Thalamic fasciculus

Zona incerta

Lenticular fasciculus

Subthalamic nucleus

Alveus of hippocampus

Ventral lateral nucleus

Mammillothalamic tract

Hippocampal formation

Cingulate gyrus

Medial longitudinal stria

Lateral longitudinal stria of indusium griseum

Fornix, body

Caudate nucleus, body

Stria terminalis

Anterior nucleus

Third ventricle

Globus pallidus

lat.

med.

Putamen

Insula

Posterior hypothalamus

Mammillary body

Internal capsule, posterior limb

Extreme capsule

Claustrum

External capsule

Optic tract

Amygdaloid nuclear complex

Lateral ventricle, inferior horn

Corticospinal fibers (somatomotor)

6-33A   Slightly oblique section of the forebrain through the *anterior nucleus of the thalamus* and the *subthalamic nucleus*. The section also includes the rostral portion of the *midbrain tegmentum*. Many of the structures labeled in this figure can be easily identified in the T1-weighted MRI adjacent to the photograph. VL = ventral lateral nucleus of thalamus; VA = ventral anterior nucleus of thalamus.

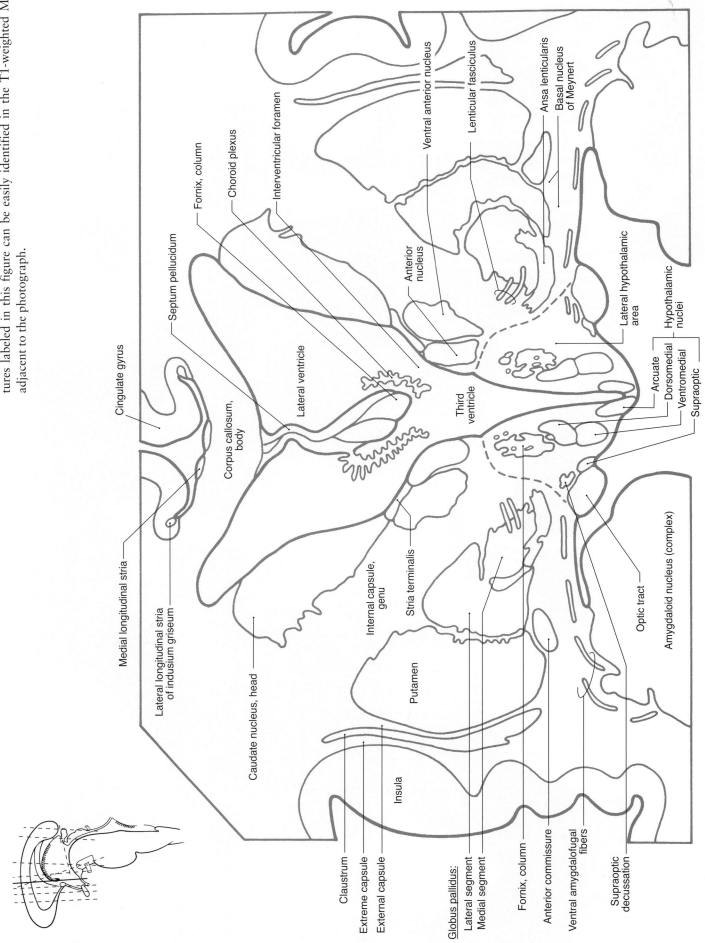

6-34A Coronal section of the forebrain through the *interventricular foramen*, *genu of the internal capsule*, rostral tip of the *dorsal thalamus*, and about the middle third of the *hypothalamus*. Many of the structures labeled in this figure can be easily identified in the T1-weighted MRI adjacent to the photograph.

Cingulate gyrus

Fornix, column

Choroid plexus

Interventricular foramen

Ventral anterior nucleus

Lenticular fasciculus

Ansa lenticularis

Basal nucleus of Meynert

Septum pellucidum

Anterior nucleus

Lateral ventricle

Lateral hypothalamic area

Hypothalamic nuclei

Third ventricle

Arcuate

Dorsomedial

Ventromedial

Supraoptic

Medial longitudinal stria

Lateral longitudinal stria of indusium griseum

Corpus callosum, body

Caudate nucleus, head

Internal capsule, genu

Stria terminalis

Putamen

Insula

Claustrum

Extreme capsule

External capsule

Globus pallidus:
Lateral segment
Medial segment

Fornix, column

Anterior commissure

Ventral amygdalofugal fibers

Supraoptic decussation

Optic tract

Amygdaloid nucleus (complex)

6-35A Coronal section of the forebrain through the *anterior commissure* and rostral aspects of the *hypothalamus*. Many of the structures labeled in this figure can be identified easily in the T1-weighted MRI.

Cingulate gyrus

Cingulum

Septum pellucidum

Fornix, column

Anterior commissure

Putamen

Globus pallidus, lateral segment

Basal nucleus of Meynert

Anterior perforated substance

Preoptic area of hypothalamus

Supraoptic decussation

Lateral ventricle, anterior horn

Infundibulum

Corpus callosum, body

Third ventricle

Optic tract

Medial longitudinal stria of indusium griseum

Lateral longitudinal stria

Supraoptic nucleus

Septal nuclei

Uncus

Caudate nucleus, head

Amygdaloid nucleus

Stria terminalis

Internal capsule, genu to anterior limb

Claustrum

Insula

Extreme capsule

External capsule

Diagonal band (of Broca)

Lateral olfactory stria

6-35B

6-36A Coronal section of the forebrain through the *head of the caudate nucleus*, rostral portions of the *optic chiasm*, and the *nucleus accumbens*. Many of the structures labeled in this figure can be easily identified in the T1-weighted MRI adjacent to the photograph.

Cingulate gyrus

Cingulum

Lateral longitudinal stria

Anterior cerebral arteries

Medial longitudinal stria of indusium griseum

Corpus callosum, body

Lateral ventricle, anterior horn

Caudate nucleus, head

Globus pallidus, lateral segment

Extreme capsule

External capsule

Claustrum

Insula

Internal capsule, anterior limb

Putamen

Nucleus accumbens

Septum pellucidum

Medial olfactory stria

Paraterminal gyrus

Optic chiasm

Diagonal band (of Broca)

Anterior cerebral artery

Lateral olfactory stria

Middle cerebral artery

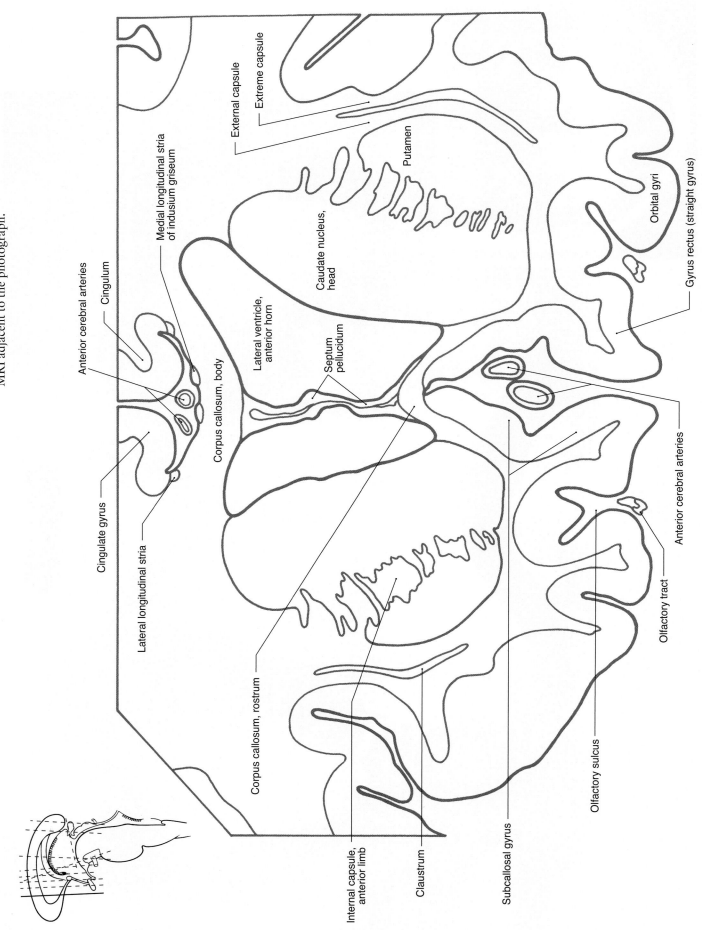

6-37A   Coronal section of the forebrain through the *head of the caudate nucleus* and the *anterior horn of the lateral ventricle.* Many of the structures labeled in this figure can be identified easily in the T1-weighted MRI adjacent to the photograph.

External capsule

Extreme capsule

Putamen

Medial longitudinal stria of indusium griseum

Caudate nucleus, head

Anterior cerebral arteries

Cingulum

Lateral ventricle, anterior horn

Corpus callosum, body

Septum pellucidum

Orbital gyri

Gyrus rectus (straight gyrus)

Cingulate gyrus

Lateral longitudinal stria

Anterior cerebral arteries

Olfactory tract

Corpus callosum, rostrum

Olfactory sulcus

Internal capsule, anterior limb

Claustrum

Subcallosal gyrus

6-37B

6-38 Semi-diagrammatic representation of the internal distribution of arteries to the diencephalon, basal nuclei, and internal capsule. Selected structures are labeled on the left side of each section; the general pattern of arterial distribution overlies these structures on the right side. The general distribution patterns of arteries in the forebrain, as shown here, may vary from patient to patient. For example, the adjacent territories served by neighboring vessels may overlap to varying degrees at their margins or the territory of a particular vessel may be larger or smaller than seen in the general pattern.

ABBREVIATIONS

APS	Anterior perforated substance	GP	Globus pallidus
		HyTh	Hypothalamus
BCorCl	Body of corpus callosum	PulNu	Pulvinar nuclear complex
CC	Crus cerebri	Put	Putamen
CM	Centromedian nucleus of thalamus	SplCorCl	Splenium of the corpus callosum
		VA	Ventral anterior nucleus of thalamus
DMNu	Dorsomedial nucleus of thalamus	VL	Ventral lateral nucleus of thalamus

Vascular Syndromes or Lesions of the Forebrain

Forebrain vascular lesions result in a wide range of deficits that include motor and sensory losses and a variety of cognitive disorders. Forebrain vessels may be occluded by a *thrombus*. This is a structure (usually a clot) formed by blood products and frequently attached to the vessel wall. Deficits may appear slowly, or wax and wane, as the blood flow is progressively restricted.

Vessels may also be occluded by *embolization*. A foreign body, or *embolus* (fat, air, piece of thrombus, piece of sclerotic plaque, clump of bacteria, etc.), is delivered from some distant site into the cerebral circulation where it lodges in a vessel. Because this is a sudden event, deficits usually appear quickly and may progress rapidly. Interruption of blood supply to a part of the forebrain results in an *infarct* of the area served by the occluded vessel.

Lesion in the Subthalamic Nucleus

Small vascular lesions occur in the subthalamic nucleus, resulting in rapid and unpredictable flailing movements of the contralateral extremities (*hemiballismus*). Movements are more obvious in the upper extremity than in the lower extremity. The clinical expression of this lesion is through corticospinal fibers; therefore, these deficits are located on the side of the body contralateral to the lesion.

Occlusion of Lenticulostriate Branches to Internal Capsule

Damage to the internal capsule may result in contralateral *hemiplegia* (corticospinal fibers) and *a loss, or diminution, of sensory perception* (pain, thermal sense, proprioception) caused by damage to thalamocortical fibers traversing the posterior limb to the overlying sensory cortex. If the lesion extends into the genu of the capsule (damaging corticonuclear fibers), *a partial paralysis of facial muscles and tongue movement may also occur contralaterally.*

Infarction of Posterior Thalamic Nuclei

Occlusion of vessels to posterior thalamic regions results in either a *complete sensory loss* (pain/thermal sense, touch, and vibratory and position sense) on the contralateral side of the body or a *dissociated sensory loss*. In the latter case, the patient may experience pain/thermal sensory losses but not position/vibratory losses, or vice versa. As the lesion resolves, the patient may experience intense persistent pain, *thalamic pain, or anesthesia dolorosa.*

Occlusion of Distal Branches of the Anterior or Middle Cerebral Arteries

Occlusion of distal branches of the anterior cerebral artery (ACA) results in motor and sensory losses in the contralateral foot, leg, and thigh owing to damage to the anterior and posterior paracentral gyri (primary motor and sensory cortices for the lower extremity). Occlusion of distal branches of the middle cerebral artery (MCA) results in contralateral motor and sensory losses of the upper extremity, trunk, and face with sparing of the leg and foot, and a consensual deviation of the eyes to the ipsilateral side. This represents damage to the precentral and postcentral gyri and the frontal eye fields.

Watershed Infarct

Sudden systemic hypotension, hypoperfusion, or embolic showers may result in infarcts at border zones between the territories served by the ACA, MCA, and posterior cerebral artery (PCA). *Anterior watershed infarcts* (at the ACA–MCA junction) result in a contralateral hemiparesis (mainly leg) and expressive language or behavioral changes. *Posterior watershed infarcts* (MCA–PCA interface) result in visual deficits and language problems.

Anterior Choroidal Artery Syndrome

Occlusion of this vessel may result from small emboli or small vessel disease. This syndrome may also occur as a complication of temporal lobectomy (removal of the temporal lobe to treat intractable epilepsy). The infarcted area usually includes the optic tract, lower portions of the basal nuclei, and lower aspects of the internal capsule. The patient experiences a contralateral *hemiplegia, hemianesthesia* (and possibly *hemihypesthesia*), and *homonymous hemianopsia* (*fibers of the optic tract*) and, *in some patients, damage to the thalamocortical fibers in the posterior limb*. These deficits are due to involvement of corticospinal fibers in the posterior limb of the internal capsule or possibly in the crus cerebri, involvement of thalamocortical fibers in the posterior limb of the internal capsule, and involvement of the fibers of the optic tract.

Parkinson Disease

Parkinson disease (paralysis agitans) results from a loss of the dopamine-containing cells in the substantia nigra. Although this part of the brain is located in the midbrain, the terminals of these nigrostriatal fibers are in the putamen and caudate nucleus. The classic signs and symptoms of this disease are a *stooped posture, resting tremor, rigidity, shuffling or festinating gait,* and difficulty initiating or maintaining movement (*akinesia, hypokinesia,* or *bradykinesia*). Initially, the tremor and walking difficulty may appear on one side of the body, but these signs usually spread to both sides with time. This is a neurodegenerative disease that has a dementia component in its later stages.

Transient Ischemic Attack

A transient ischemic attack, commonly called TIA, is a temporary (and frequently focal) neurological deficit that usually resolves within 10 to 30 minutes from the onset of symptoms. The cause is temporary occlusion of a vessel or inadequate perfusion of a restricted vascular territory. TIAs that last 60 minutes may result in some permanent deficits. This vascular event may take place anywhere in the central nervous system but is more common in the cerebral hemisphere.

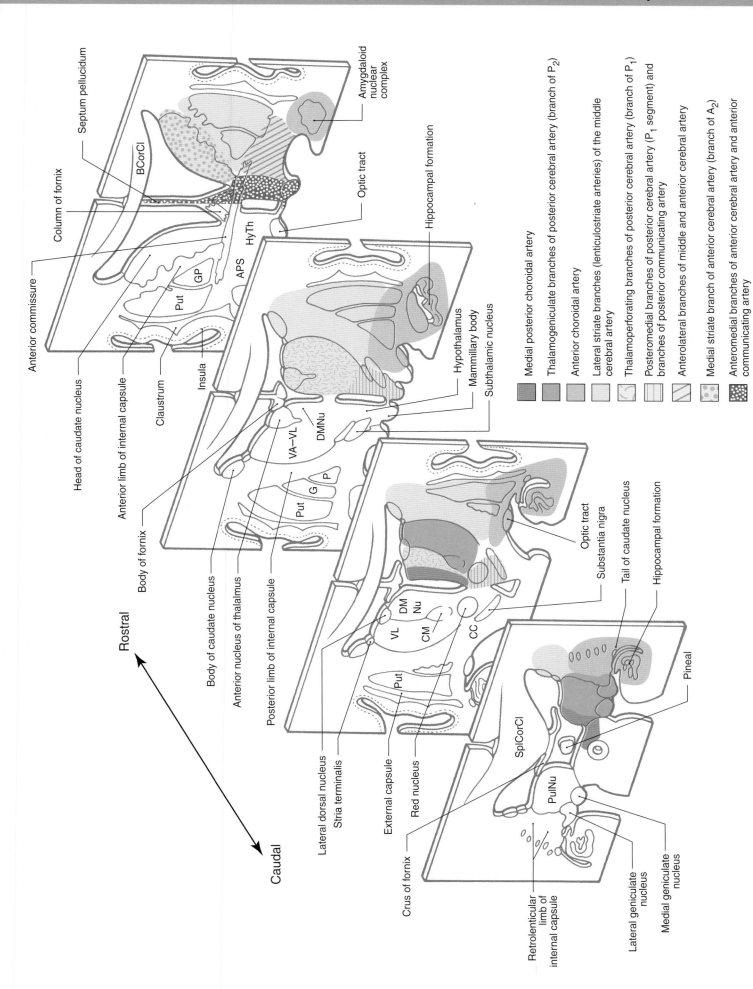

Rostral

Caudal

Septum pellucidum

Amygdaloid nuclear complex

BCorCl

Column of fornix

Optic tract

Anterior commissure

Hippocampal formation

HyTh

APS

Head of caudate nucleus

Put

GP

Anterior limb of internal capsule

Hypothalamus

Mammillary body

Subthalamic nucleus

Claustrum

Insula

DMNu

VA–VL

Put

G

P

Optic tract

Body of fornix

Substantia nigra

Tail of caudate nucleus

Hippocampal formation

Body of caudate nucleus

Anterior nucleus of thalamus

VL

DM Nu

CM

Posterior limb of internal capsule

Put

CC

Pineal

Lateral dorsal nucleus

Stria terminalis

External capsule

Red nucleus

SplCorCl

PulNu

Crus of fornix

Retrolenticular limb of internal capsule

Lateral geniculate nucleus

Medial geniculate nucleus

Medial posterior choroidal artery

Thalamogeniculate branches of posterior cerebral artery (branch of P_2)

Anterior choroidal artery

Lateral striate branches (lenticulostriate arteries) of the middle cerebral artery

Thalamoperforating branches of posterior cerebral artery (branch of P_1)

Posteromedial branches of posterior cerebral artery (P_1 segment) and branches of posterior communicating artery

Anterolateral branches of middle and anterior cerebral artery

Medial striate branch of anterior cerebral artery (branch of A_2)

Anteromedial branches of anterior cerebral artery and anterior communicating artery

6-38

NOTES

Internal Morphology of the Brain in Stained Sections: Axial–Sagittal Correlations with MRI

Although the general organization of Chapter 7 has been described in Chapter 1 (the reader may wish to refer back to this section), it is appropriate to reiterate its unique features at this point. Each set of facing pages has photographs of an axial stained section (left-hand page) and a sagittal stained section (right-hand page). In addition to individually labeled structures, a heavy line appears on each photograph. This prominent line on the axial section represents the approximate plane of the sagittal section located on the facing page. On the sagittal section, this line signifies the approximate plane of the corresponding axial section. The reader can identify features in each photograph and then, using this line as a reference point, visualize structures that are located either above or below that plane (axial-to-sagittal comparison) or medial or lateral to that plane (sagittal-to-axial comparison). This method of presentation provides a useful format that will form the basis for a three-dimensional understanding of structures and relationships within the central nervous system.

The magnetic resonance image (MRI) placed on every page in this chapter gives the reader an opportunity to compare internal brain anatomy, as seen in stained sections, with those structures as visualized in clinical images generated in the same plane. Even a general comparison reveals that many features, as seen in the stained section, can be readily identified in the adjacent MRI.

This chapter is also organized so that one can view structures in either the axial or the sagittal plane only. Axial photographs appear on left-hand pages and are sequenced from dorsal to ventral (odd-numbered Figures 7-1 through 7-9), whereas sagittal photographs are on the right-hand pages and progress from medial to lateral (even-numbered Figures 7-2 through 7-10). Consequently, the user can identify and follow structures through an axial series by simply flipping through the left-hand pages or through a sagittal series by flipping through the right-hand pages. The inherent flexibility in this chapter should prove useful in a wide variety of instructional/learning situations. The drawings shown in the following illustrate the axial and sagittal planes of the photographs in this chapter.

Axial Planes

Fig. 7-1
Fig. 7-3
Fig. 7-5
Fig. 7-7
Fig. 7-9

Fig. 7-6
Fig. 7-4   Fig. 7-8
Fig. 7-2   Fig. 7-10

Sagittal Planes

Corpus
callosum

Anterior horn of
lateral ventricle

Septum
pellucidum

Caudate
nucleus,
head

Putamen

Fornix,
column

Anterior
nucleus
of thalamus

Habenular
nucleus

Pulvinar nuclear
complex

Hippocampal
commissure

Atrium of
lateral ventricle

Hippocampal formation

Internal capsule, anterior limb

Internal capsule, genu

Internal capsule, posterior limb

Claustrum

Ventral anterior nucleus of thalamus

Ventral lateral nucleus of thalamus

Dorsomedial nucleus of thalamus

External medullary lamina and
thalamic reticular nucleus

Centromedian nucleus of thalamus

Ventral posterolateral nucleus

Stria terminalis

Caudate nucleus, tail

Choroid plexus

Hippocampus, fimbria

Optic radiations

7-1 Axial section through the *head of the caudate nucleus* and several key *thalamic nuclei (anterior, centromedian, pulvinar, and habenular)*. At this plane of section, the *internal medullary lamina* conveniently divides the dorsal thalamus into an anterior part (*anterior thalamic nucleus*), a posterior part (the large *pulvinar*), a medial area (*dorsomedial nucleus*), and a lateral area (containing the *ventral anterior, ventral lateral,* and *ventral posterolateral nuclei*). The *centromedian nucleus* is located within the internal medullary lamina and is the largest of the intralaminar nuclei. The heavy red line represents the approximate plane of the sagittal section shown in Figure 7-2 (facing page). Many of the structures labeled in this photograph can be clearly identified in the adjacent T1-weighted MRI.

Fornix, body
Lateral dorsal nucleus
Dorsomedial nucleus of thalamus
Corpus callosum, splenium
Anterior nucleus of thalamus
Corpus callosum, genu
Pretectal nuclei
Anterior commissure
Fornix, column
Mammillo-thalamic tract
Hypothalamus
Optic nerve
Mammillary body
Oculomotor nerve
Superior cerebellar peduncle, decussation
Basilar pons
Medial lemniscus
Pyramid
Principal olivary nucleus
Hypoglossal nucleus
Lateral corticospinal tract
RNu
Stria medullaris thalami
Habenular nuclei
Superior colliculus
Posterior commissure
Inferior colliculus
Trochlear nerve
Medial longitudinal fasciculus
Fastigial nucleus (medial cerebellar nucleus)
Abducens nucleus
Nucleus gracilis

7-2 Sagittal section through the *column of the fornix, anterior thalamic nucleus, red nucleus,* and medial portions of the *pons (abducens nucleus),* cerebellum *(fastigial nucleus),* and *medulla (nucleus gracilis).* As the fornix (body to column) arches around the anterior thalamic nucleus, the space formed between the column of the fornix and the anterior thalamic nucleus is the *interventricular foramen* (see Figure 7-1 on the facing page). The column of the fornix continues immediately caudal to the anterior commissure, as the post-commissural fornix, to end in the mammillary body. Note the relative positions of the red nucleus and decussation of the superior cerebellar peduncle within the midbrain. The heavy red line represents the approximate plane of the axial section shown in Figure 7-1 (facing page). Many of the structures labeled in this photograph can be clearly identified in the adjacent T1-weighted MRI (RNu = red nucleus).

Internal capsule, anterior limb

Globus pallidus, lateral segment

Claustrum

Anterior horn of lateral ventricle

Septum pellucidum

Caudate nucleus, head

Putamen   Insula

Fornix, column

Mammillothalamic tract

Dorsomedial nucleus of thalamus

Habenular commissure

Superior colliculus

Ventral anterior nucleus of thalamus

External capsule

Internal capsule, posterior limb

Ventral lateral nucleus of thalamus

Ventral posteromedial nucleus of thalamus

Ventral posterolateral nucleus of thalamus

Centromedian nucleus of thalamus

Stria terminalis

Caudate nucleus, tail

Optic radiations

Tapetum

Superior colliculus, brachium

Pulvinar nuclear complex

Hippocampal formation

Medial geniculate nucleus

7-3 Axial section through the *head of the caudate nucleus, centromedian nucleus, medial geniculate body,* and *superior colliculus.* In this more inferior plane of section, the lateral-to-medial relationship of the *ventral posterolateral* and *ventral posteromedial thalamic nuclei,* and the apposition of the latter to the centromedian, are clear. Also, the lateral three main thalamic nuclei (*ventral anterior, ventral lateral, ventral posterolateral*) appear as relatively clear cell groups. As seen here, and in Figure 7-1, all the major portions of the internal capsule are obvious in axial views. The heavy red line represents the approximate plane of the sagittal section shown in Figure 7-4 (facing page). Many of the structures labeled in this photograph can be clearly identified in the adjacent T2-weighted MRI.

Anterior nucleus of thalamus
Ventral lateral nucleus of thalamus
Mammillothalamic tract
Ventral anterior nucleus of thalamus
Corpus callosum, body
Lateral dorsal nucleus
Dorsomedial nucleus of thalamus
Fornix, body
Centromedian nucleus
Corpus callosum, splenium
Lateral ventricle, anterior horn
Anterior commissure
Thalamic fasciculus
Lenticular fasciculus
Olfactory tract
Ansa lenticularis
Optic tract
Hypothalamus
Crus cerebri
Substantia nigra
Medial lemniscus
Basilar pons
Facial nucleus
Principal olivary nucleus
Solitary nuclei and tract
Nucleus cuneatus
Pulvinar nuclear complex
Superior colliculus
Inferior colliculus
Superior cerebellar peduncle (brachium conjunctivum)
Fourth ventricle
Nucleus gracilis
H
RNu

7-4 Sagittal section through *anterior* and *ventral anterior thalamic nuclei, red nucleus*, and central areas of the *pons, cerebellum (and superior peduncle)*, and *medulla (solitary nuclei and tract)*. Note the position of the *facial motor nucleus* at the pons–medulla junction. In this sagittal plane, several of the thalamic nuclei are clearly demarcated, and the important relationships between the *red nucleus, substantia nigra*, and *crus* cerebri are seen. The teardrop shape of the anterior thalamic nucleus, which is clearly seen in this image, illustrates how the anterior nucleus may be seen in some coronal sections that also include the ventral lateral thalamic nucleus (see Figure 6-32**A,B**). Many clinically significant structures in the brainstem also stand out. The heavy red line represents the approximate plane of the axial section shown in Figure 7-3 (facing page). Many of the structures labeled in this photograph can be clearly identified in the adjacent T1-weighted MRI (H = Forel field H [prerubral area]; RNu = red nucleus).

Caudate nucleus, head

Putamen

Anterior commissure

Lamina terminalis

Fornix, column

Hypothalamus

Mammillothalamic tract

Ventral posteromedial nucleus of thalamus

Central gray (periaqueductal gray)

Superior colliculus

Medial geniculate nucleus

Hippocampal formation

Pulvinar nuclear complex

Atrium of lateral ventricle

Internal capsule, anterior limb

Globus pallidus, lateral segment

Globus pallidus, medial segment

Claustrum

Insula

Internal capsule, posterior limb

Ventral lateral nucleus of thalamus

Ventral posterolateral nucleus of thalamus

Centromedian nucleus of thalamus

Internal capsule, retrolenticular limb

Hippocampus, fimbria

Optic radiations

Choroid plexus

7-5 Axial section through the *head of the caudate nucleus, ventral posteromedial nucleus, medial geniculate body,* and ventral parts of the *pulvinar.* This axial section is through the upper portions of the *hypothalamus* and the lower, and widest, portions of the lenticular nucleus. The anterior limb of the internal capsule is beginning to disappear (the caudate head and putamen will join), and inferior portions of the *ventral lateral, ventral posterolateral,* and *pulvinar nuclei* are still present. The heavy red line represents the approximate plane of the sagittal section shown in Figure 7-6 (facing page). Many of the structures labeled in this photograph can be clearly identified in the adjacent T1-weighted MRI.

7-6 Sagittal section through central regions of the *diencephalon (centromedian nucleus)* and *midbrain (red nucleus)*, and through lateral areas of the *pons (trigeminal motor nucleus)* and *medulla (nucleus cuneatus)*. A clear separation of the thalamic nuclei is seen in this sagittal plane along with the characteristics of the interface of midbrain structures with the diencephalon. Note how the fibers of the *crus cerebri* splay out into the basilar pons (see also Figure 7-4), and also note the clarity of the *crus cerebri* and *substantia nigra* in the MRI. The heavy red line represents the approximate plane of the axial section shown in Figure 7-5 (facing page). Many of the structures labeled in this photograph can be clearly identified in the adjacent T1-weighted MRI (H = Forel field H [prerubral area]; RNu = red nucleus).

Caudate nucleus

Insula

Lamina terminalis

Hypothalamus

Fornix

Mammillothalamic tract

Red nucleus

Medial lemniscus

Inferior colliculus, brachium

Inferior colliculus

Anterior commissure

Optic tract

Crus cerebri

Lateral geniculate nucleus

Stria terminalis

Caudate nucleus, tail

Lateral ventricle, inferior (temporal) horn

Hippocampal formation

Optic radiation (geniculocalcarine fibers)

Medial geniculate nucleus

7-7 Axial section through the *hypothalamus, red nucleus, inferior colliculus,* and *lateral geniculate body*. This axial plane is through lower portions of the *hypothalamus* (the *fornix* and *mammillothalamic tract* are meeting just superior to the mammillary body), the *red nucleus*, and portions of the geniculate nuclei. Note that the caudate head and putamen have joined. The optic tract is always located on the surface of the crus cerebri (see also Figure 7-8 on the facing page) no matter what the plane of section. The heavy red line represents the approximate plane of the sagittal section shown in Figure 7-8 (facing page). The axial plane through the hemisphere, when continued into the midbrain, represents a slightly oblique section through the mesencephalon. Compare the appearance of the midbrain in this axial section with that in Figure 6-26 on pp. 144–145. The position of the lamina terminalis is indicated by the double-dashed lines. Many of the structures labeled in this photograph can be clearly identified in the adjacent T1-weighted MRI.

Globus pallidus, medial segment
Globus pallidus, lateral segment
Putamen
Anterior commissure
Thalamic fasciculus
Ventral lateral nucleus of thalamus
Zona incerta
Lenticular fasciculus
Ventral posterolateral nucleus of thalamus
Pulvinar nuclear complex
Brachium of superior colliculus
Caudate nucleus
Subthalamic nucleus
SN
Medial geniculate nucleus
Optic tract
Hippocampal formation
Crus cerebri
Dentate nucleus (lateral cerebellar nucleus)
Amygdaloid nucleus (complex)
Middle cerebellar peduncle (brachium pontis)
Posterior cochlear nucleus

7-8 Sagittal section through the *caudate nucleus*, central parts of the *diencephalon (ventral posteromedial nucleus)*, and lateral portions of the *pons* and *cerebellum (dentate nucleus)*. In this sagittal plane, several important relationships are seen. First, the head of the caudate and putamen coalesce in the rostral and ventral area of the hemisphere. Second, the important structures in the immediate vicinity of the *zona incerta* and *subthalamic nucleus* are obvious. Third, the *medial geniculate nucleus* is characteristically located just inferior to the *pulvinar* and separated from it by the *brachium of the superior colliculus*. The heavy red line represents the approximate plane of the axial section shown in Figure 7-7 (facing page). Compare the appearance of the midbrain in this axial section with those in Figure 6-23 and 6-24 on pp. 138 and 140. Many of the structures labeled in this photograph can be clearly identified in the adjacent T1-weighted MRI.

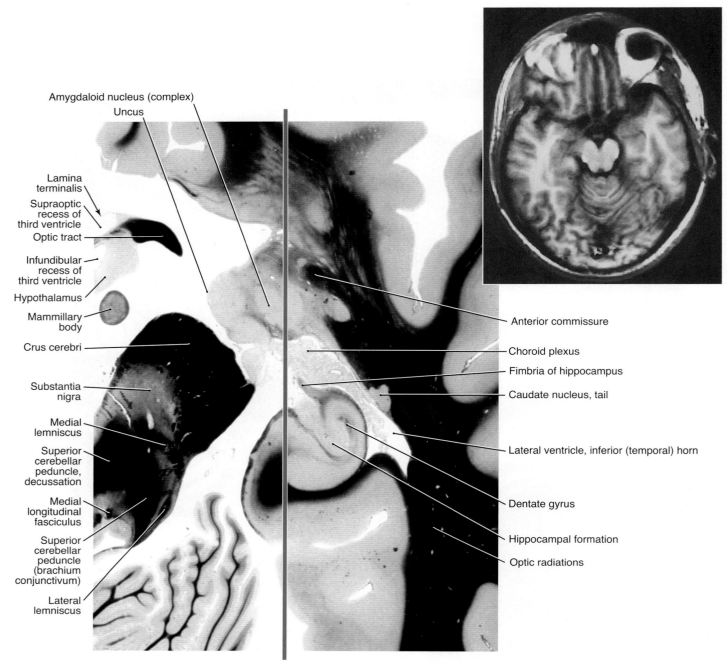

Amygdaloid nucleus (complex)

Uncus

Lamina terminalis

Supraoptic recess of third ventricle

Optic tract

Infundibular recess of third ventricle

Hypothalamus

Mammillary body

Crus cerebri

Substantia nigra

Medial lemniscus

Superior cerebellar peduncle, decussation

Medial longitudinal fasciculus

Superior cerebellar peduncle (brachium conjunctivum)

Lateral lemniscus

Anterior commissure

Choroid plexus

Fimbria of hippocampus

Caudate nucleus, tail

Lateral ventricle, inferior (temporal) horn

Dentate gyrus

Hippocampal formation

Optic radiations

7-9 Axial section through ventral portions of the *hypothalamus* (*supraoptic recess* and *mammillary body*) and forebrain (*amygdaloid nucleus*), and through the *superior cerebellar peduncle decussation* in the midbrain. This axial section is through the lowest portions of the *hypothalamus* as evidenced by the presence of the *supraoptic* and *infundibular recesses*, a very small amount of hypothalamic tissue, and a tip of the *mammillary body*. Note the relationship of the *uncus* to the *crus cerebri* (also in the MRI) and the fact that the amygdaloid nucleus is internal to the uncus and in the rostral wall of the temporal horn of the lateral ventricle. The *tail of the caudate* is in the lateral wall of the ventricle and the *hippocampus* is medially located. The heavy red line represents the approximate plane of the sagittal section shown in Figure 7-10 (facing page). The axial plane through the hemisphere, when continued into the midbrain, represents a slightly oblique section through the mesencephalon. Many of the structures labeled in this photograph can be clearly identified in the adjacent T1-weighted MRI.

Globus pallidus, medial segment
Globus pallidus, lateral segment
Anterior commissure

External medullary lamina
and thalamic reticular
nuclei

Optic
tract

Ventral lateral nucleus of thalamus and
ventral posterolateral nucleus of thalamus

Caudate nucleus,
body

Atrium of lateral ventricle
Pulvinar nuclear complex

Calcarine sulcus

Hippocampal
formation

Optic radiations

Lateral geniculate
nucleus

Fimbria of
hippocampus

Dentate gyrus

Dentate nucleus

Putamen

CP

Hippocampal
formation

Amygdaloid nucleus
(complex)

Lateral ventricle,
inferior (temporal) horn

7-10 Sagittal section through the *putamen, amygdaloid nucleus,* and *hippocampus* and through the most lateral portions of the *diencephalon (external medullary lamina and ventral posterolateral nucleus).* The relationship of the *amygdaloid nucleus,* anterior to the space of the temporal horn within the rostromedial portion of the temporal lobe, is clearly seen. In this sagittal section, the *optic tract* is seen entering the *lateral geniculate*

nucleus which, as was the case for its medial counterpart (see Figure 7-8), is also located immediately inferior to the *pulvinar.* This plane also passes through the long axis of the *hippocampal formation.* The heavy red line represents the approximate plane of the axial section shown in Figure 7-9 (facing page). Many of the structures labeled in this photograph can be clearly identified in the adjacent T1-weighted MRI.

NOTES

8

Synopsis of Functional Components, Tracts, Pathways, and Systems: Examples in Anatomical and Clinical Orientation

The study of *regional neurobiology* (brain structures in gross specimens, brain slices, stained sections, and MRI and CT) is the basis for the study of *systems neurobiology* (tracts, pathways, and cranial nerves and their functions), which in turn is the basis for understanding and diagnosing the neurologically impaired patient. Building on the concepts learned in earlier chapters, this chapter explores *systems neurobiology*, with a particular emphasis on clinical correlations.

The modifications made in this chapter recognize an essential reality for users of this book who are preparing for a career in medicine, as broadly defined. Although it is common to teach the anatomy of the brain in an *Anatomical Orientation* (e.g., in the medulla, the pyramid is "down" in the image and the fourth ventricle is "up"), this information should be *viewed and used*, in the clinical years and beyond, in a *Clinical Orientation* (pyramid "up" in the image, fourth ventricle "down"). Therefore, it is essential to present systems information in a format that resembles, as closely as reasonably possible, how these systems (and dysfunctions thereof) are viewed in the clinical setting. To this end selected systems are illustrated in the *Clinical Orientation*.

■ Anatomical Orientation ■

Major pathways, including those important to diagnosis of the neurologically compromised patient, are illustrated in line drawings in an *Anatomical Orientation*. The format of each set of these facing pages is designed to summarize, accurately and concisely, the relationships of a given tract or pathway. This includes, but is not limited to: 1) the location of the cells of origin for a given tract or pathway; 2) its entire course throughout the neuraxis and cerebrum; 3) the location of the decussation of these fibers, if applicable; 4) the neurotransmitters associated with the neurons comprising the tract or pathway; 5) a brief review of its blood supply; and 6) a summary of a number of deficits seen as a result of lesions at various points in the tract or pathway.

■ Clinical Orientation ■

Twelve of the systems pathways, with particular emphasis on those essential to understanding the patient with neurological problems, are illustrated in *Clinical Orientation*. These new pathway illustrations do not replace their counterparts shown in *Anatomical Orientation*, but are designed to complement these existing drawings. These sets of new facing pages are formatted to show the pathway superimposed on MRI at representative levels of the central nervous system (CNS) (left page) and summarize the deficits seen following lesions at various

CNS levels that involve the pathway (right page). The new illustrations show: 1) the position of the tract/fibers in MRI at representative levels; 2) the somatotopy (if applicable) of the tract as it appears in MRI/clinical orientation; 3) the trajectory of the tract/fibers through the CNS; 4) deficits correlated with the location of lesions at various locations and levels; and 5) the laterality (R/L) of the deficit as dictated by the position of the lesion in the MRI.

Intra-axial brainstem lesions *frequently result in both sensory and motor deficits*. Recognizing this fact, both types of deficits are listed for those lesions illustrated on the MRI pathways. However, for sensory pathways, sensory deficits are listed first and motor deficits are listed last. For motor pathways, the reverse is used: motor deficits are listed first, and sensory deficits listed last. This approach emphasizes the particular pathway being described but, at the same time, acknowledges the multiplicity of deficits resulting from CNS lesions.

■ Additional Points ■

The structure of an atlas does not allow a detailed definition of each clinical term on the printed page. However, as in other chapters, the full definition of each clinical term or phrase, when used, is available from the online resources that come with this atlas; these are taken from the current edition of *Stedman's Medical Dictionary*. In this respect, the full definitions are actually available in this book. Researching the full definition of a clinical term or phrase is a powerful and effective learning tool. Also, each clinical term or phrase is available in any standard medical dictionary or comprehensive neurology text.

The layout of the illustrations in this chapter clearly shows the laterality of the tract or pathway. That is, the relationship between the location of the cell of origin and the termination of the fibers making up a tract or pathway or the projections of cranial nerve nuclei. Although this is clear in the anatomical drawings, it is particularly relevant to the clinical setting, as shown in the MRI pathway illustrations. *This information is absolutely essential to understand the position of a lesion and correlate this fact with the deficits seen in the neurologically compromised patient*. For example, is the deficit on the same side as the lesion (ipsilateral), the opposite side (contralateral), or both sides (bilateral)? The concept of laterality is expressed as "right," "left," or "bilateral" in reference to the side of the deficit(s) when written on the patient's chart.

This chapter is designed to maximize the correlation between structure and function, provide a range of clinical examples for each tract or pathway, and help the user develop a knowledge base that can be easily integrated into the clinical setting.

■ Functional Components in the Neural Tube, Spinal Cord, and Brainstem (Figures 8-1 and 8-2) ■

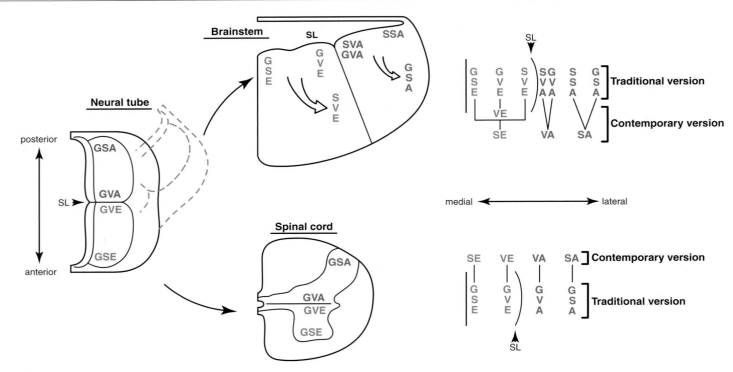

8-1 The concept of *functional components* (of both spinal and cranial nerves) recognizes that primary afferent fibers entering, and the efferent fibers leaving, the spinal cord or brainstem convey specific types of information. There are two versions of *functional components*: 1) a traditional version that originated early in the 20th century and was the standard for many decades; and 2) a contemporary version that reflects recent discoveries in head and neck development. Both of these plans are complementary, one to the other.

Traditional version: In this version (Figures 8-1, 8-2), the components seen in the developing neural tube (left), that are associated with the alar plate (GSA, GVA), are located posterior (dorsal) to the sulcus limitans (SL); those associated with the basal plate (GVE, GSE) are located anterior (ventral) to the SL (Figure 8-1, left). These are general features also seen in the contemporary version. In the adult spinal cord, this general posterior/anterior relationship is maintained (Figure 8-1, lower center).

At the spinal cord–brainstem transition, two important changes occur. First, as the central canal enlarges into the fourth ventricle, and the cerebellum develops, the alar (sensory) portion of the neural tube is rotated laterally. The SL is present in the adult brainstem and separates the medially located basal plate derivatives (motor nuclei) from the laterally located alar plate derivatives (sensory nuclei). Second, in the brainstem, special functional components, as traditionally identified (SVE to muscles of the pharyngeal arches; SVA to taste; SSA to vestibular and auditory), form cell columns that are restricted to the brainstem and not represented in the spinal cord.

Within the brainstem, there are transpositions of the SVE and GSA components. Early in development, cells associated with the SVE component (nucleus ambiguus, facial and trigeminal motor nuclei) appear in the floor of the ventricle, but then migrate ventrolaterally to their

adult locations. In like manner, cells with the GSA component (spinal trigeminal, principal sensory) that appear in the ventricular floor in the alar area also migrate ventrolaterally to their adult locations. Cells of the mesencephalic nucleus arise from the neural crest and migrate into the brainstem to become part of the GSA cell column. The border between motor and sensory areas of the brainstem is represented by an oblique line beginning at the SL. The relative positions, and color coding, of the various components shown in the above image (right) is directly translatable to Figure 8-2 on the facing page.

Contemporary version: This version (Figure 8-1 right), as was the traditional version, is based on development, but incorporates more detailed data concerning neuron and muscle origin and their respective migration patterns. For example, striated muscles innervated by cranial nerves (CNs) III, IV, V, VI, VII, IX, X, and XII all arise from the epimere (paraxial mesoderm) which segments into somitomeres. Consequently, the cells of all of these motor nuclei are designated as an SE (Somatic Efferent) functional component. The neurons of CN III that influence orbital smooth muscles, the cells of CNs VII and IX which influence vascular smooth muscle and glandular epithelium in the head, and cells of CN X that influence the same tissues in the thorax and abdomen, are all designated as VE (Visceral Efferent). All visceral afferent information (traditionally divided into *General* and *Special*) is associated with the solitary tract and nuclei and is designated VA (Visceral Afferent). The components traditionally associated with the vestibulocochlear nuclei (SSA) and with the trigeminal sensory nuclei (GSA) are consolidated into an SA (Somatic Afferent) category. The correlation between the traditional and contemporary versions is shown in Figure 8-1, far right.

ABBREVIATIONS

GSA	General Somatic Afferent	SVE	Special Visceral Efferent
GSE	General Somatic Efferent	SL	Sulcus Limitans
GVA	General Visceral Afferent	SA	Somatic Afferent
GVE	General Visceral Efferent	SE	Somatic Efferent
SSA	Special Somatic Afferent	VA	Visceral Afferent
SVA	Special Visceral Afferent	VE	Visceral Efferent

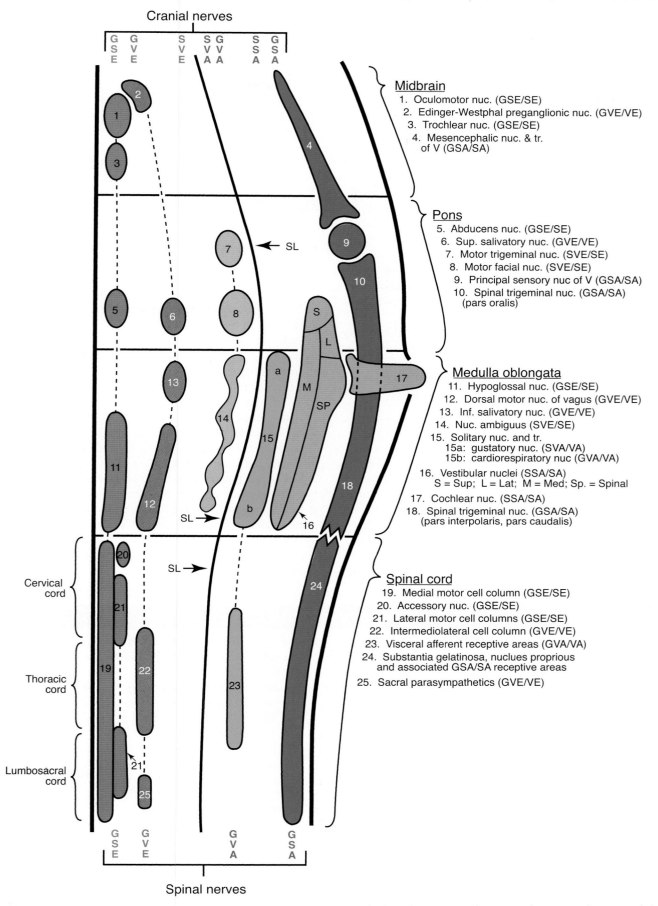

Cranial nerves

1. Oculomotor nuc. (GSE/SE)
2. Edinger-Westphal preganglionic nuc. (GVE/VE)
3. Trochlear nuc. (GSE/SE)
4. Mesencephalic nuc. & tr. of V (GSA/SA)

Midbrain

1. Oculomotor nuc. (GSE/SE)
2. Edinger-Westphal preganglionic nuc. (GVE/VE)
3. Trochlear nuc. (GSE/SE)
4. Mesencephalic nuc. & tr. of V (GSA/SA)

Pons

5. Abducens nuc. (GSE/SE)
6. Sup. salivatory nuc. (GVE/VE)
7. Motor trigeminal nuc. (SVE/SE)
8. Motor facial nuc. (SVE/SE)
9. Principal sensory nuc of V (GSA/SA)
10. Spinal trigeminal nuc. (GSA/SA) (pars oralis)

Medulla oblongata

11. Hypoglossal nuc. (GSE/SE)
12. Dorsal motor nuc. of vagus (GVE/VE)
13. Inf. salivatory nuc. (GVE/VE)
14. Nuc. ambiguus (SVE/SE)
15. Solitary nuc. and tr.
    15a: gustatory nuc. (SVA/VA)
    15b: cardiorespiratory nuc (GVA/VA)
16. Vestibular nuclei (SSA/SA)
    S = Sup; L = Lat; M = Med; Sp. = Spinal
17. Cochlear nuc. (SSA/SA)
18. Spinal trigeminal nuc. (GSA/SA) (pars interpolaris, pars caudalis)

Spinal cord

19. Medial motor cell column (GSE/SE)
20. Accessory nuc. (GSE/SE)
21. Lateral motor cell columns (GSE/SE)
22. Intermediolateral cell column (GVE/VE)
23. Visceral afferent receptive areas (GVA/VA)
24. Substantia gelatinosa, nucleus proprious and associated GSA/SA receptive areas
25. Sacral parasympathetics (GVE/VE)

Spinal nerves

8-2 The medial-to-lateral positions of brainstem cranial nerve and spinal cord nuclei as shown here are the same as in Figure 8-1. This diagrammatic posterior (dorsal) view shows: 1) the relative positions and names of specific cell groups and their associated functional components; 2) the approximate location of particular nuclei in their specific division of brainstem and/or spinal cord; and 3) the rostrocaudal continuity of cell columns (either as contin-uous or discontinuous cell groups) from one division of the brainstem to the next or from brainstem to spinal cord. The nucleus ambiguus is a column of cells composed of distinct cell clusters interspersed with more diffusely arranged cells, much like a string of beads. Nuclei associated with CNs I and II are not shown. The color coding used on this figure correlates with that on Figure 8-1 (facing page).

■ Orientation Drawing for Pathways in Anatomical Orientation ■

8-3 Orientation drawing for pathways. The trajectories of pathways in the *Anatomical Orientation* are illustrated in Chapter 8 on individualized versions of this representation of the central nervous system (CNS). Although slight changes are made in each drawing, so as to more clearly diagram a specific pathway, the basic configuration of the CNS is as represented here. This allows the user to move from pathway to pathway without being required to learn a different representation or drawing for each pathway; also, laterality of the pathway, a feature essential to diagnosis (see Introduction), is inherently evident in each illustration. In addition, many pathways, particularly those that are clinically important, are also shown on MRI and are, therefore, shown in a *Clinical Orientation*.

The forebrain (telencephalon and diencephalon) is shown in the coronal plane, and the midbrain, pons, medulla, and spinal cord are represented through their longitudinal axes. The internal capsule is represented in the axial plane in an effort to show the rostrocaudal distribution of fibers located therein.

The reader should become familiar with the structures and regions as shown here because their locations and relationships are easily transferable to subsequent illustrations. Also, it may be helpful to refer back to this illustration when using subsequent sections of this chapter.

Neurotransmitters

Three important facts are self-evident in the descriptions of neurotransmitters that accompany each pathway drawing. These are illustrated by noting, as an example, that glutamate is found in corticospinal fibers (see Figure 8-13). First, the *location of neuronal cell bodies* containing a specific transmitter is indicated (glutamate-containing cell bodies are found in cortical areas that project to the spinal cord). Second, the *trajectory of fibers* containing a particular neurotransmitter is obvious from the route taken by the tract (glutaminergic corticospinal fibers are found in the internal capsule, crus

cerebri, basilar pons, pyramid, and lateral corticospinal tract). Third, the *location of terminals* containing specific neurotransmitters is indicated by the site(s) of termination of each tract (glutaminergic terminals of corticospinal fibers are located in the spinal cord gray matter). In addition, the action of most neuroactive substances is indicated as excitatory (+) or inhibitory (−). This level of neurotransmitter information, as explained here for glutaminergic corticospinal fibers, is repeated for each pathway drawing.

Clinical Correlations

The clinical correlations are designed to give the user an overview of specific deficits (i.e., *hemiplegia, athetosis*) seen in lesions of each pathway and to provide examples of some syndromes or diseases (e.g., *Brown-Séquard syndrome, Wilson disease*) in which these deficits are seen. Although purposefully brief, these correlations highlight examples of deficits for each pathway and provide a built-in mechanism for expanded study. For example, the words in *italics* in each correlation are clinical terms and phrases that are defined in *Stedman's*, any standard medical dictionary, and in clinical neuroscience textbooks. An especially useful feature of this Atlas is the fact that the full definition of all clinical terms that are indicated in *italics* (*PICA syndrome, hemiplegia, resting tremor*, etc.) is easily available when using the online resources through thePoint; instructions to access thePoint are in the inside of the front cover. Consulting these sources, especially the online resources, will significantly enhance understanding of the deficits seen in the neurologically compromised patient. Expanded information, based on the deficits mentioned in this chapter, is integrated into some of the questions for Chapter 8. Referring to such sources allows the user to glean important clinical points that correlate with the pathway under consideration, and enlarge his or her knowledge and understanding by researching the italicized words and phrases.

ABBREVIATIONS

CE	Cervical enlargement of spinal cord		**IntCap,PL**	Internal capsule, posterior limb
Cer	Cervical levels of spinal cord		**LatSul**	Lateral sulcus (Sylvian sulcus)
CinSul	Cingulate sulcus		**LatVen**	Lateral ventricle
CaNu	Caudate nucleus (+ Put = neostriatum)		**LSE**	Lumbosacral enlargement of spinal cord
CM	Centromedian (and intralaminar) nuclei		**LumSac**	Lumbosacral level of spinal cord
CorCl	Corpus callosum		**L-VTh**	Lateral and ventral thalamic nuclei excluding VPM and VPL
Dien	Diencephalon		**Mes**	Mesencephalon
DMNu	Dorsomedial nucleus of thalamus		**Met**	Metencephalon
For	Fornix		**Myelen**	Myelencephalon
GP	Globus pallidus (paleostriatum)		**Put**	Putamen (+ CaNu = neostriatum)
GPl	Globus pallidus, lateral segment		**SThNu**	Subthalamic nucleus
GPm	Globus pallidus, medial segment		**Telen**	Telencephalon
HyTh	Hypothalamic area		**Thor**	Thoracic levels of spinal cord
IC	Internal capsule		**VPL**	Ventral posterolateral nucleus of thalamus
IntCap,AL	Internal capsule, anterior limb		**VPM**	Ventral posteromedial nucleus of thalamus
IntCap,G	Internal capsule, genu			

■ 8-3 Orientation Drawing for Pathways in Anatomical Orientation ■

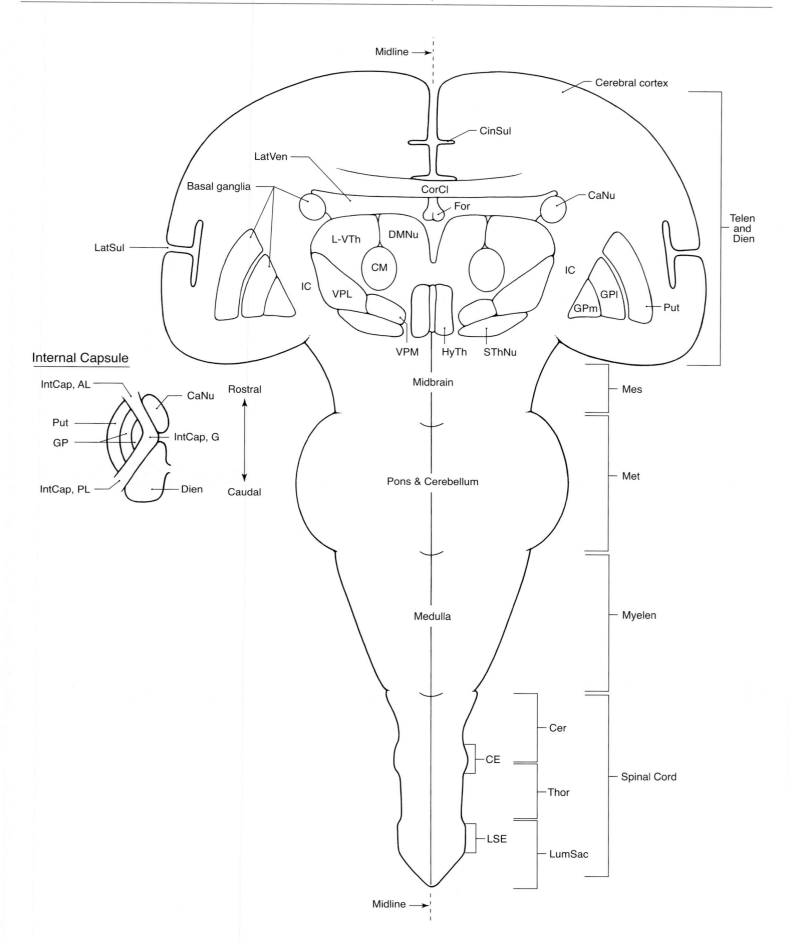

■ Posterior (Dorsal) Column–Medial Lemniscus System in Anatomical Orientation ■

8-4 The origin, course, and distribution of fibers comprising the posterior (dorsal) column–medial lemniscus (PC–ML) system. This illustration shows the longitudinal extent, positions in representative cross sections of brainstem and spinal cord, and somatotopy of fibers in both the posterior column (PC) and medial lemniscus (ML) portions of this system. The ML undergoes positional changes as it courses from the myelencephalon (medulla) rostrally toward the mesencephalic–diencephalic junction. In the medulla, ML and anterolateral system (ALS) fibers are widely separated and receive different blood supplies, whereas they are served by a common arterial source in the midbrain. As the ML makes positional changes, the somatotopy therein follows accordingly. Fibers of the postsynaptic posterior column system (shown in green) are considered in detail in Figure 8-8 on p. 197.

Neurotransmitters

Acetylcholine and the excitatory amino acids, glutamate and aspartate, are associated with some of the large-diameter, heavily myelinated fibers of the posterior horn and posterior columns.

Clinical Correlations

Damage to posterior column fibers on one side of the spinal cord (e.g., the *Brown-Séquard syndrome*) results in an ipsilateral loss of vibratory sensation, position sense, and discriminative touch (*astereognosis, stereoagnosis*) below the level of the lesion. The term *stereoanesthesia* is frequently used to specify a lesion of peripheral nerves that results in an inability to perceive proprioceptive and tactile sensations. The term *tactile agnosia* is sometimes considered to be synonymous with these preceding three terms. However, *tactile agnosia* is also used to describe deficits seen in lesions of the parietal cortex. Bilateral damage (e.g., *tabes dorsalis* or *subacute combined degeneration of the spinal cord*) produces bilateral losses. Although *ataxia* is the most common feature in patients with tabes dorsalis, they also have a loss of *muscle stretch reflexes*, severe *lancinating pain* over the body below the head (more common in the lower extremity), and bladder dysfunction. The *ataxia* that may be seen in patients with posterior column lesions (*sensory ataxia*) is due to a lack of proprioceptive input and position sense. These individuals tend to forcibly place their feet to the floor in an attempt to stimulate the missing sensory input. A patient with mild ataxia due to posterior column disease may compensate for the motor deficit by using visual cues. Patients with *subacute combined degeneration of the spinal cord* first have signs and symptoms of posterior column involvement, followed later by signs of corticospinal tract damage (*spastic weakness of legs, increased muscle stretch reflexes [hyperreflexia], Babinski sign*).

Rostral to the sensory decussation, medial lemniscus lesions result in contralateral losses that include the entire body, excluding the head. Brainstem lesions involving medial lemniscus fibers usually include adjacent structures, result in motor and additional sensory losses, and may reflect the distribution patterns of vessels (e.g., *medial medullary* or *medial pontine syndromes*). Large lesions in the forebrain may result in a complete contralateral loss of modalities carried in the posterior columns and anterolateral systems, or may produce *pain* (e.g., the *thalamic syndrome*).

ABBREVIATIONS

ALS	Anterolateral system	NuGr	Gracile nucleus
BP	Basilar pons	PC	Posterior column
CC	Crus cerebri	PO	Principal olivary nucleus
CTT	Central tegmental tract	PoCGy	Postcentral gyrus
FCu	Cuneate fasciculus	PPGy	Posterior paracentral gyrus
FGr	Gracile fasciculus	PRG	Posterior (dorsal) root ganglia
IAF	Internal arcuate fibers	Py	Pyramid
IC	Internal capsule	RB	Restiform body
ML	Medial lemniscus	RNu	Red nucleus
MLF	Medial longitudinal fasciculus	SN	Substantia nigra
NuCu	Cuneate nucleus	VPL	Ventral posterolateral nucleus of thalamus

SOMATOPY OF BODY AREAS

A	Fibers conveying input from upper extremity (UE)	C2	Fibers from approximately the second cervical level
L	Fibers conveying input from lower extremity (LE)	S5	Fibers from approximately the fifth sacral level
N	Fibers conveying input from neck	T5	Fibers from approximately the fifth thoracic level
T	Fibers conveying input from trunk		

Review of Blood Supply to PC–ML System

STRUCTURES	ARTERIES
PC in Spinal Cord	Penetrating branches of arterial vasocorona (see Figure 6-6)
ML in Medulla	Anterior spinal (see Figure 6-14)
ML in Pons	Overlap of paramedian and long circumferential branches of basilar (see Figure 6-21)
ML in Midbrain	Short circumferential branches of posterior cerebral, quadrigeminal, choroidal arteries (see Figure 6-27)
VPL	Thalamogeniculate branches of posterior cerebral (see Figure 6-38)
Posterior Limb of IC	Lateral striate branches of middle cerebral (see Figure 6-38)

■ 8-4 Posterior (Dorsal) Column–Medial Lemniscus System in Anatomical Orientation ■

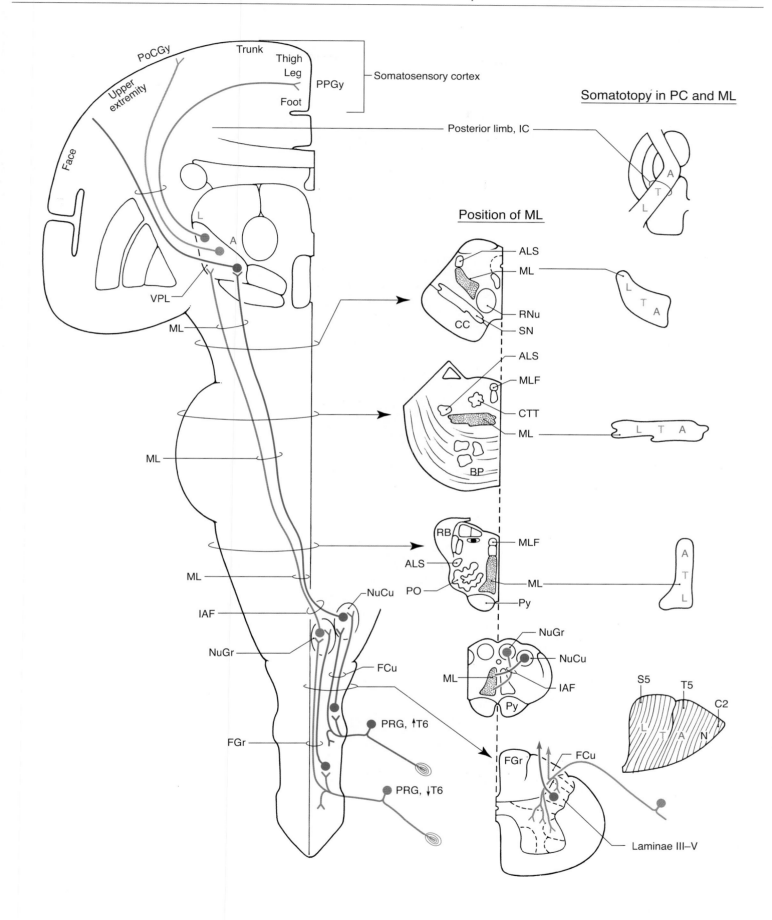

Somatotopy in PC and ML

Position of ML

■ Posterior Column–Medial Lemniscus System in Clinical Orientation ■

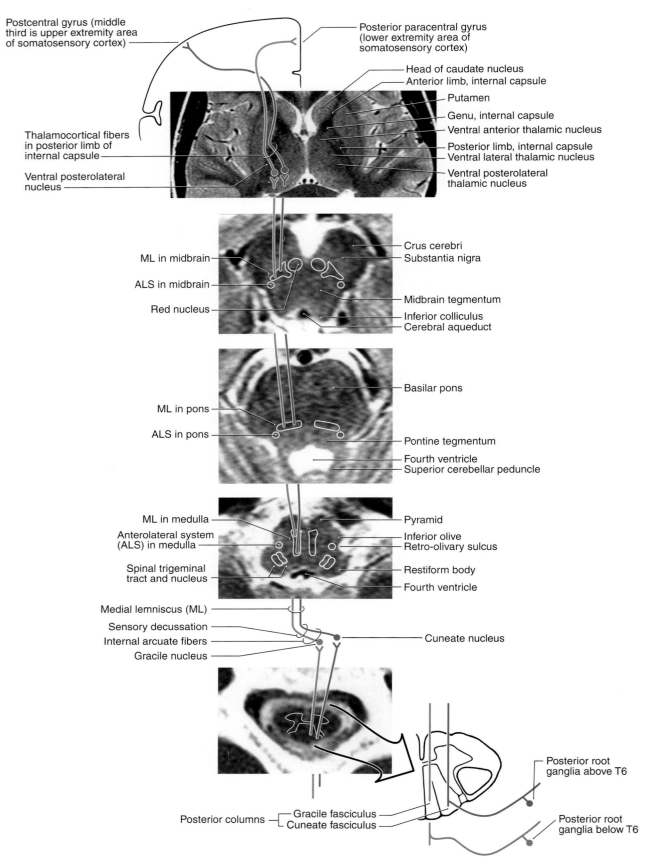

8-5A The posterior column–medial lemniscus (PC–ML) system superimposed on CT (spinal cord, myelogram) and MRI (brainstem and forebrain, T2-weighted MRI) showing the location, topography, and trajectory of this pathway in a clinical orientation. The red and blue fibers correlate with those of the same color in Figure 8-4.

■ Posterior Column–Medial Lemniscus System in Clinical Orientation: Representative Lesions and Deficits ■

Postcentral gyrus (middle third is upper extremity area of somatosensory cortex)

Posterior paracentral gyrus (lower extremity area of somatosensory cortex)

Thalamocortical fibers in posterior limb of internal capsule

Ventral posterolateral nucleus

- Diminution/loss proprioception, discriminative touch, vibratory sense, pain, and thermal sense on right UE and LE plus face and oral cavity if VPM involved
- Paresthesias
- Transient right hemiplegia

ML in midbrain

ALS in midbrain

Red nucleus

- Loss of proprioception, discriminative touch, and vibratory sense on right LE (plus UE if medial part of ML involved)
- Loss of pain and thermal sensation on right UE and LE

Mid-to-rostral pons
- Loss of proprioception; discriminative touch; and vibratory, pain, and thermal senses on right UE and LE
- Loss of discriminative touch, pain, and thermal sense on left side of face; paralysis of masticatory muscles (trigeminal nuclei involved)

Caudal pons
- Proprioception and pain/thermal loss as in mid-to-rostral pons
- Left-sided facial and lateral rectus paralysis (facial/abducens nucleus/nerve)
- Loss pain/thermal sense on left face
- Left ptosis, miosis, and anhidrosis (Horner)

ML in pons

ALS in pons

ML in medulla

Anterolateral system (ALS) in medulla

Spinal trigeminal tract and nucleus

- Loss of proprioception, discriminative touch, and vibratory sense of right UE/LE
- Tongue weakness: Deviates to left on attempted protrusion
- Hemiplegia of right UE and LE

Medial lemniscus (ML)

Sensory decussation

Internal arcuate fibers

Gracile nucleus

Cuneate nucleus

Spinal cord hemisection
- Right-sided loss of proprioception, discriminative touch, and vibratory sense below lesion
- Left-sided loss of pain/thermal sensation beginning about two levels below lesion
- Right-sided paralysis below lesion
- Right Horner, if lesion at cervical levels

Posterior column lesion
- Right-sided loss of proprioception, discriminative touch, and vibratory sense below lesion

Posterior root ganglia above T6

Posterior columns — Gracile fasciculus / Cuneate fasciculus

Posterior root ganglia below T6

8-5B Representative lesions within the CNS that involve the PC–ML system and the deficits that correlate with the level and laterality of each lesion. Note that the laterality (R/L) of the deficits is determined by whether the lesion is on the left or right side of the MRI/CT; this reinforces important clinical concepts.

■ Anterolateral System in Anatomical Orientation ■

8-6 The longitudinal extent and somatotopy of fibers comprising the anterolateral system (ALS). The ALS is a composite bundle containing ascending fibers that terminate in the reticular formation (spinoreticular fibers), mesencephalon (spinotectal fibers to deep layers of the superior colliculus, spinoperiaqueductal fibers to the periaqueductal gray), hypothalamus (spinohypothalamic fibers), and sensory relay nuclei of the dorsal thalamus (spinothalamic fibers). Other fibers in the ALS include spinoolivary projections to the accessory olivary nuclei. Spinothalamic fibers terminate primarily in the VPL and reticulothalamic fibers terminate in some intralaminar nuclei and medial areas of the posterior thalamic complex.

Descending fibers from the PAG and nucleus raphe dorsalis enter the nucleus raphe magnus and adjacent reticular area. These latter sites, in turn, project to laminae I, II, and V of the spinal cord via raphespinal and reticulospinal fibers that participate in the modulation of pain transmission in the spinal cord.

Neurotransmitters

Glutamate (+), calcitonin gene-related peptide, and substance P (+) containing posterior (dorsal) root ganglion cells project into laminae I, II (heavy), V (moderate), and III, IV (sparse). Some spinoreticular and spinothalamic fibers contain enkephalin (−), somatostatin (−), and cholecystokinin (+). In addition to enkephalin and somatostatin, some spinomesencephalic fibers contain vasoactive intestinal polypeptide (+). Neurons in the PAG and nucleus raphe dorsalis containing serotonin and neurotensin project into the nuclei raphe magnus and adjacent reticular formation. Cells in these latter centers that contain serotonin and enkephalin send processes to spinal cord laminae I, II, and V. Serotonergic raphespinal or enkephalinergic reticulospinal fibers may inhibit primary sensory fibers or projection neurons, conveying nociceptive (pain) information.

Clinical Correlations

Spinal lesions involving the anterolateral system (e.g., the *Brown-Séquard syndrome*) result in a loss of pain and temperature sensations on the contralateral side of the body beginning usually two levels caudal to the lesion. *Syringomyelia* produces bilateral sensory losses restricted to adjacent dermatomes because of damage to the anterior (ventral) white commissure. Vascular lesions in the spinal cord (e.g., *acute central cervical cord syndrome*) may result in a bilateral and splotchy loss of pain and thermal sense below the lesion because the ALS has a dual vascular supply.

Vascular lesions in the lateral medulla *(posterior inferior cerebellar artery syndrome)* or lateral pons *(anterior inferior cerebellar artery occlusion)* result in a loss of pain and thermal sensations over the entire contralateral side of the body (ALS) as well as on the ipsilateral face (spinal trigeminal tract and nucleus), coupled with other motor and/or sensory deficits based on damage to structures these vessels serve. Note that the ALS and PC–ML systems are separated in the medulla (in different vascular territories) but are adjacent to each other in the midbrain (basically in the same vascular territory). Consequently, medullary lesions will not result in deficits related to both pathways, whereas a lesion in the midbrain may result in a contralateral loss of pain, thermal, vibratory, and discriminative touch sensations on the body, excluding the head.

Profound loss of posterior column and anterolateral system modalities, or *intractable pain* and/or *paresthesias* (e.g., the *thalamic syndrome*), may result from vascular lesions in the posterolateral thalamus. So-called thalamic pain also may be experienced by patients who have brainstem lesions.

ABBREVIATIONS

A	Input from upper extremity (UE) regions		**PRG**	Posterior (dorsal) root ganglion
ALS	Anterolateral system		**Py**	Pyramid
AWCom	Anterior (ventral) white commissure		**RaSp**	Raphespinal fibers
CC	Crus cerebri		**RB**	Restiform body
IC	Internal capsule		**RetF**	Reticular formation (of midbrain)
L	Input from lower extremity (LE) regions		**RetTh**	Reticulothalamic fibers
MCP	Middle cerebellar peduncle		**RNu**	Red nucleus
ML	Medial lemniscus		**S**	Input from sacral regions
MLF	Medial longitudinal fasciculus		**SC**	Superior colliculus
Nu	Nuclei		**SpRet**	Spinoreticular fibers
NuDark	Nucleus of Darkschewitsch		**SpTec**	Spinotectal fibers
NuRa,d	Nucleus raphe, dorsalis		**SpTh**	Spinothalamic fibers (rostral midbrain and above)
NuRa,m	Nucleus raphe, magnus		**T**	Input from thoracic regions
PAG	Periaqueductal gray		**VPL**	Ventral posterolateral nucleus of thalamus
PoCGy	Postcentral gyrus		**I–VIII**	Laminae I–VIII of Rexed
PPGy	Posterior paracentral gyrus			

Review of Blood Supply to ALS

STRUCTURES	ARTERIES
ALS in Spinal Cord	Penetrating branches of arterial vasocorona and branches of anterior spinal (see Figures 6-6 and 6-14)
ALS in Medulla	Caudal third, vertebral; rostral two-thirds, posterior inferior cerebellar (see Figure 6-14)
ALS in Pons	Long circumferential branches of basilar (see Figure 6-21)
ALS in Midbrain	Short circumferential branches of posterior cerebral, superior cerebellar (see Figure 6-27)
VPL	Thalamogeniculate branches of posterior cerebral (see Figure 6-38)
Posterior Limb of **IC**	Lateral striate branches of middle cerebral (see Figure 6-38)

■ 8-6 Anterolateral System in Anatomical Orientation ■

Somatosensory cortex

Somatotopy of ALS fibers

Position of ALS fibers

■ Anterolateral System in Clinical Orientation ■

Postcentral gyrus (middle third is upper extremity area of somatosensory cortex)

Posterior paracentral gyrus (lower extremity area of somatosensory cortex)

Anterior limb, internal capsule

Genu, internal capsule

Ventral anterior thalamic nucleus

Ventral lateral thalamic nucleus

Thalamocortical fibers in posterior limb of internal capsule

Posterior limb, internal capsule

Ventral posterolateral nucleus

Ventral posterolateral thalamic nucleus

Crus cerebri

ALS in midbrain

Substantia nigra

ML in midbrain
Red nucleus

Midbrain tegmentum

Cerebral aqueduct

Basilar pons

ALS in pons

ML in pons

Pontine tegmentum

Superior cerebellar peduncle

Fourth ventricle

Pyramid

Inferior olive

ALS in medulla

Spinal trigeminal tract and nucleus

ML in medulla

Restiform body

Anterolateral system (ALS)

Input from upper extremity

Anterior white commissure (AWC)

ALS in spinal cord

Posterior root ganglia

Posterior horn

Input from lower extremity

AWC

8-7A The anterolateral system (ALS) superimposed on CT (spinal cord, myelogram) and MRI (brainstem and forebrain, T2-weighted MRI) showing the location, topography, and trajectory of this pathway in a clinical orientation. The blue and green fibers correlate with those of the same color in Figure 8-6.

■ Anterolateral System in Clinical Orientation: Representative Lesions and Deficits ■

Postcentral gyrus (middle third is upper extremity area of somatosensory cortex)

Posterior paracentral gyrus (lower extremity area of somatosensory cortex)

Thalamocortical fibers in posterior limb of internal capsule

Ventral posterolateral nucleus

- Diminution/loss pain, thermal, and vibratory senses; discriminative touch; and proprioception on right face and oral cavity (if VPM included), and on right UE and LE
- Paresthesias on right face, trunk, UE/LE
- Transient right hemiplegia

- Loss of pain and thermal sensation on right UE and LE
- Loss of proprioception, discriminative touch, and vibratory sense on right LE (plus UE if medial part of ML involved)

ALS in midbrain

ML in midbrain
Red nucleus

Mid-to-rostral pons
- Loss of pain, thermal, and vibratory sense; discriminative touch; and proprioception on right UE/LE
- Loss of pain/thermal sense and discriminative touch on left side of face; paralysis of masticatory muscles (trigeminal nuclei involved)

Caudal pons
- Pain/thermal sense and proprioception loss as in mid-to-rostral pons
- Left-sided facial and lateral rectus paralysis (facial/abducens nucleus/nerve)
- Left-sided loss pain/thermal sense of face
- Left ptosis/miosis/anhidrosis (Horner)

ALS in pons

ML in pons

- Loss of pain/thermal sense on right UE, LE, and on left side of face (alternating hemianesthesia)
- Dysarthria and dysphagia (nu. ambiguus)
- Vertigo, ataxia, and nystagmus (vestibular nucleus; restiform body)
- Nausea, vomiting, and singultus (area postrema, reticular formation)
- Left ptosis/miosis/anhidrosis (Horner)

ALS in medulla

Spinal trigeminal tract and nucleus

ML in medulla

Anterolateral quadrant lesion
- Loss of pain/thermal sensation begining about two levels below lesion on right side of body

Anterolateral system (ALS)

Spinal cord hemisection
- Right-sided loss of pain/thermal sensation beginning about two levels below lesion
- Left-sided loss of proprioception, discriminative touch, and vibratory sense below lesion
- Left-sided paralysis below lesion
- Left Horner if lesion at cervical levels

Input from upper extremity

Anterior white commissure (AWC)

ALS in spinal cord

Posterior root ganglia

Posterior horn

Input from lower extremity

AWC

8-7B Representative lesions within the CNS that involve the ALS and the deficits that correlate with the level and laterality of each lesion. Note that the laterality (R/L) of the deficits is determined by whether the lesion is on the left or right side of the MRI/CT; this reinforces important clinical concepts.

■ Postsynaptic–Posterior (Dorsal) Column System and the Spinocervicothalamic Pathway in Anatomical Orientation ■

8-8 The origin, course, and distribution of fibers comprising the postsynaptic–posterior column system (upper) and the spinocervicothalamic pathway (lower). Postsynaptic–posterior column fibers originate primarily from cells in lamina IV (some cells in laminae III and V–VII also contribute), ascend in the ipsilateral dorsal fasciculi, and end in their respective nuclei in the caudal medulla. Moderate-to-sparse collaterals project to a few other medullary targets.

Fibers of the spinocervical part of the spinocervicothalamic pathway also originate from cells in lamina IV (less so from III and V). The axons of these cells ascend in the posterior part of the lateral funiculus (this is sometimes called the dorsolateral funiculus) and end in a topographic fashion in the lateral cervical nucleus: lumbosacral projections terminate posterolaterally and cervical projections anteromedially. Axons arising from cells of the lateral cervical nucleus decussate in the anterior white commissure, and ascend to targets in the midbrain and thalamus. Cells of the posterior column nuclei also convey information to the contralateral thalamus via the medial lemniscus.

Neurotransmitters

Glutamate (+) and possibly substance P (+) are present in some spinocervical projections. Because some cells in laminae III–V have axons that collateralize to both the lateral cervical nucleus *and* the dorsal column nuclei, glutamate (and substance P) also may be present in some postsynaptic dorsal column fibers.

Clinical Correlations

The postsynaptic–posterior column and spinocervicothalamic pathways are not known to be major circuits in the human nervous system. However, the occurrence of these fibers may explain a well-known clinical observation. Patients who have received an *anterolateral cordotomy* (this lesion is placed just ventral to the denticulate ligament) for *intractable pain* may experience complete or partial relief, or there may be a recurrence of pain perception within days or weeks. Although the cordotomy transects fibers of the anterolateral system (the main pain pathway), this lesion spares the posterior horn, posterior columns, and spinocervical fibers. Consequently, the recurrence of pain perception (or even the partial relief of pain) in these patients may be explained by these postsynaptic–dorsal column and spinocervicothalamic projections. Through these connections, some nociceptive (pain) information may be transmitted to the ventral posterolateral nucleus and on to the sensory cortex, via circuits that bypass the anterolateral system and are spared in a cordotomy.

ABBREVIATIONS	
ALS	Anterolateral system
AWCom	Anterior (ventral) white commissure
FCu	Cuneate fasciculus
FGr	Gracile fasciculus
IAF	Internal arcuate fibers
LCerNu	Lateral cervical nucleus
ML	Medial lemniscus
NuCu	Cuneate nucleus
NuGr	Gracile nucleus
PRG	Posterior (dorsal) root ganglion

Review of Blood Supply to Posterior Horn, FGr, Fcu, and LcerNu	
STRUCTURES	**ARTERIES**
FGr, FCu in Spinal Cord	Penetrating branches of arterial vasocorona and some branches from central (sulcal) (see Figure 6-6)
LCerNu	Penetrating branches of arterial vasocorona and branches from central (see Figure 6-6)
NuGr NuCu	Posterior spinal (see Figure 6-14)

■ 8-8 Postsynaptic–Posterior (Dorsal) Column System and the Spinocervicothalamic Pathway in Anatomical Orientation ■

■ Trigeminal Pathways in Anatomical Orientation ■

8-9 The distribution of general sensory GSA or SA information originating on CNs V (trigeminal), VII (facial), IX (glossopharyngeal), and X (vagus). Some of these primary sensory fibers end in the principal sensory nucleus, but many form the spinal trigeminal tract and end in the spinal trigeminal nucleus.

Neurons in the spinal trigeminal nucleus and in ventral parts of the principal sensory nucleus give rise to crossed anterior (ventral) trigeminothalamic fibers. Collaterals of these ascending fibers influence the hypoglossal, facial *(corneal reflex, supraorbital, or trigeminofacial reflex)*, and trigeminal motor nuclei; mesencephalic collaterals are involved in the *jaw reflex*, also called the *jaw-jerk reflex*. Collaterals also enter the dorsal motor vagal nucleus *(vomiting reflex)*, the superior salivatory nucleus *(tearing/lacrimal reflex)*, and the nucleus ambiguus and adjacent reticular formation *(sneezing reflex)*. Uncrossed posterior (dorsal) trigeminothalamic fibers arise from posterior regions of the principal sensory nucleus.

Neurotransmitters

Substance P (+)-containing and cholecystokinin (+)-containing trigeminal ganglion cells project to the spinal trigeminal nucleus, especially its caudal part (pars caudalis). Glutamate (+) is found in many trigeminothalamic fibers arising from the principal sensory nucleus and the pars interpolaris of the spinal nucleus. It is present in fewer trigeminothalamic fibers from the pars caudalis and in almost none from the pars oralis. The locus ceruleus (noradrenergic fibers) and the raphe nuclei (serotonergic fibers) also project to the spinal nucleus. Enkephalin (−)-containing cells are present in caudal regions of the spinal nucleus, and enkephalinergic fibers are found in the nucleus ambiguus and in the hypoglossal, facial, and trigeminal motor nuclei.

Clinical Correlations

Lesions of the trigeminal ganglion or nerve proximal to the ganglion result in: 1) a loss of pain, temperature, and tactile sensation from the ipsilateral face, oral cavity, and teeth; 2) ipsilateral paralysis of masticatory muscles; and 3) ipsilateral loss of the corneal reflex. Damage to peripheral portions of the trigeminal nerve may be traumatic (skull fracture, especially of supraorbital and infraorbital branch), inflammatory (e.g., *herpes zoster*), or result from tumor growth. The deficit would reflect the peripheral portion of the trigeminal nerve damaged.

Trigeminal neuralgia (tic douloureux) is a severe burning pain restricted to the peripheral distribution of the trigeminal nerve, usually its V_2 (maxillary) division. This pain may be initiated by any contact to areas of the face, such as the corner of the mouth, nose, lips, or cheek (e.g., shaving, putting on make-up, chewing, or even smiling). The attacks frequently occur without warning, may happen only a few times a month to many times in a single day, and are usually seen in patients 40 years of age or older. One probable cause of trigeminal neuralgia is compression of the trigeminal root by aberrant vessels, most commonly a loop of the superior cerebellar artery (see p. 45). Other causes may include tumor, *multiple sclerosis*, and ephaptic transmission *(ephapse)* in the trigeminal ganglion. This is the most common type of neuralgia.

In the medulla, fibers of the spinal trigeminal tract and ALS are served by the posterior inferior cerebellar artery (PICA). Consequently, an *alternating (alternate) hemianesthesia* is one characteristic feature of the *PICA syndrome*. This is a loss of pain and thermal sensations on one side of the body and the opposite side of the face. Pontine gliomas may produce a paralysis of masticatory muscles (motor trigeminal damage) and some loss of tactile input (principal sensory nucleus damage), as well as other deficits based on the adjacent structures involved.

ABBREVIATIONS

ALS	Anterolateral system	OpthV	Ophthalmic division of trigeminal nerve	VPM	Ventral posteromedial nucleus of thalamus
CC	Crus cerebri			VTTr	Ventral (anterior) trigeminothalamic tract
DTTr	Dorsal (posterior) trigeminothalamic tract	PSNu	Principal (chief) sensory nucleus		
FacNu	Facial nucleus	RB	Restiform body		
GSA	General somatic afferent	RetF	Reticular formation		**Ganglia**
HyNu	Hypoglossal nucleus	RNu	Red nucleus		
IC	Internal capsule	SpTNu	Spinal trigeminal nucleus	1	Trigeminal ganglion
ManV	Mandibular division of trigeminal nerve	SpTTr	Spinal trigeminal tract	2	Geniculate ganglion
		TriMoNu	Trigeminal motor nucleus	3	Superior of glossopharyngeal
MaxV	Maxillary division of trigeminal nerve	TMJ	Temporomandibular joint	4	Superior of vagus
		VPL	Ventral posterolateral nucleus of thalamus		
MesNu	Mesencephalic nucleus				
ML	Medial lemniscus				

Review of Blood Supply to SpTT, SpTNu, and Trigeminothalamic Tracts

STRUCTURES	ARTERIES
SpTTr and SpTNu in Medulla	Caudal third, vertebral; rostral two-thirds, posterior inferior cerebellar (see Figure 6-14)
SpTTr and SpTNu in Pons	Long circumferential branches of basilar (see Figure 6-21)
Trigeminothalamic Fibers in Midbrain	Short circumferential branches of posterior cerebral and superior cerebellar (see Figure 6-27)
VPM	Thalamogeniculate branches of posterior cerebral (see Figure 6-38)
Posterior Limb of IC	Lateral striate branches of middle cerebral (see Figure 6-38)

■ 8-9 Trigeminal Pathways in Anatomical Orientation ■

Trunk

Thigh

Leg

Foot

Somatosensory cortex

Upper extremity

Face

Posterior limb, IC

VPM

DTTr

VTTr

MesNu

PSNu

1

Position of trigeminal tracts

MesNu

ALS

VTTr

DTTr

ML

RNu

CC

TriMoNu

TriMoNu

SpTTr

SpTNu

FacNu

RetF

VTTr

Origin of SA data

GSA, skin of face; forehead and part of scalp; membranes of nose and of nasal, maxillary, and frontal sinuses; oral cavity; teeth; anterior two thirds of tongue; muscles of mastication; TMJ; cornea and conjunctiva; and dura of middle and anterior cranial fossae

GSA, external auditory meatus and medial and lateral surfaces of ear (conchae)

2

GSA, small area on ear

3

GSA, medial and lateral surfaces of ear (conchae); posterior wall and floor of external auditory meatus; tympanic membrane; and dura of posterior cranial fossa

4

SpTTr

Somatotopy in SpTTr and SpTNu

Input from VII, IX, X

RB

SpTTr

ManV

MaxV

SpTNu

OpthV

ALS

SpTTr

SpTNu

HyNu

SpTNu

■ Trigeminal Pathways in Clinical Orientation ■

8-10A Spinal trigeminal and trigeminothalamic fibers superimposed on MRI (brainstem and forebrain, T2-weighted MRI) showing the location, topography, and trajectory of these fibers in a clinical orientation. The red and blue fibers correlate with those of the same color in Figure 8-9.

Trigeminal Pathways in Clinical Orientation: Representative Lesions and Deficits

Postcentral gyrus (lateral third is face area of somato-sensory cortex

Genu, internal capsule

Posterior limb, internal capsule

Putamen

Thalamocortical fibers in posterior limb of internal capsule

Ventral posteromedial nucleus

- Diminution/loss pain, thermal sense, and discriminative touch on left side of face plus UE/LE if VPL involved
- Paresthesias; dysesthesias
- Possible transient left hemiplegia

Red nucleus

Crus cerebri

Substantia nigra

ML in midbrain

ALS in midbrain

TriThalFib in midbrain

Trigeminal ganglion

Trigeminal nerve root

Middle cerebellar peduncle

Pontine tegmentum

Damage to trigeminal root
- Left-sided loss pain, thermal sense, and discriminative touch on face and in oral cavity (including teeth)
- Loss of corneal reflex on left: Damage to afferent limb
- Paralysis of masticatory muscles on left and slight deviation of jaw to right on closure

Irritation of trigeminal root
- Trigeminal neuralgia (tic douloureux) on left side of face

Inferior olivary eminence

Restiform body

Medial lemniscus (ML) in medulla

Ganglia of cranial nerves VII, IX, X

Spinal trigeminal tract

Spinal trigeminal fibers to dorsolateral tract in upper cervical spinal cord

Spinal trigeminal nucleus, pars caudalis

Trigeminothalamic fibers (TriThalFib) in medulla

- Loss of pain/thermal sense on left side of face and on right UE and LE (alternating hemianesthesia)
- Dysarthria, dysphagia, and hoarseness (nucleus ambiguus)
- Vertigo, ataxia, and nystagmus (vestibular nucleus; restiform body)
- Nausea, vomiting, and singultus (area postrema; reticular formation)
- Left ptosis/miosis/anhidrosis (Horner)

8-10B Representative lesions of the brainstem and thalamus that involve elements of the trigeminal system and the deficits that correlate with the level and laterality of each lesion.

Note that the laterality (R/L) of the deficits is determined by whether the lesion is on the left or right side of the MRI; this reinforces important clinical concepts.

■ Solitary Pathways in Anatomical Orientation ■

8-11 Visceral afferent input (SVA, taste; GVA, general visceral sensation) on CNs VII (facial), IX (glossopharyngeal), and X (vagus) enters the solitary nuclei via the solitary tract. Recall that the SVA and GVA functional components may be collectively grouped as VA (Visceral Afferent) functional components. What is commonly called the solitary "nucleus" is actually a series of small nuclei that collectively form this rostrocaudal-oriented cell column.

Solitary cells project to the salivatory, hypoglossal, and dorsal motor vagal nuclei and the nucleus ambiguus. Solitary projections to the nucleus ambiguus are largely bilateral and are the intermediate neurons in the pathway for the *gag reflex*. The afferent limb of the *gag reflex* is carried on the glossopharyngeal nerve, and the efferent limb originates from the nucleus ambiguus. In this respect, the efferent limb travels on both the glossopharyngeal and vagus nerves. Although not routinely tested, the *gag reflex* should be evaluated in patients with *dysarthria, dysphagia,* or *hoarseness.* Solitariospinal fibers are bilateral with a contralateral preponderance and project to the phrenic nucleus, intermediolateral cell column, and ventral horn. The VPM is the thalamic center through which visceral afferent information is relayed onto the cerebral cortex.

Neurotransmitters

Substance P (+)-containing and cholecystokinin (+)-containing cells in the geniculate ganglion (facial nerve) and the inferior ganglia of the glossopharyngeal and vagus nerves project to the solitary nucleus. Enkephalin (−), neurotensin, and GABA (+) are present in some solitary neurons that project into the adjacent dorsal motor vagal nucleus. Cholecystokinin (+), somatostatin (−), and enkephalin (−) are present in solitary neurons, cells of the parabrachial nuclei, and some thalamic neurons that project to taste and other visceral areas of the cortex.

Clinical Correlations

Lesions of the geniculate ganglion, or facial nerve proximal to the ganglion, result in: 1) ipsilateral loss of taste *(ageusia)* from the anterior two-thirds of the tongue; and 2) an ipsilateral *facial (Bell) palsy.* Although a glossopharyngeal nerve lesion will result in *ageusia* from the posterior third of the tongue on the ipsilateral side, this loss is difficult to test. On the other hand, *glossopharyngeal neuralgia* (this may also be called *glossopharyngeal tic*) is an idiopathic pain localized to the peripheral sensory branches of the ninth nerve in the posterior pharynx, posterior tongue, and tonsillar area. Although comparatively rare, glossopharyngeal neuralgia may be aggravated by talking or even swallowing. Occlusion of the posterior inferior cerebellar artery (e.g., the *posterior inferior cerebellar artery* or *lateral medullary syndrome*), in addition to producing an *alternate hemianesthesia,* also results in *ageusia* from the ipsilateral side of the tongue because the posterior inferior cerebellar artery serves the solitary tract and nuclei in the medulla.

Interestingly, lesions of the olfactory nerves or tract (*anosmia,* loss of olfactory sensation; *dysosmia,* distorted olfactory sense) may affect how the patient perceives taste. Witness the fact that the nasal congestion accompanying a severe cold markedly affects the sense of taste.

ABBREVIATIONS

AmyNu	Amygdaloid nucleus (complex)		**SalNu**	Salivatory nuclei
CardResp	Cardiorespiratory portion (caudal) of solitary nucleus		**SolTr and Nu**	Solitary tract and nuclei
			SVA	Special visceral afferent
GustNu	Gustatory nucleus (rostral portion of solitary nucleus)		**Tr**	Tract
			VA	Visceral afferent
GVA	General visceral afferent		**VPM**	Ventral posteromedial nucleus of thalamus
HyNu	Hypoglossal nucleus			
HyTh	Hypothalamus			**Number Key**
InfVNu	Inferior (or spinal) vestibular nucleus			
MVNu	Medial vestibular nucleus		1	Geniculate ganglion of facial
NuAm	Nucleus ambiguus		2	Inferior ganglion of glossopharyngeal
PBNu	Parabrachial nuclei		3	Inferior ganglion of vagus
RB	Restiform body		4	Dorsal motor vagal nucleus

Review of Blood Supply to SolNu and SolTr

STRUCTURES	ARTERIES
SolNu and Tr in Medulla	Caudal medulla, anterior spinal; rostral medulla, posterior inferior cerebellar (see Figure 6-14)
Ascending Fibers in Pons	Long circumferential branches of basilar and branches of superior cerebellar (see Figure 6-21)
VPM	Thalamogeniculate branches of posterior cerebral (see Figure 6-38)
Posterior Limb of IC	Lateral striate branches of middle cerebral (see Figure 6-38)

■ 8-11 Solitary Pathways in Anatomical Orientation ■

Thigh
Trunk
Leg
Foot
Upper extremity
Face

HyTh

VPM

AmyNu

PBNu

to HyNu, SalNu

Origin of VA data

SVA, taste, anterior two thirds of tongue

GVA, submandibular, sublingual, and lacrimal glands

1

SVA, taste, posterior third of tongue

GVA, parotid gland; mucosa of pharynx; tonsillar sinus; posterior third of tongue; carotid body

SVA
(GustNu)

SolTr and Nu

2

4

3

GVA
(CardResp)

SVA, taste buds at root of tongue and on epiglottis

NuAm

GVA, pharynx; larynx; aortic bodies; and thoracic and abdominal viscera

Solitariospinal tract

Position of SolTr and Nu

MVNu

InfVNu

RB

SolTr and Nu

■ Blank Master Drawing for Sensory Pathways ■

8-12   Blank master drawing for sensory pathways. This illus-   understanding, for the instructor to expand on sensory pathways
tration is provided for self-evaluation of sensory pathway   not covered in the atlas, or both.

NOTES

■ 8-12 Blank Master Drawing for Sensory Pathways ■

■ Corticospinal Tracts in Anatomical Orientation ■

8-13 The longitudinal extent of corticospinal fibers and their position and somatotopy at representative levels within the neuraxis. The somatotopy of corticospinal fibers in the basilar pons is less obvious than in the internal capsule, crus cerebri, pyramid, or spinal cord. In the motor decussation (pyramidal decussation), fibers originating from upper extremity areas of the cerebral cortex cross rostral to those that arise from lower extremity areas. In addition to fibers arising from the somatomotor area of the cerebral cortex (area 4), a significant contingent also originates from the postcentral gyrus (areas 3, 1, 2); the former terminate primarily in laminae VI–IX, whereas the latter end mainly in laminae IV and V. Prefrontal regions, especially area 6, and parietal areas 5 and 7 also contribute to the corticospinal tract.

Neurotransmitters

Acetylcholine, γ-aminobutyric acid (−), and substance P (+, plus other peptides) are found in small cortical neurons presumed to function as local circuit cells or in cortico-cortical connections. Glutamate (+) is present in cortical efferent fibers that project to the spinal cord. Glutaminergic corticospinal fibers and terminals are found in all spinal levels, but are especially concentrated in cervical and lumbosacral enlargements. This correlates with the fact that approximately 55% of all corticospinal fibers terminate in cervical levels of the spinal cord, approximately 20% in thoracic levels, and approximately 25% in lumbosacral levels. Some corticospinal fibers may branch and terminate at multiple spinal levels. Lower motor neurons are influenced by corticospinal fibers, either directly or indirectly, via interneurons. Acetylcholine and calcitonin gene-related peptides are present in these large motor cells and in their endings in skeletal muscle.

Clinical Correlations

Myasthenia gravis, a disease characterized by moderate to profound weakness of skeletal muscles, is caused by circulating antibodies that react with postsynaptic nicotinic acetylcholine receptors. Progressive muscle fatigability throughout the day is a hallmark of this disease. Ocular muscles are affected first in about 45% of patients (*diplopia, ptosis*) and ultimately in about 85% of individuals. In over 50% of patients, facial and oropharyngeal muscles are commonly affected (*facial weakness, dysphagia, dysarthria*). Weakness also may be seen in limb muscles, but almost always in combination with facial/oral weaknesses.

Injury to corticospinal fibers on one side of the cervical spinal cord (e.g., the *Brown-Séquard syndrome*) results in paralysis (*hemiplegia*) of the ipsilateral upper and lower extremities. With time, these patients may also exhibit features of an *upper motor neuron lesion* (*hyperreflexia, spasticity,* loss of superficial *abdominal reflexes,* and the *Babinski sign*). Bilateral cord damage above C4–C5 may result in *quadriplegia*; at C1–C2, respiratory arrest is an additional complication. Unilateral cord lesions in thoracic levels may result in paralysis of the ipsilateral lower extremity (*monoplegia*). If the thoracic spinal cord damage is bilateral both lower extremities may be paralyzed (*paraplegia*). Small lesions within the decussation of the pyramids may result in a bilateral paresis of the upper extremities (lesion in rostral portions) or a bilateral paresis of the lower extremities (lesion in caudal portions) based on the crossing patterns of fibers within the decussation. Recall that *-plegia*, as in *hemiplegia*, refers to a paralysis whereas *-paresis*, as in *hemiparesis*, refers to a weakness or incomplete paralysis.

Rostral to the pyramidal decussation, vascular lesions in the medulla (the *medial medullary syndrome*), pons (the *Millard-Gubler* or *Foville syndromes*), or midbrain (the *Weber syndrome*) all produce *alternating (crossed) hemiplegias*. These present as a contralateral hemiplegia of the upper and lower extremities, coupled with an ipsilateral paralysis of the tongue (medulla), facial muscles or lateral rectus muscle (pons), and most eye movements (midbrain). Sensory deficits are frequently seen as part of these syndromes. Lesions in the internal capsule (*lacunar strokes*) produce contralateral hemiparesis sometimes coupled with various cranial nerve signs due to corticonuclear fiber involvement. Bilateral weakness, indicative of corticospinal involvement, is also present in *amyotrophic lateral sclerosis*.

ABBREVIATIONS

ACSp	Anterior corticospinal tract	**ML**	Medial lemniscus		
ALS	Anterolateral system	**MLF**	Medial longitudinal fasciculus		
APGy	Anterior paracentral gyrus				
BP	Basilar pons	**PO**	Principal olivary nucleus		
CC	Crus cerebri	**PrCGy**	Precentral gyrus		
CNu	Corticonuclear (corticobulbar) fibers	**Py**	Pyramid		
		RB	Restiform body		
CSp	Corticospinal fibers	**RNu**	Red nucleus		
IC	Internal capsule	**SN**	Substantia nigra		
LCSp	Lateral corticospinal tract				

Somatotopy of CSp Fibers

A — Position of fibers coursing to upper extremity (UE) regions of spinal cord
L — Position of fibers coursing to lower extremity (LE) regions of spinal cord
T — Position of fibers coursing to thoracic regions of spinal cord

---

Review of Blood Supply to Corticospinal Fibers

STRUCTURES	ARTERIES
Posterior Limb of **IC**	Lateral striate branches of middle cerebral (see Figure 6-38)
Crus Cerebri in Midbrain	Paramedian and short circumferential branches of basilar and posterior communicating (see Figure 6-27)
CSp in **BP**	Paramedian branches of basilar (see Figure 6-21)
Py in Medulla	Anterior spinal (see Figure 6-14)
LCSp in Spinal Cord	Penetrating branches of arterial vasocorona (LE fibers), branches of central artery (UE fibers) (see Figure 6-6)

■ 8-13 Corticospinal Tracts in Anatomical Orientation ■

Somatomotor cortex

Somatotopy of CSp

Posterior limb, IC

Position of CSp

PrCGy
Upper extremity
Trunk
Thigh
Leg APGy
Foot
Face

ALS
ML
RNu
SN
CC

CSp fibers in CC

Face (CNu Fibers)

VesNu
ALS
MLF
ML
BP
CSp

CSp fibers in BP

CSp fibers in Py

RB
MLF
ALS
ML
PO
Py

Pyramidal (motor) decussation
LCSp

ACSp

LCSp
Laminae IV–IX
ALS
ACSp

■ Corticospinal Tracts in Clinical Orientation ■

Precentral gyrus (middle third is upper extremity area of somatomotor cortex)

Anterior paracentral gyrus (lower extremity area of somatomotor cortex)

Head of caudate nucleus
Anterior limb, internal capsule

Putamen

Corticospinal (CSp) fibers in posterior limb of the internal capsule

Thalamus

CSp fibers in crus cerebri

Frontopontine fibers

Parieto-, occipito-, and temporopontine fibers

Midbrain tegmentum

Cerebral aqueduct

CSp fibers in basilar pons

Basilar pons

Pontine tegmentum

Superior cerebellar peduncle

Fourth ventricle

CSp fibers in pyramid of medulla

Medial lemniscus

Inferior olive

Restiform body

Fourth ventricle

CSp fibers

Motor (pyramidal) decussation

Lateral CSp tract (LCSp)

LCSp fibers

Cervical spinal cord at C7–C8

LCSp tract

LCSp fiber termination in anterior horn at cervical levels

LCSp fiber termination in anterior horn at lumbosacral levels

8-14A The corticospinal system superimposed on CT (spinal cord, myelogram) and MRI (brainstem and forebrain, T2-weighted MRI) showing the location, topography, and trajec- tory of this pathway in a clinical orientation. The blue and green fibers correlate with those of the same color in Figure 8-13.

■ Corticospinal Tracts in Clinical Orientation: Representative Lesions and Deficits ■

Precentral gyrus (middle third is upper extremity area of somatomotor cortex)

Anterior paracentral gyrus (lower extremity area of somatomotor cortex)

Corticospinal (CSp) fibers in posterior limb of the internal capsule

- Hemiplegia of right UE and LE
- Reduced sensation (pain, thermal sense, proprioception, discriminative touch, and vibratory sense on right side of face and on right UE and LE)

CSp fibers in crus cerebri

- Hemiplegia of right UE and LE
- Paralysis of most eye movement on left; eye oriented down and out: Superior oblique and lateral rectus preserved
- Dilated left pupil
- Paralysis of lower face on right
- Tongue weakness: Deviates to the right on attempted protrusion

CSp fibers in basilar pons

Mid-to-rostral pons
- Hemiplegia of right UE and LE
- Loss of all sensation on left side of face/oral cavity, paralysis of left masticatory muscles (if trigeminal nerve involved)
- Loss of proprioception, discriminative touch, and vibratory sense if ML involved

Caudal pons
- Hemiplegia of right UE and LE
- Abducens (lateral rectus) paralysis on left
- Paralysis of upper/lower facial muscles on left (if facial nerve involved)
- Loss of proprioception, discriminative touch, and vibratory sense if ML involved

CSp fibers in pyramid of medulla

Medial lemniscus

- Hemiplegia of right UE and LE
- Loss of proprioception, discriminative touch, and vibratory sense on right UE/LE
- Tongue weakness: Deviates to left on attempted protrusion

CSp fibers

- Bilateral paralysis of UE and/or LE depending on position and extent of midline lesion

Cervical spinal cord at C7–C8

Lateral CSp tract (LCSp)

LCSp fibers

Spinal cord hemisection
- Right-sided paralysis below lesion
- Right-sided loss of proprioception, discriminative touch, and vibratory sense below lesion
- Left-sided loss of pain/thermal sensation beginning about two levels below lesion
- Right ptosis/miosis/anhidrosis (Horner) if lesion at cervical levels

LCSp tract

LCSp fiber termination in anterior horn at cervical levels

LCSp fiber termination in anterior horn at lumbosacral levels

8-14B Representative lesions within the CNS that involve the corticospinal system and the deficits that correlate with the level and laterality of teach lesion. Note that the laterality (R/L) of the deficits is determined by whether the lesion is on the left or right side of the MRI/CT; this reinforces important clinical concepts.

■ Corticonuclear (Corticobulbar) Fibers in Anatomical Orientation ■

8-15 The origin, course, and distribution of corticonuclear (corticobulbar) fibers to brainstem motor nuclei. These fibers influence—either directly or through neurons in the immediately adjacent reticular formation—the motor nuclei of oculomotor, trochlear, trigeminal, abducens, facial, glossopharyngeal and vagus (both via nucleus ambiguus), accessory, and hypoglossal nerves.

Corticonuclear fibers arise in the frontal eye fields (areas 6 and 8 in caudal portions of the middle frontal gyrus), the precentral gyrus (somatomotor cortex, area 4), and some originate from the postcentral gyrus (areas 3, 1, and 2). Fibers from area 4 occupy the genu of the internal capsule, but those from the frontal eye fields (areas 8 and 6) may traverse caudal portions of the anterior limb, and some (from areas 3, 1, and 2) may occupy the most rostral portions of the posterior limb. Fibers that arise in areas 8 and 6 terminate in the *rostral interstitial nucleus of the medial longitudinal fasciculus (vertical gaze center)* and the *paramedian pontine reticular formation (horizontal gaze center)*; these areas, in turn, project respectively to the third, fourth, and sixth nuclei. Fibers from area 4 terminate in, or adjacent to, cranial nerve motor nuclei excluding those of III, IV, and VI.

Although not illustrated here, the superior colliculus receives cortical input from area 8 and from the parietal eye field (area 7) and also projects to the riMLF and PPRF. In addition, it is important to note that descending cortical fibers (many arising in areas 3, 1, and 2) project to sensory relay nuclei of some cranial nerves and to other sensory relay nuclei in the brainstem, such as those of the posterior column system.

Neurotransmitters

Glutamate (+) is found in many corticofugal axons that directly innervate cranial nerve motor nuclei and in those fibers that terminate near, but not in, the various motor nuclei (indirect).

Clinical Correlations

Lesions involving the motor cortex (e.g., cerebral artery occlusion) or the internal capsule (e.g., *lacunar strokes* or occlusion of lenticulostriate branches of M_1) give rise to a contralateral *hemiplegia* of the upper and lower extremities (corticospinal fiber involvement) coupled with certain cranial nerve signs. Strictly cortical lesions may produce a transient *gaze palsy* in which the eyes deviate toward the lesioned side and away from the side of the hemiplegia. In addition to a contralateral *hemiplegia*, common cranial nerve findings in capsular lesions may include: 1) deviation of the tongue toward the side of the weakness and away from the side of the lesion when protruded; and 2) paralysis of facial muscles on the contralateral lower half of the face (*central facial palsy*). This reflects the fact that corticonuclear fibers to genioglossus motor neurons and to facial motor neurons serving the lower face are primarily crossed. Interruption of corticonuclear fibers to the nucleus ambiguus may result in weakness of palatal muscles contralateral to the lesion; the uvula will deviate toward the ipsilateral (lesioned) side on attempted phonation. In addition, a lesion involving corticonuclear fibers to the accessory nucleus may result in drooping of the ipsilateral shoulder (or an inability to elevate the shoulder against resistance) due to trapezius weakness, and difficulty in turning the head (against resistance) to the contralateral side due to weakness of the sternocleidomastoid muscle. In contrast to the *alternating hemiplegia* seen in some brainstem lesions, hemisphere lesions result in spinal and cranial nerve deficits that are generally, but not exclusively, contralateral to the cerebral injury.

Brainstem lesions, especially in the midbrain or pons, may result in the following: 1) *vertical gaze palsies* (midbrain); 2) the *Parinaud syndrome*—paralysis of upward gaze (tumors in area of pineal); 3) *internuclear ophthalmoplegia* (lesion in the MLF between motor nuclei of III and VI); 4) *horizontal gaze palsies* (lesion in abducens nucleus + PPRF); or 5) *the one-and-a-half syndrome*. In the latter case, the lesion is adjacent to the midline and involves the abducens nucleus and adjacent PPRF, internuclear fibers from the ipsilateral abducens that are crossing to enter the contralateral MLF, and internuclear fibers from the contralateral abducens nucleus that cross to enter the MLF on the ipsilateral (lesioned) side. The result is a loss of ipsilateral abduction (lateral rectus) and adduction (medial rectus, the "one") and a contralateral loss of adduction (medial rectus, the "half"); the only remaining horizontal movement is contralateral abduction via the intact abducens motor neurons.

ABBREVIATIONS

AbdNu	Abducens nucleus	**OcNu**	Oculomotor nucleus
AccNu	Accessory nucleus	**PPRF**	Paramedian pontine reticular formation
EWpgNu	Edinger-Westphal nucleus	**riMLF**	Rostral interstitial nucleus of the medial longitudinal
FacNu	Facial nucleus		fasciculus
HyNu	Hypoglossal nucleus	**TriMoNu**	Trigeminal motor nucleus
IC	Internal capsule	**TroNu**	Trochlear nucleus
NuAm	Nucleus ambiguus		

Review of Blood Supply to Cranial Nerve Motor Nuclei

Structures	Arteries
OcNu and EWpgNu	Paramedian branches of basilar bifurcation and medial branches of posterior cerebral and posterior communicating (see Figure 6-27)
TriMoNu	Long circumferential branches of basilar (see Figure 6-21)
AbdNu and FacNu	Long circumferential branches of basilar (see Figure 6-21)
NuAm	Posterior inferior cerebellar (see Figure 6-14)
HyNu	Anterior spinal (see Figure 6-14)

■ 8-15 Corticonuclear (Corticobulbar) Fibers in Anatomical Orientation ■

Motor cortex, precentral gyrus

Frontal eye fields

Genu of IC

Bilateral for upper face

riMLF
OcNu
TroNu

TriMoNu
PPRF
AbdNu
FacNu

Crossed for lower face

NuAm

Crossed for uvula (soft palate)

Crossed for genioglossus muscle

HyNu

AccNu

= Direct to motor neurons of nucleus

= Indirect to motor neurons via adjacent reticular formation

= Bilateral projections

= Primarily crossed projections

■ Corticonuclear (Corticobulbar) Fibers in Clinical Orientation ■

Precentral gyrus (lateral third is face area of somatomotor cortex)

Corticonuclear fibers (CortNuFib) in genu of internal capsule

Head of caudate nucleus

Anterior limb, internal capsule

Genu, internal capsule

Putamen

Posterior limb, internal capsule

Dorsal thalamus

CortNuFib in crus cerebri

Corticospinal fibers in crus cerebri

Substantia nigra

Cerebral aqueduct

Frontopontine fibers

Parieto-, occipito-, and temporopontine fibers

Interpeduncular fossa

Midbrain tegmentum

Portion of facial nucleus innervating lower face

Portion of facial nucleus innervating upper face

CortNuFib in pons

Facial colliculus

Basilar pons

Facial (motor) nucleus

Fourth ventricle

Nucleus ambiguus

CortNuFib in medulla

Hypoglossal nucleus

Inferior olive

Restiform body

Fourth ventricle

Corticospinal fibers/Pyramid

Nucleus ambiguus

Hypoglossal nucleus

Preolivary sulcus

Retro-olivary sulcus

Fourth ventricle

CortNuFib to accessory nucleus

Accessory nucleus (C1–C5 cord levels)

8-16A Fibers comprising the corticonuclear (corticobulbar) system superimposed on MRI (brainstem and forebrain, T2-weighted MRI) showing their location, topography, and trajectory in a clinical orientation. The main projection is indicated by the larger diameter branches. The red fibers correlate with those of the same color in Figure 8-15.

■ Corticonuclear (Corticobulbar) Fibers in Clinical Orientation: Representative Lesions and Deficits ■

Precentral gyrus (lateral third is face area of somatomotor cortex)

Head of caudate nucleus

Anterior limb, internal capsule

Genu, internal capsule

Putamen

Posterior limb, internal capsule

Dorsal thalamus

- Lesion in genu of internal capsule on right: deficits predominantly on left; see below

CortNuFib in crus cerebri

Corticospinal fibers in crus cerebri

Substantia nigra

Cerebral aqueduct

Frontopontine fibers

Parieto-, occipito-, and temporopontine fibers

Interpeduncular fossa

Midbrain tegmentum

- No effect on masticatory muscles; corticonuclear input to motor V is bilateral

Portion of facial nucleus innervating lower face

Portion of facial nucleus innervating upper face

CortNuFib in pons

Facial colliculus

- Paralysis of lower facial muscles on left; predominant input from right motor cortex
- Upper facial muscles normal; bilateral input from motor cortex

Nucleus ambiguus

CortNuFib in medulla

Hypoglossal nucleus

- Dysphagia, dysarthria, and deviation of uvula to right on phonation; hoarseness

- Deviation of tongue to left on protrusion; predominant input from right motor cortex

Corticospinal fibers/Pyramid

Nucleus ambiguus

Hypoglossal nucleus

- Dysphagia, dysarthria, and deviation of uvula to right on phonation; hoarseness

- Deviation of tongue to left on protrusion; predominant input from right motor cortex

CortNuFib to accessory nucleus

Accessory nucleus (C1– C5 cord levels)

- Unable to rotate head to left against resistance
- Unable to elevate right shoulder against resistance

8-16B Representative lesion of corticonuclear fibers in the genu of the internal capsule that results in deficits related to the motor function of certain cranial nerves. Note that the laterality (R/L) of the deficits is determined by the location of the lesion in the genu on the right; this reinforces important clinical concepts.

■ Tectospinal and Reticulospinal Tracts in Anatomical Orientation ■

8-17 The origin, course, and position in representative cross-sections of brainstem and spinal cord, and the general distribution of tectospinal and reticulospinal tracts. Tectospinal fibers originate from deeper layers of the superior colliculus, cross in the posterior (dorsal) tegmental decussation, and distribute to cervical cord levels. Several regions of cerebral cortex (e.g., frontal, parietal, temporal) project to the tectum, but the most highly organized corticotectal projections arise from the visual cortex. Pontoreticulospinal fibers (medial reticulospinal) tend to be uncrossed, whereas those from the medulla (bulboreticulospinal or lateral reticulospinal) are bilateral, but with a pronounced ipsilateral preponderance. Corticoreticular fibers are bilateral with a slight contralateral preponderance and originate from several cortical areas.

Neurotransmitters

Corticotectal projections, especially those from the visual cortex, use glutamate (+). This substance is also present in most corticoreticular fibers. Some neurons of the gigantocellular reticular nucleus that send their axons to the spinal cord, as reticulospinal projections, contain enkephalin (−) and substance P (+). Enkephalinergic reticulospinal fibers may be part of the descending system that modulates pain transmission at the spinal level. Many reticulospinal fibers influence the activity of lower motor neurons.

Clinical Correlations

Isolated lesions of only tectospinal and reticulospinal fibers are essentially never seen. Tectospinal fibers project to upper cervical levels where they influence reflex movement of the head and neck. Such movements may be diminished or slowed in patients with damage to these fibers. Pontoreticulospinal (medial reticulospinal) fibers are excitatory to extensor motor neurons and to neurons innervating axial musculature; some of these fibers also may inhibit flexor motor neurons. In contrast, some bulboreticulospinal (lateral reticulospinal) fibers are primarily inhibitory to extensor motor neurons and neurons innervating muscles of the neck and back; these fibers also may excite flexor motor neurons via interneurons. Reticulospinal (and vestibulospinal) fibers contribute to the *spasticity* that develops in patients having lesions of corticospinal fibers. These fibers, particularly reticulospinal fibers (see Figure 8-18 on p. 216) also contribute to the tonic extension of the arms and legs seen in *decerebrate rigidity* when spinal motor neurons are released from descending cortical control. The sudden increase in extensor rigidity, seen in decerebrate patients when a noxious stimulus is applied to, for example, the skin between the toes, is mediated via spinoreticular fibers (traveling in the ALS) that end on reticulospinal neurons whose axons descend to increase the level of excitation to extensor motor neurons.

ABBREVIATIONS

ALS	Anterolateral system	PO	Principal olivary nucleus
ATegDec	Anterior tegmental decussation (rubrospinal fibers)	PTegDec	Posterior tegmental decussation (tectospinal fibers)
BP	Basilar pons	Py	Pyramid
CC	Crus cerebri	RB	Restiform body
CRet	Corticoreticular fibers	RetNu	Reticular nuclei
CTec	Corticotectal fibers	RetSp	Reticulospinal tract(s)
GigRetNu	Gigantocellular reticular nucleus	RNu	Red nucleus
LCSp	Lateral corticospinal tract	RuSp	Rubrospinal tract
ML	Medial lemniscus	SC	Superior colliculus
MLF	Medial longitudinal fasciculus	SN	Substantia nigra
MVNu	Medial vestibular nucleus	SpVNu	Spinal (or inferior) vestibular nucleus
OcNu	Oculomotor nucleus	TecSp	Tectospinal tract

Review of Blood Supply to SC, Reticular Formation of Pons and Medulla, and TecSp and RetSp Tracts in Cord	
Structures	**Arteries**
SC	Long circumferential branches (quadrigeminal branch) of posterior cerebral plus some from superior cerebellar and posterior choroidal (see Figure 6-27)
Pontine Reticular Formation	Long circumferential branches of basilar plus branches of superior cerebellar in rostral pons (see Figure 6-21)
Medullary Recticular Formation	Branches of vertebral plus paramedian branches of basilar at medulla–pons junction (see Figure 6-14)
TecSp and **RetSp**	Branches of central artery (TecSp and Medullary RetSp); tracts penetrating branches of arterial vasocorona (Pontine RetSp) (see Figures 6-14 and 6-6)

■ 8-17 Tectospinal and Reticulospinal Tracts in Anatomical Orientation ■

Position of TecSp and RetSp

Medullary RetSp
to laminae VII
(VI, VIII, IX)

Pontine RetSp
to laminae VIII
(VII, IX)

TecSp
to laminae VI, VII (VIII)
of cervical levels

■ Rubrospinal and Vestibulospinal Tracts in Anatomical Orientation ■

8-18 The origin, course, and position in representative cross sections of brainstem and spinal cord, and the general distribution of rubrospinal and vestibulospinal tracts. Rubrospinal fibers cross in the anterior (ventral) tegmental decussation and distribute to all spinal levels, although projections to cervical levels clearly predominate. Cells in dorsomedial regions of the red nucleus receive input from upper extremity areas of the motor cortex and project to cervical levels, but those in ventrolateral areas of the nucleus receive some fibers from lower extremity areas of the motor cortex and may project in sparse numbers to lumbosacral levels. The red nucleus also projects, via the central tegmental tract, to the ipsilateral inferior olivary complex (rubro-olivary fibers).

Medial and lateral vestibular nuclei give rise to the medial and lateral vestibulospinal tracts, respectively. The former tract is primarily ipsilateral, projects to upper spinal levels, and is considered a component of the medial longitudinal fasciculus in the spinal cord. The latter tract is ipsilateral and somatotopically organized; fibers to lumbosacral levels originate from dorsal and caudal regions of the lateral nucleus, whereas those to cervical levels arise from its rostral and more ventral areas.

Neurotransmitters

Glutamate (+) is present in corticorubral fibers. Some lateral vestibulospinal fibers contain aspartate (+), whereas glycine (−) is present in a portion of the medial vestibulospinal projection. There are numerous γ-aminobutyric acid (−)-containing fibers in the vestibular complex; these represent the endings of cerebellar corticovestibular fibers.

Clinical Correlations

Isolated injury to rubrospinal and vestibulospinal fibers is really not seen in humans. Deficits in fine distal limb movements seen in monkeys following experimental rubrospinal lesions may be present in humans. However, these deficits are overshadowed by the *hemiplegia* associated with injury to the adjacent corticospinal fibers. The contralateral tremor seen in patients with the *Claude syndrome* (a lesion of the medial midbrain) is partially related to damage to the red nucleus as well as the adjacent cerebellothalamic fibers. These patients also may have a paucity of most eye movement on the ipsilateral side and a dilated pupil (*mydriasis*) due to concurrent damage to exiting rootlets of the oculomotor nerve. The sudden increase in extensor rigidity, seen in decerebrate patients when a noxious stimulus is applied to, for example, the skin between the toes, is mediated via spinoreticular fibers (traveling in the ALS) that end on reticulospinal neurons whose axons descend to excite extensor motor neurons.

Medial vestibulospinal fibers primarily inhibit motor neurons innervating extensors and neurons serving muscles of the back and neck. Lateral vestibulospinal fibers may inhibit some flexor motor neurons, but they mainly facilitate spinal reflexes via their excitatory influence on spinal motor neurons innervating extensors. Vestibulospinal and reticulospinal (see Figure 8-17 on p. 214) fibers contribute to the *spasticity* seen in patients with damage to corticospinal fibers or to the tonic extension of the extremities in patients with *decerebrate rigidity*. In the case of decerebrate rigidity, the descending influences on spinal flexor motor neurons (corticospinal, rubrospinal) are removed; the descending brainstem influence on spinal extensor motor neurons predominates; this is augmented by excitatory spinoreticular input (via ALS) to some of the centers giving rise to reticulospinal fibers (see also Figure 8-17 on p. 214). See Figures 8-19 for lesions that influence the activity of rubrospinal, and reticulospinal fibers.

ABBREVIATIONS

ATegDec	Anterior tegmental decussation (rubrospinal fibers)	MVesSp	Medial vestibulospinal tract
CC	Crus cerebri	MVNu	Medial vestibular nucleus
CorRu	Corticorubral fibers	OcNu	Oculomotor nucleus
FacNu	Facial nucleus	PTegDec	Posterior tegmental decussation (tectospinal fibers)
InfVNu	Inferior (or spinal) vestibular nucleus	Py	Pyramid
LCSp	Lateral corticospinal tract	RNu	Red nucleus
LRNu	Lateral reticular nucleus	RuSp	Rubrospinal tract
LVNu	Lateral vestibular nucleus	SC	Superior colliculus
LVesSp	Lateral vestibulospinal tract	SVNu	Superior vestibular nucleus
ML	Medial lemniscus	TecSp	Tectospinal tract
MLF	Medial longitudinal fasciculus	VesSp	Vestibulospinal tracts

---

Review of Blood Supply to RNu, Vestibular Nuclei, MFL and RuSp, and Vestibulospinal Tracts in Cords

Structures	Arteries
RNu	Medial branches of posterior cerebral and posterior communicating plus some from short circumferential branches of posterior cerebral (see Figure 6-27)
Vestibular Nuclei	Posterior inferior cerebellar in medulla (see Figure 6-14) and long circumferential branches in pons (see Figure 6-21)
MLF	Long circumferential branches of basilar in pons (see Figure 6-21) and anterior spinal in medulla (see Figure 6-14)
MVesSp	Branches of central artery (see Figures 6-6 and 6-14)
LVesSp and RuSp	Penetrating branches of arterial vasocorona plus terminal branches of central artery (see Figure 6-6)

■ 8-18 Rubrospinal and Vestibulospinal Tracts in Anatomical Orientation ■

Position of RuSp and VesSp

■ Rubrospinal, Reticulospinal, and Vestibulospinal Fibers: Clinical Orientation ■

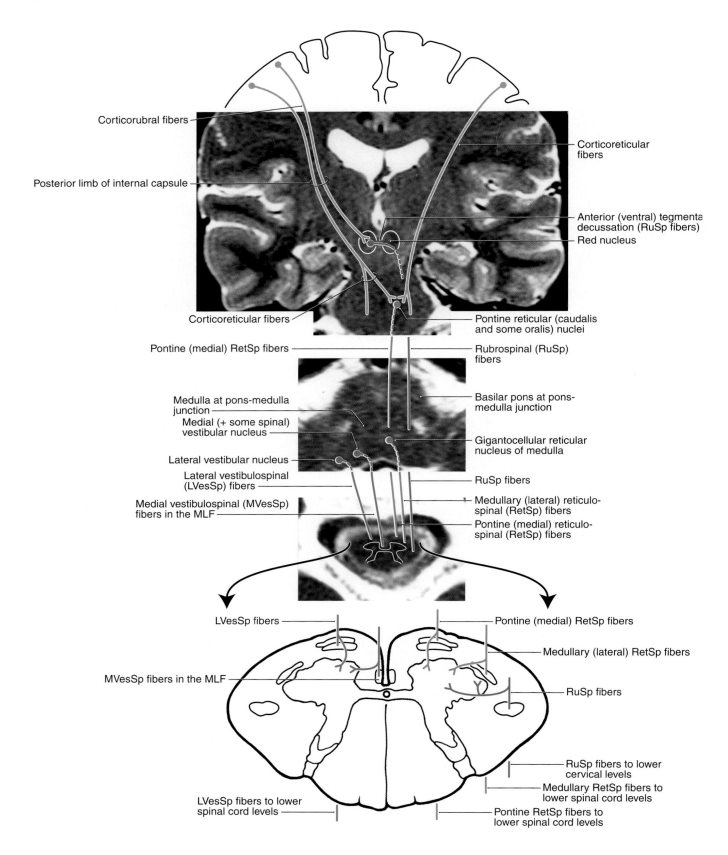

Corticorubral fibers

Posterior limb of internal capsule

Corticoreticular fibers

Pontine (medial) RetSp fibers

Medulla at pons-medulla junction

Medial (+ some spinal) vestibular nucleus

Lateral vestibular nucleus

Lateral vestibulospinal (LVesSp) fibers

Medial vestibulospinal (MVesSp) fibers in the MLF

LVesSp fibers

MVesSp fibers in the MLF

LVesSp fibers to lower spinal cord levels

Corticoreticular fibers

Anterior (ventral) tegmental decussation (RuSp fibers)

Red nucleus

Pontine reticular (caudalis and some oralis) nuclei

Rubrospinal (RuSp) fibers

Basilar pons at pons-medulla junction

Gigantocellular reticular nucleus of medulla

RuSp fibers

Medullary (lateral) reticulo-spinal (RetSp) fibers

Pontine (medial) reticulo-spinal (RetSp) fibers

Pontine (medial) RetSp fibers

Medullary (lateral) RetSp fibers

RuSp fibers

RuSp fibers to lower cervical levels

Medullary RetSp fibers to lower spinal cord levels

Pontine RetSp fibers to lower spinal cord levels

8-19A Rubrospinal, reticulospinal, and vestibulospinal fibers superimposed on CT (spinal cord, myelogram) and MRI (brainstem and forebrain, T2-weighted MRI) showing their origin, location, and trajectory in clinical orientation.

■ Rubrospinal, Reticulospinal, and Vestibulospinal Fibers: Clinical Orientation— Lesions Affecting Their Influence on Spinal Motor Neurons ■

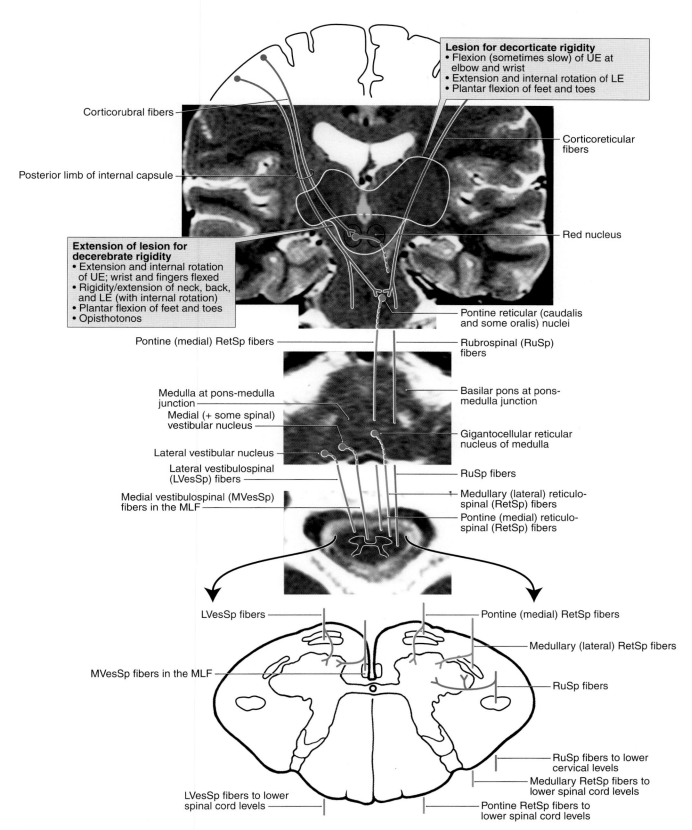

Corticorubral fibers

Posterior limb of internal capsule

Lesion for decorticate rigidity
- Flexion (sometimes slow) of UE at elbow and wrist
- Extension and internal rotation of LE
- Plantar flexion of feet and toes

Corticoreticular fibers

Red nucleus

Extension of lesion for decerebrate rigidity
- Extension and internal rotation of UE; wrist and fingers flexed
- Rigidity/extension of neck, back, and LE (with internal rotation)
- Plantar flexion of feet and toes
- Opisthotonos

Pontine reticular (caudalis and some oralis) nuclei

Pontine (medial) RetSp fibers

Rubrospinal (RuSp) fibers

Medulla at pons-medulla junction

Basilar pons at pons-medulla junction

Medial (+ some spinal) vestibular nucleus

Lateral vestibular nucleus

Gigantocellular reticular nucleus of medulla

Lateral vestibulospinal (LVesSp) fibers

RuSp fibers

Medial vestibulospinal (MVesSp) fibers in the MLF

Medullary (lateral) reticulospinal (RetSp) fibers

Pontine (medial) reticulospinal (RetSp) fibers

LVesSp fibers

Pontine (medial) RetSp fibers

Medullary (lateral) RetSp fibers

MVesSp fibers in the MLF

RuSp fibers

RuSp fibers to lower cervical levels

Medullary RetSp fibers to lower spinal cord levels

LVesSp fibers to lower spinal cord levels

Pontine RetSp fibers to lower spinal cord levels

8-19B Representative lesions in the forebrain that are supratentorial (located above the tentorial notch) and then extend downward through the notch and become infratentorial. These lesions alter the activity of rubrospinal, vestibulospinal, and reticulospinal fibers that results in the characteristic deficits seen in these patients. In a large supratentorial lesion (*decorticate*), all brainstem nuclei (including the red nucleus) are intact. When the lesion becomes infratentorial, the red nucleus influence is removed, the extensor rigidity predominates, and is exacerbated by incoming signals from the anterolateral system; the patient becomes *decerebrate*.

■ Blank Master Drawing for Motor Pathways ■

8-20 Blank master drawing for motor pathways. This illustration is provided for self-evaluation of motor pathways understanding, for the instructor to expand on motor pathways not covered in this atlas, or both.

NOTES

■ 8-20 Blank Master Drawing for Motor Pathways ■

■ Cranial Nerve Efferents (III, IV, VI, XI–AccNu, XII) in Anatomical Orientation ■

8-21 The origin and peripheral distribution of GSE or SE fibers from the oculomotor, trochlear, abducens, accessory, and hypoglossal nuclei. Edinger-Westphal cells adjacent to the oculomotor nucleus are organized into the *Edinger-Westphal centrally projecting nucleus* (EWcpNu) and the *Edinger-Westphal preganglionic nucleus* (EWpgNu). Neurons of the EWcpNu project to the spinal cord and a variety of brainstem nuclei (such as parabrachial, inferior olivary, dorsal raphe) that are involved in stress and food/drink intake behaviors. Neurons of the EWpgNu are the origin of the GVE/VE preganglionic parasympathetic input to the ciliary ganglion traveling on the third nerve; this is part of the *pupillary light reflex* pathway. Internuclear abducens neurons (in green) project, via the MLF, to contralateral oculomotor neurons that innervate the medial rectus muscle (*internuclear ophthalmoplegia* pathway).

The trapezius and sternocleidomastoid muscles originate from cervical somites located caudal to the last pharyngeal arch; they are designated here as GSE or SE. In addition, animal experiments reveal that motor neurons innervating these same muscles are found in cervical cord levels C1 to about C6.

Neurotransmitters

Acetylcholine (and probably calcitonin gene-related peptide, CGRP) is found in the motor neurons of cranial nerve nuclei and in their peripheral endings. This substance is also found in cells of the Edinger-Westphal nucleus and the ciliary ganglion.

Clinical Correlations

Myasthenia gravis (MG) is a disease caused by autoantibodies that may directly block nicotinic acetylcholine receptors or damage the postsynaptic membrane (via complement-mediated lysis) thereby reducing the number of viable receptor sites. Ocular movement disorders (*diplopia, ptosis*) are the initial deficits observed in approximately 50% of patients and are present in approximately 85% of all MG patients. Movements of the neck and tongue also may be impaired, with the latter contributing to *dysphagia* and *dysarthria*.

Lesions of the third nerve (e.g., the *Weber syndrome* or in *carotid cavernous aneurysms*) may result in: 1) *ptosis*; 2) lateral and downward deviation of the eye; and 3) *diplopia* (except on ipsilateral lateral gaze). In addition, the pupil may be unaffected (pupillary sparing) or dilated and fixed. Lesions in the midbrain that involve the root of the third nerve and the crus cerebri give rise to a *superior alternating (crossed) hemiplegia*. This is a paralysis of most eye movement and a dilated pupil on the ipsilateral side and a contralateral hemiplegia of the extremities.

Damage to the MLF (e.g., *multiple sclerosis* or small vessel occlusion) between the sixth and third nuclei results in *internuclear ophthalmoplegia*; on attempted lateral gaze, the opposite medial rectus muscle will not adduct. A lesion of the fourth nerve (frequently caused by trauma) produces *diplopia* on downward and inward gaze (tilting the head may give some relief), and the eye is slightly elevated when the patient looks straight ahead.

Diabetes mellitus, trauma, or *pontine gliomas* are some causes of sixth nerve dysfunction. In these patients, the affected eye is slightly adducted, and *diplopia* is pronounced on attempted gaze to the lesioned side. Damage in the caudal and medial pons may involve the fibers of the sixth nerve and the adjacent corticospinal fibers in the basilar pons, giving rise to a *middle alternating (crossed) hemiplegia*. The deficits are an ipsilateral paralysis of the lateral rectus muscle and a contralateral hemiplegia of the extremities. The eleventh nerve may be damaged centrally (e.g., *syringobulbia* or *amyotrophic lateral sclerosis*) or at the jugular foramen with resultant paralysis of the ipsilateral sternocleidomastoid and upper parts of the trapezius muscle.

Central injury to the twelfth nucleus or fibers (e.g., the *medial medullary syndrome* or in *syringobulbia*) or to its peripheral parts (e.g., *polyneuropathy*, trauma, or tumor) results in deviation of the tongue toward the lesioned side on attempted protrusion. A lesion in the medial aspects of the medulla will give rise to an *inferior alternating (crossed) hemiplegia*. This is characterized by a paralysis of the ipsilateral side of the tongue (twelfth root damage) and contralateral hemiplegia of the extremities (damage to corticospinal fibers in the pyramid).

ABBREVIATIONS

AbdNr	Abducens nerve	OcNu	Oculomotor nucleus
AbdNu	Abducens nucleus	PO	Principal olivary nucleus
AccNr	Accessory nerve	Py	Pyramid
AccNu	Accessory nucleus	RNu	Red nucleus
BP	Basilar pons	SC	Superior colliculus
CC	Crus cerebri	SCP,Dec	Superior cerebellar peduncle, decussation
EWpgNu	Edinger-Westphal preganglionic nucleus	TroDec	Trochlear decussation
FacCol	Facial colliculus	TroNr	Trochlear nerve
HyNr	Hypoglossal nerve	TroNu	Trochlear nucleus
HyNu	Hypoglossal nucleus		
ML	Medial lemniscus		**Ganglion**
MLF	Medial longitudinal fasciculus	1 Ciliary	
OcNr	Oculomotor nerve		

Review of Blood Supply to OcNu, TroNu, AbdNu, and HyNu and the Internal Course of Their Fibers

Structures	Arteries
OcNu and Fibers	Medial branches of posterior cerebral and posterior communicating (see Figure 6-27)
TroNu	Paramedian branches of basilar bifurcation (see Figure 6-27)
AbdNu	Long circumferential branches of basilar (see Figure 6-21)
Abducens Fibers in **BP**	Paramedian branches of basilar (see Figure 6-21)
HyNu and Fibers	Anterior spinal (see Figure 6-14)

■ 8-21 Cranial Nerve Efferents (III, IV, VI, XI—AccNu, and XII) in Anatomical Orientation ■

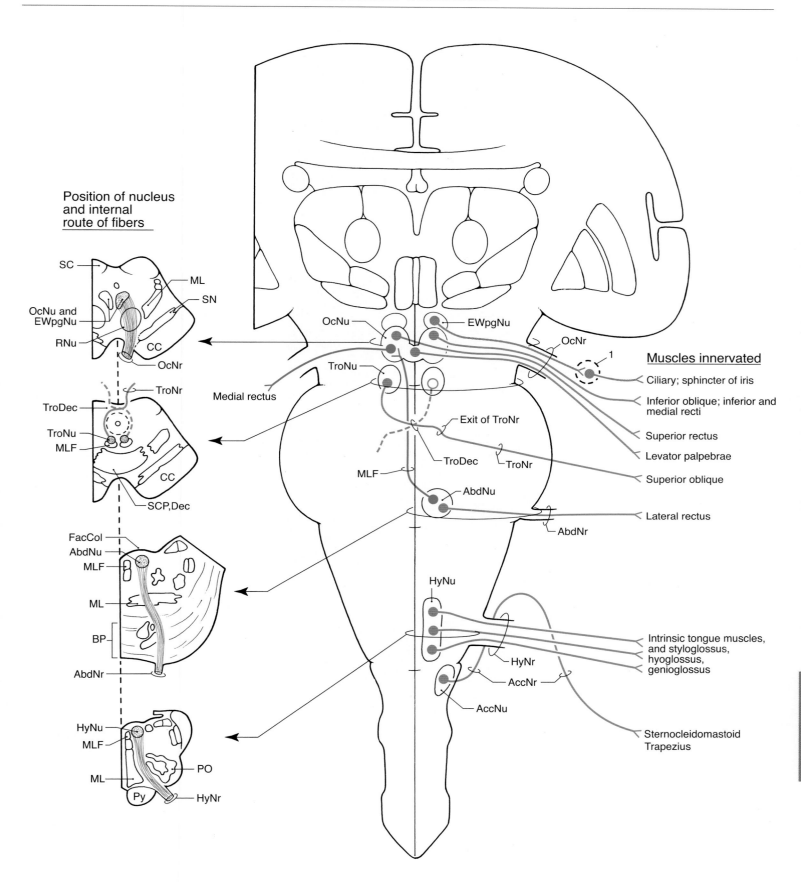

Position of nucleus and internal route of fibers

Muscles innervated

Ciliary; sphincter of iris

Inferior oblique; inferior and medial recti

Superior rectus

Levator palpebrae

Superior oblique

Lateral rectus

Intrinsic tongue muscles, and styloglossus, hyoglossus, genioglossus

Sternocleidomastoid Trapezius

■ Cranial Nerve Efferents (III, IV, VI, and XII) in Clinical Orientation ■

Mammillary body/nuclei

Interpeduncular fossa

Oculomotor nerve

Corticospinal and corticonuclear fibers

Red nucleus

Oculomotor nucleus (GSE and GVE cells)

Cerebral aqueduct and periaqueductal grey

Frontopontine fibers

Red nucleus

Substantia nigra

Midbrain tegmentum

Superior colliculus

Medial longitudinal fasciculus

Substantia nigra

Decussation of superior cerebellar peduncle

Trochlear nucleus

Cerebral aqueduct

Trochlear nerve exit

Superior oblique muscle →

Parieto- occipito- and temporopontine fibers

Inferior colliculus

Medial longitudinal fasciculus

Lateral rectus muscle →
Abducens nerve

ML in pons

Abducens nucleus

Facial colliculus

Corticospinal fibers in basilar pons

Basilar pons

Pontine tegmentum

Sulcus limitans

Pyramid
Intrinsic tongue muscles and stylo-, hyo-, and genio- → glossus muscles
Hypoglossal nerve

Anterolateral system

Spinal trigeminal tract and nucleus

Hypoglossal nucleus

Inferior olive

Medial lemniscus (ML) in medulla

Fourth ventricle

8-22A The nuclei and efferent fibers of CNs III, IV, VI, and XII superimposed on MRI (brainstem, T2-weighted MRI) shown in a clinical orientation. Also shown is the internuclear pathway from the sixth nucleus on one side to the third nucleus on the contralateral side. The red and green fibers correlate with those of the same color in Figure 8-21.

■ Cranial Nerve Efferents (III, IV, VI, and XII) in Clinical Orientation: Representative Lesions and Deficits ■

Mammillary body/nuclei

Interpeduncular fossa

Oculomotor nerve

Corticospinal and corticonuclear fibers

Red nucleus

Oculomotor nucleus (GSE and GVE cells)

Cerebral aqueduct and periaqueductal grey

Medial longitudinal fasciculus

Substantia nigra

Decussation of superior cerebellar peduncle

Trochlear nucleus

Cerebral aqueduct

Trochlear nerve exit

Superior oblique muscle →

Lateral rectus muscle →
Abducens nerve

ML in pons

Abducens nucleus

Facial colliculus

Pyramid

Intrinsic tongue muscles and stylo-, hyo-, and genio- →
glossus muscles

Hypoglossal nerve

Anterolateral system

Spinal trigeminal tract and nucleus

Hypoglossal nucleus

Damage to oculomotor root
• Paralysis of most eye movement on left; eye oriented down and out: Superior oblique and lateral rectus preserved
• Ptosis of left upper eyelid
• Left pupil dilated; diplopia

Oculomotor deficits from other causes
• Cerebral peduncle/Weber syndrome on left = left-sided oculomotor paralysis: Right-sided hemiplegia of UE/LE: Paralysis of lower face on right: deviation of tongue to right on protrusion
• Red nucleus/Claude syndrome on left = left-sided oculomotor paralysis: Right-sided loss of proprioception, discriminative touch, and vibratory sense on UE: Right-sided hyperkinesia (red nucleus): Right-sided akinesia (substantia nigra)
• Benedikt syndrome = Weber + Claude

Damage to trochlear root
• Paralysis of left superior oblique muscle
• Diplopia; head-tilt to healthy right side

Lesion in medial longitudinal fasciculus
• Lesion on left = left internuclear ophthalmoplegia (INO)

Damage to abducens root
• Paralysis of left lateral rectus muscle
• Diplopia on left lateral gaze

Abducens deficits from other causes
• Caudal pontine base/Foville syndrome on left = paralysis of left lateral rectus: Right-sided hemiplegia UE/LE: Diplopia
• Lesion of facial colliculus on left = paralysis of facial muscle on left and left gaze palsy consisting of paralysis of left lateral rectus muscles and right internuclear ophthalmoplegia
• Lesion of abducens nucleus and adjacent MLF = one-and-a-half syndrome

Damage to hypoglossal root
• Deviation of the tongue to the left on protrusion

Hypoglossal deficits from other causes
• Medial medullary/Déjèrine syndrome on left = deviation of the tongue to the left on protrusion: Right-sided hemiplegia: Right-sided loss of proprioception, discriminative touch, and vibratory sense on UE and LE
• Lesion of genu of internal capsule on right = deviation of the tongue to left on protrusion

8-22B Representative lesions of the roots of CNs III, IV, VI, and XII and the deficits that correlate with each lesion. Also shown is a lesion of the medial longitudinal fasciculus.

Additional examples of the causes of deficits related to these particular cranial nerves are also indicated. Note that lesions of these cranial nerve roots result in motor deficits on the side of the lesion.

■ Cranial Nerve Efferents (V, VII, IX, and X) in Anatomical Orientation ■

8-23 The origin and peripheral distribution of fibers arising from the motor nuclei of the trigeminal, facial, and glossopharyngeal and vagus (via the nucleus ambiguus) nerves. Also shown is the origin of GVE or VE preganglionic parasympathetic fibers from the superior (to facial nerve) and inferior (to glossopharyngeal nerve) salivatory nuclei and from the dorsal motor vagal nucleus. The SVE functional component traditionally specified cranial nerve motor nuclei innervating muscles arising from pharyngeal arches; these may also be classified as SE neurons (see Figure 8-1, p. 184). Muscles innervated by the trigeminal nerve (V) come from the first arch, those served by the facial nerve (VII) from the second arch; the stylopharyngeal muscle originates from the third arch and is innervated by the glossopharyngeal nerve (IX), and the muscles derived from the fourth arch are served by the vagus nerve (X).

Neurotransmitters

The transmitter found in the cells of cranial nerve motor nuclei, and in their peripheral endings, is acetylcholine; CGRP is also colocalized in these motor neurons. This substance is also present in preganglionic and postganglionic parasympathetic neurons.

Clinical Correlations

Patients with *myasthenia gravis* frequently have oropharyngeal symptoms and complications that result in *dysarthria*, and *dysphagia*. These individuals have difficulty chewing and swallowing, their jaw may hang open, and the mobility of facial muscles is decreased. Impaired hearing (weakness of tensor tympani) and *hyperacusis* (increased hearing sensitivity caused by weakness of the stapedius muscle) also may be present.

Lesions of the fifth nerve (e.g., *meningiomas* or trauma) result in: 1) loss of pain, temperature, and touch on the ipsilateral face and in the oral and nasal cavities; 2) *paralysis* of ipsilateral masticatory muscles (jaw deviates to the lesioned side when closed); and 3) loss

of the afferent limb of the *corneal reflex*. If especially large, a *vestibular schwannoma* may compress the trigeminal nerve root and result in a hemifacial sensory loss that may include the oral cavity. *Trigeminal neuralgia (tic douloureux)* is an intense, sudden, intermittent pain emanating from the area of the cheek, oral cavity, or adjacent parts of the nose (distribution of V_2 or V_3, see also Figure 8-9 on p. 198).

Tumors (e.g., *chordoma* or *vestibular schwannoma*), trauma, or *meningitis* may damage the seventh nerve, resulting in: 1) an ipsilateral *facial palsy* (or *Bell palsy*); 2) loss of taste from the ipsilateral two-thirds of the tongue; and 3) decreased secretion from the ipsilateral lacrimal, nasal, and sublingual and submandibular glands. Injury distal to the chorda tympani produces only an ipsilateral *facial palsy*. A paralysis of the muscles on one side of the face with no paralysis of the extremities is a *facial hemiplegia*, whereas intermittent and involuntary contraction of the facial muscles is called *hemifacial spasm*. One cause of hemifacial spasm is compression of the facial root by an aberrant loop from the anterior inferior cerebellar artery. These patients also may have *vertigo, tinnitus,* or *hearing loss* suggesting involvement of the adjacent vestibulocochlear nerve.

Because of their common origin from NuAm, adjacent exit from the medulla, and passage through the jugular foramen, the ninth and tenth nerves may be damaged together (e.g., *amyotrophic lateral sclerosis* or in *syringobulbia*). The results are *dysarthria, dysphagia, dyspnea,* loss of taste from the ipsilateral caudal tongue, and loss of the *gag reflex*. Damage to structures at, or traversing, the jugular foramen gives rise to combinations of deficits generally called *jugular foramen syndromes* (or the *Avellis syndrome*); examples of some of these are the *Collet-Sicard syndrome, Schmidt syndrome, Tapia syndrome,* and *Vernet syndrome*. These syndromes describe deficits reflecting damage to CNs IX, X, XI, and the adjacent root of XII. Bilateral lesions of the tenth nerve may be life-threatening because of the resultant total paralysis (and closure) of the muscles in the vocal folds (vocalis muscle).

ABBREVIATIONS

AbdNu	Abducens nucleus	**SpTNu**	Spinal trigeminal nucleus
ALS	Anterolateral system	**SpTTr**	Spinal trigeminal tract
BP	Basilar pons	**SSNu**	Superior salivatory nucleus
DVagNu	Dorsal motor nucleus of vagus	**TecSp**	Tectospinal tract
FacNr	Facial nerve	**TriMoNu**	Trigeminal motor nucleus
FacNu	Facial nucleus	**TriNr**	Trigeminal nerve
GlNr	Glossopharyngeal nerve	**VagNr**	Vagus nerve
HyNu	Hypoglossal nucleus		
ISNu	Inferior salivatory nucleus		
MesNu	Mesencephalic nucleus		**Ganglia**
ML	Medial lemniscus	1	Pterygopalatine
MLF	Medial longitudinal fasciculus	2	Submandibular
NuAm	Nucleus ambiguus	3	Otic
PSNu	Principal (chief) sensory nucleus	4	Terminal and/or intramural

---

Review of Blood Supply to TriMoNu, FacNu, DMNu, and NuAm and the Internal Course of Their Fibers

Structures	Arteries
TriMoNu and Trigeminal Root	Long circumferential branches of basilar (see Figure 6-21)
FacNu and Internal Genu	Long circumferential branches of basilar (see Figure 6-21)
DMNu and **NuAm**	Branches of vertebral and posterior inferior cerebellar (see Figure 6-14)

■ 8-23 Cranial Nerve Efferents (V, VII, IX, and X) in Anatomical Orientation ■

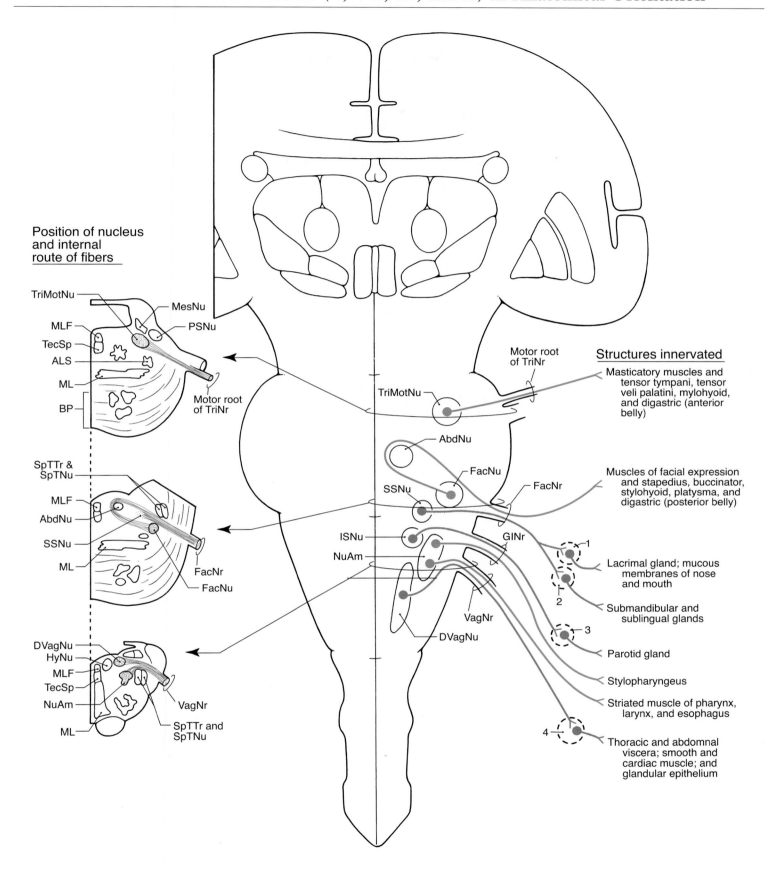

Position of nucleus
and internal
route of fibers

TriMotNu
MesNu
MLF
PSNu
TecSp
ALS
ML
BP
Motor root
of TriNr

SpTTr &
SpTNu
MLF
AbdNu
SSNu
ML
FacNr
FacNu

DVagNu
HyNu
MLF
TecSp
NuAm
VagNr
ML
SpTTr and
SpTNu

Motor root
of TriNr
TriMotNu
AbdNu
FacNu
SSNu
FacNr
ISNu
NuAm
GlNr
VagNr
DVagNu

Structures innervated

Masticatory muscles and
tensor tympani, tensor
veli palatini, mylohyoid,
and digastric (anterior
belly)

Muscles of facial expression
and stapedius, buccinator,
stylohyoid, platysma, and
digastric (posterior belly)

1

Lacrimal gland; mucous
membranes of nose
and mouth

2

Submandibular and
sublingual glands

3

Parotid gland

Stylopharyngeus

Striated muscle of pharynx,
larynx, and esophagus

4

Thoracic and abdomnal
viscera; smooth and
cardiac muscle; and
glandular epithelium

■ Cranial Nerve Efferents (V, VII, IX, and X) in Clinical Orientation ■

Masticatory muscles (including medail and lateral pterygoids), tensor tympani, tensor veli palatini, mylohyoid, digastric (anterior belly)

Trigeminal nerve

Basilar pons

Corticospinal (CSp) fibers

Middle cerebellar peduncle

Medial lemniscus (ML)

Principal sensory trigeminal nucleus

Anterolateral system (ALS)

Trigeminal motor nucleus

Fourth ventricle

Superior cerebellar peduncle

Pons-medulla junction

ML at pons-medulla junction

CSp fibers

Facial nucleus

Muscles of facial expression, stapedius, buccinator, stylohyoid, platysma, digastric (posterior belly)

ALS in medulla

Facial nerve

Spinal trigeminal tract (SpTTr) and nucleus (SpTNu)

Abducens nucleus

CSP fibers in pyramid

ML in medulla

Inferior olive
ALS in medulla

Stylopharyngeus muscle

Glossopharyngeal nerve

Nucleus ambiguus

Restiform body

SpTTr + SpTNu

ALS in medulla

ML in medulla

Striated muscles of pharynx, larynx, including vocalis muscle and of upper esophagus

Nucleus ambiguus

Vagus nerve

SpTTr + SpTNu

Nucleus ambiguus

Fourth ventricle

8-24A The nuclei and efferent fibers of CNs V, VII, IX, and X superimposed on MRI (brainstem, T2-weighted MRI) shown in clinical orientation. The red fibers correlate with those of the same color on Figure 8-23.

Cranial Nerve Efferents (V, VII, IX, and X) in Clinical Orientation: Representative Lesions and Deficits

Masticatory muscles (including medial and lateral pterygoids), tensor tympani, tensor veli palatini, mylohyoid, and digastric (anterior belly)

Trigeminal nerve

Basilar pons

Middle cerebellar peduncle

Principal sensory trigeminal nucleus

Trigeminal motor nucleus

Superior cerebellar peduncle

Damage to trigeminal root
• Paralysis of masticatory muscles on left and slight deviation of jaw to right on closure
• Left-sided loss of pain, thermal sense, and discriminative touch on face and in oral cavity (including teeth)
• Loss of afferent limb of corneal reflex on left

Irritation of trigeminal root
• Trigeminal neuralgia (tic douloureux) on left side of face

ML at pons–medulla junction

Pons–medulla junction

Facial nucleus

Muscles of facial expression, stapedius, buccinator, stylo-hyoid, platysma, and digastric (posterior belly)

Facial nerve

Abducens nucleus

Damage to facial root
• Paralysis of upper and lower facial muscles on left
• Left-sided loss of pain/thermal sensation on posterior surface of ear and part of auditory canal
• Loss of taste on anterior two thirds of tongue on left
• Decreased secretions of lacrimal, sublingual, and submaxillary glands and mucous membranes of mouth

Facial deficits from other causes
• Lesion of genu of internal capsule on right = left lower facial paralysis
• Lesion of right internal facial genu = paralysis of upper and lower facial muscles on right
• Irritation of facial root = facial tic on that side

CSP fibers in pyramid

ML in medulla

Stylopharyngeus muscle

Glossopharyngeal nerve

Nucleus ambiguus

SpTTr and SpTNu

Damage to roots of IX and X
• Left-sided loss of pain/thermal sense on tympanic membrane, external auditory meatus, and posterior ear (small)
• Loss of taste (not testable)
• Loss of sensation on tonsils, hard/soft palate, posterior pharyngeal wall, posterior/root of tongue, fauces, and eustachian tube opening
• Dysphagia, dysarthria, and hoarseness
• Glossopharyngeal neuralgia
• Loss of gag, palatal/uvular reflexes
• Lowering of left palatal arch, deviation of uvula to right on phonation

ALS in medulla

Striated muscles of pharynx, larynx, including vocalis ms. and ofand upper esophagus

Vagus nerve

Nucleus ambiguus

8-24B Representative lesions of the roots of CNs V, VII, IX, and X and the deficits that correlate with each lesion. Also indicated are deficits related to the fifth and seventh cranial nerves that may originate from other causes. Note that lesions of these cranial nerve roots result in motor deficits on the side of the lesion.

■ Spinal and Cranial Nerve Reflexes ■

Examining *reflexes* is an essential part of any neurological examination because it provides information critical to the diagnosis of the neurologically compromised patient. All reflexes have an *afferent limb* (usually a *primary sensory fiber* with a cell body in a ganglion) and an *efferent limb* (usually a fiber innervating skeletal muscle) originating from a motor nucleus. The afferent fiber may synapse directly on the efferent neuron, in which case it is a *monosynaptic reflex*, or there may be one, or more, interneurons insinuated between the afferent and efferent limbs; these are *polysynaptic reflexes*. In many reflexes, the influence on the motor neuron may be both monosynaptic and polysynaptic. In the case of cranial nerves, polysynaptic reflexes may also be mediated through the immediately adjacent reticular formation of the brainstem.

The *primary sensory fiber* is regarded as the *first-order neuron* in a pathway. Although the first-order neuron may participate in a reflex, it also contributes information to ascending pathways. The primary sensory fiber may synapse directly on a tract cell, or may communicate through interneurons. In either case, this *tract cell* is regarded as the *second order neuron* in the pathway.

Spinal reflexes may rely on *sensory/afferent* information that arises from the body, enters the spinal cord, influences lower motor neurons, and results in an appropriate response. The same principle applies to *cranial nerve reflexes*. The *afferent input* enters the brainstem on a cranial nerve and influences motor neurons, and the *efferent outflow* exits the brainstem on the same, or another, cranial nerve. Because of these structural/functional features, the reflex pathways are placed at this location in Chapter 8, following "Sensory and Motor Pathways and Cranial Nerves." The circuits for the more routinely tested reflexes are described; this is not intended as an all-inclusive list.

Particularly brisk or hyperactive reflexes, commonly demonstrated in muscle stretch reflexes, are specified as *hyperreflexia*. Decreased or hypoactive reflexes are described as *hyporeflexia*. A complete absence of reflex activity is *areflexia*. These deviations from normal may be seen in spinal reflexes as well as in cranial nerve reflexes. The aberrations from normal reflex activity may indicate peripheral nerve disease or injury/disease of the brainstem, spinal cord, or forebrain.

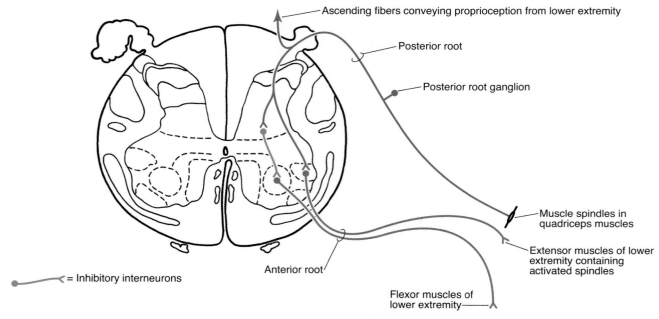

8-25   The *muscle stretch reflex* (also called a *stretch* or *myotatic reflex*) is sometimes called the *tendon reflex* or *deep tendon reflex* (these are actually misnomers); the receptor for this reflex is the *muscle spindle* (within the muscle itself, hence *muscle stretch*). The afferent limb is activated by tapping the tendon of a muscle and momentarily stretching *muscles spindles* (*primary* or *secondary*) within the muscle. These action potentials are propagated on *A-alpha* (*13–20 μm in diameter, 80–120 m/s conduction velocity*) or *A-beta* (*6–12 μm, 35–75 m/s*) *fibers*. Their cell bodies are in *posterior root ganglia*; these fibers *monosynaptically* excite motor neurons innervating the muscle from which the afferent volley

arose, and the muscle contracts, precipitating the reflex. Collaterals of the afferent axons synapse on interneurons that, in turn, inhibit motor neurons innervating antagonistic muscles.

Muscle stretch reflexes test the functional integrity of different spinal levels. Examples of these *reflexes*, and their corresponding levels are: *triceps (C7–C8), biceps (C5–C6), brachioradialis (C5–C6), Achilles/ankle jerk (S1), patellar/knee jerk (L2–L4),* and the *finger flexor (C7–C8)*. Concurrent with the reflex, the central processes send ascending collaterals that relay information to the *nuclei gracilis or cuneatus*, depending on the level of the input, and the sensation is perceived. The *patellar reflex* is shown here.

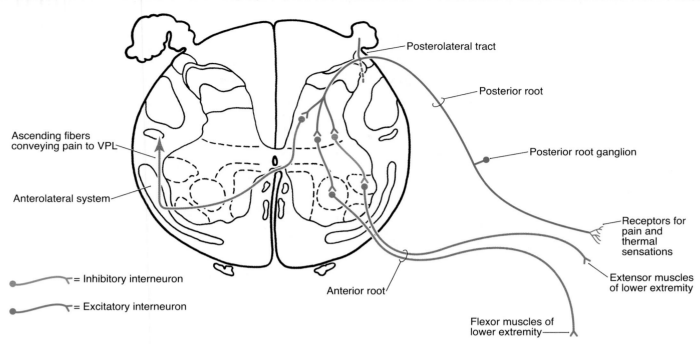

Labels for image 1:
- Posterolateral tract
- Posterior root
- Ascending fibers conveying pain to VPL
- Posterior root ganglion
- Anterolateral system
- Receptors for pain and thermal sensations
- = Inhibitory interneuron
- = Excitatory interneuron
- Extensor muscles of lower extremity
- Anterior root
- Flexor muscles of lower extremity

8-26 The *nociceptive reflex* (also called a *withdrawal reflex* or *flexor reflex*) is activated by tissue damage; action potentials are propagated on *A-delta (1–5 μm in diameter, 5–30 m/s conduction velocity)* and *C (0.2–5.0 μm, 0.5–2 m/s) fibers*. These afferent fibers have cell bodies in the *posterior root ganglion* and they terminate on *inhibitory* and/or *excitatory* spinal interneurons. When a patient steps on a nail, flexor motor neurons of the lower extremity are *excited*, extensor motor neurons of the LE are *inhibited*, and the extremity is pulled away from the noxious stimulus. The same arrangement of circuits applies when the hand encounters a noxious stimulus and the upper extremity is withdrawn. Concurrent with this reflex, the recognition of pain is achieved via second order neurons that ascend in the ALS of the spinal cord.

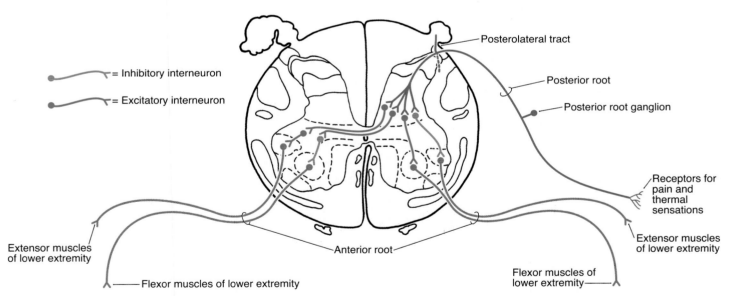

Labels for image 2:
- Posterolateral tract
- = Inhibitory interneuron
- = Excitatory interneuron
- Posterior root
- Posterior root ganglion
- Receptors for pain and thermal sensations
- Extensor muscles of lower extremity
- Extensor muscles of lower extremity
- Anterior root
- Flexor muscles of lower extremity
- Flexor muscles of lower extremity

8-27 The *crossed extension reflex* affects extremities on both sides of the body. The afferent fibers, their input to spinal interneurons, and their respective action (excitatory/inhibitory) on flexor and extensor spinal motor neurons *on the side of the noxious stimulus is the same as in the nociceptive reflex* (see Figure 8-26). The stimulus occurs and the extremity on that side is withdrawn. In an effort to maintain stability, when an injured foot is withdrawn on the side of the stimulus, the opposite LE is extended. Consequently, on the side opposite the stimulus, flexor motor neurons are *inhibited* and extensor motor neurons are *excited* and the relative posture of the patient is maintained. This reflex also gives rise to ascending information that reaches a conscious level of perception.

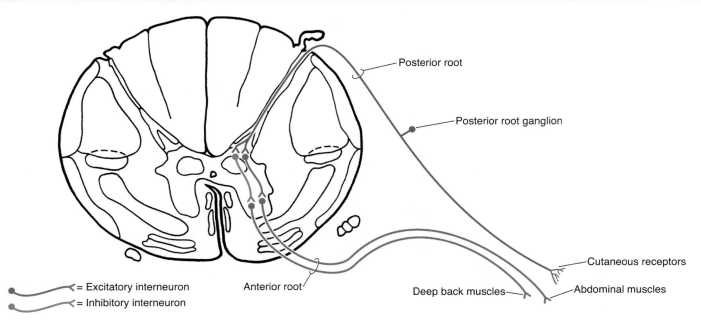

8-28 The *abdominal reflex* is a cutaneous reflex; the afferent limb arises from receptors on *A-delta and C fibers*. It is mediated through *lower thoracic spinal levels (T8–T11)* and is activated by lightly stroking the abdomen about 4–5 cm lateral to, and parallel with, the midline. The afferent fibers enter the *posterior root* and synapse on interneurons. Some of these are excitatory interneurons that, in turn, excite lower motor neurons that innervate the abdominal musculature; the muscles of the abdomen contract and the trunk flexes slightly. Other interneurons inhibit the alpha motor neurons that are innervating deep back muscles; inactivation of these motor neurons decreases the tension in the deep back muscles and increases the efficacy of the abdominal reflex. These deep back muscles extend the trunk. A normal response is occurring when the abdominal muscles contract and the umbilicus rotates slightly to the stimulated side. The sensations created by stroking the abdominal wall will also enter ascending spinal cord pathways and are consciously perceived.

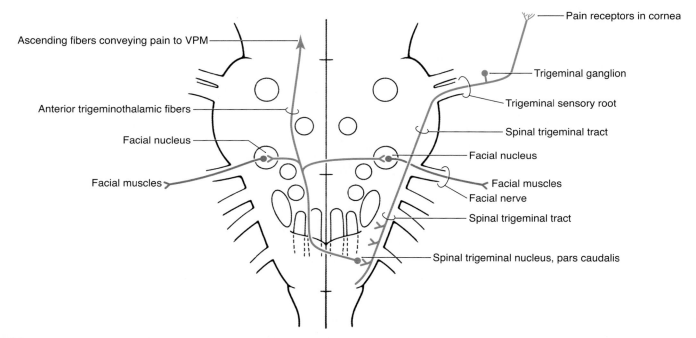

8-29 The *corneal reflex* (also called the *lid reflex*) has its afferent limb in the *trigeminal nerve* (CN V) and its efferent limb in the *facial nerve* (CN VII). An irritating stimulus to the cornea activates C fibers, the cell bodies of which are in the *trigeminal ganglion*. These axons enter the brainstem on the trigeminal nerve, descend in the *spinal trigeminal tract*, and terminate in the *spinal trigeminal nucleus, pars caudalis. Pars caudalis* neurons project to the contralateral *ventral posteromedial thalamic nucleus* and, en route, send collaterals to the *facial motor nucleus* bilaterally; the facial response is generally more active on the side of the stimulation. Axons of the motor neurons in the *facial nucleus* exit in the *facial nerve* to eventually exit the skull via the *stylomastoid foramen*. Axons in the *zygomatic branch of the facial nerve* innervate the *orbicularis oculi muscle* and the eyelids close in response to a noxious stimulus of the cornea. The noxious information being relayed via ascending fibers eventually reaches conscious perception via ascending fibers is the ALS.

8-30 The *jaw jerk reflex* (also called the *jaw jerk* or *mandibular reflex*) is a cranial nerve version of a spinal *muscle stretch reflex*; this reflex is mediated through the *trigeminal nerve* (CN V). The axons of the afferent limb synapse on the motor neurons that innervate skeletal muscles (it is a *monosynaptic reflex*). A gentle tap on the chin stretches *muscle spindles* in the *temporalis and masseter muscles*, initiating action potentials on *A-alpha (primary muscle spindles)* and *A-beta (secondary muscle spindles)* fibers. These fibers enter the brain on the *sensory root of the trigem-* *inal nerve*, and have their primary afferent cell bodies in the *mesencephalic nucleus*. Collaterals of these afferent fibers project directly, and bilaterally, to the *trigeminal motor nucleus*; axons of these motor cells exit via *the motor root of the trigeminal nerve* to innervate the *temporalis and masseter muscles*, resulting in jaw closure in response to the tap on the chin. This information also reaches a conscious level: the patient perceives the tap on the chin. The jaw-jerk reflex is often increased/brisk (*hyperreflexia*) in patients with amyotrophic lateral sclerosis.

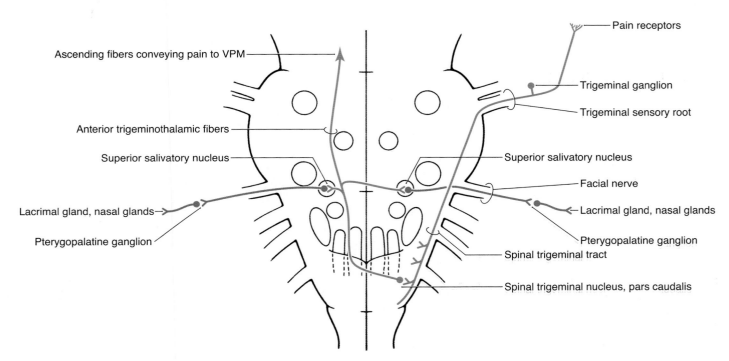

8-31 There are a variety of reflexes in which sensory input results in a visceral motor response. Examples are the *lacrimal (tearing)* and the *salivatory reflexes*. The *lacrimal reflex* is used here as an example of a *somato-visceral reflex*. The afferent limb is activated by stimulation of *C fibers* and *A-delta receptors/ fibers* in the cornea and sclera. This afferent message enters the brainstem on the *trigeminal nerve* (cell bodies in the *trigeminal ganglion*), descends within the *spinal trigeminal tract*, and synapses in the *spinal trigeminal nucleus, pars caudalis*. Collaterals of ascending *trigeminothalamic fibers* (en route to the ventral posteromedial thalamic nucleus) synapse in the *superior salivatory nucleus* (SSN) either directly (shown here) or through interneurons. Parasympathtic preganglionic fibers from the SSN exit on the *facial nerve*, travel to the *pterygopalatine ganglion*, where they synapse, and the postganglionic fibers course to the *lacrimal gland* and to *mucous membranes of the nose*. A nocuous stimulus to the cornea results in tearing and increased nasal secretions and the discomfort is perceived through ascending fibers that eventually influence the sensory cortex.

8-32 The *gag reflex* (also called the *faucial reflex)* is mediated through the *glossopharyngeal (CN IX)* and the *vagus (CN X)* nerves. The afferent limb is activated by cutaneous stimulation of *A-delta* and probably *C fibers* on the caudal base of the tongue and/or caudal roof of the mouth (soft palate). This space between the mouth and pharynx is the *fauces,* hence the term *faucial reflex.* The afferent limb is via CN IX with its cell bodies in the superior ganglion of CN IX; the central terminations are in the *nucleus ambiguus,* either directly or through interneurons (both shown here). The efferent limb from the *nucleus ambiguus* travels on CNs IX and X to the *stylopharyngeous muscle* (via IX), to the *pharyngeal constricter muscles,* and to *muscles that move the palate* (via X). In response to irritation in the caudal oral cavity, the pharynx constricts and elevates in an attempt to extrude the offending object, and the discomfort is perceived through pathways to the cerebral cortex.

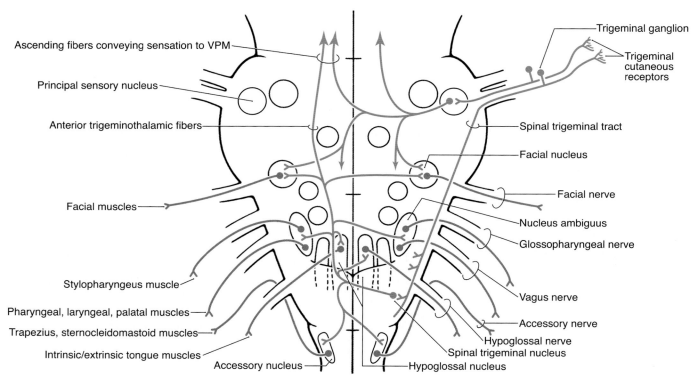

8-33 There are a variety of reflexes seen in infants mediated by CNs V, VII, IX, or XI and XII. Examples of these are the *snout, sucking,* and *rooting reflexes;* they usually disappear by about 1 year of age. These are commonly referred to as "primitive reflexes." However, these reflexes may reappear in patients with dementia, or in individuals with degenerative diseases, or dysfunction, of the frontal lobe.

The afferent limb for these reflexes is via CN V and is activated by touching around (snout, rooting), or in (sucking), the mouth opening. These afferent fibers enter the brainstem via CN V and have cell bodies in the *trigeminal ganglion.* They terminate in the *spinal trigeminal nucleus* (information relayed on *A-delta fibers* from *free nerve endings*) and in the *principal sensory nucleus* (information relayed on *A-beta fibers* from endings such as *Meissner corpuscles* and *Merkel cell complexes*).

Secondary trigeminal fibers, en route to the *ventral posteromedial nucleus* of the thalamus from both the *spinal trigeminal* and *principal sensory nuclei,* send collaterals to the *facial nucleus,* the *nucleus ambiguus,* the *accessory nucleus,* and the *hypoglossal nucleus,* either directly, or via interneurons located in the reticular formation (only the direct are shown here). In response to stimulation around, or in, the mouth opening, the infant's facial muscles respond (via the facial nucleus), the head orients toward or away from the source of the stimulus (accessory nucleus), the laryngeal and pharyngeal muscles contract during sucking (nucleus ambiguus), and the tongue moves in and out of the mouth or protrudes toward the stimulus (hypoglossal nucleus). These reflexes are absolutely essential to survival (orienting toward nutrition, sucking, tongue and facial muscle responses).

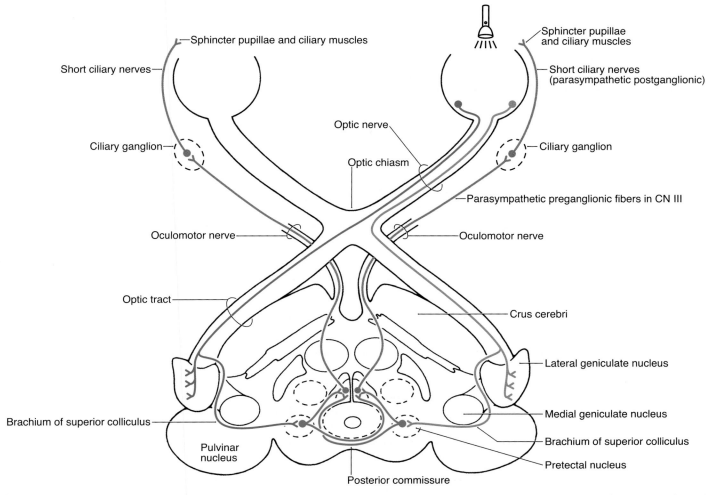

Short ciliary nerves—

—Sphincter pupillae and ciliary muscles

Sphincter pupillae
and ciliary muscles

Short ciliary nerves
(parasympathetic postganglionic)

Ciliary ganglion—

Optic nerve

Optic chiasm

Ciliary ganglion

Parasympathetic preganglionic fibers in CN III

Oculomotor nerve—

Oculomotor nerve

Optic tract—

Crus cerebri

Lateral geniculate nucleus

Medial geniculate nucleus

Brachium of superior colliculus—

Brachium of superior colliculus

Pulvinar
nucleus

Pretectal nucleus

Posterior commissure

8-34 The *pupillary light reflex* (also called the *pupillary reflex* or *light reflex*) has its afferent limb in the *optic nerve* (CN II) and its efferent limb in the *oculomotor nerve* (CN III). Light shined in the eye results in neural activity conveyed on fibers of the *optic nerve, optic chiasm* (where some cross), *optic tract,* and the *brachium of the superior colliculus,* which synapse bilaterally in the *pretectal area/nucleus.* Both pretectal areas project bilaterally to the *Edinger-Wesphal (E-W) nucleus.* The E-W nucleus sends *parasympathetic preganglionic fibers* on the oculomotor nerve to the *ciliary ganglion,* which in turn sends *postganglionic fibers,* as *short ciliary* nerves, to the *sphincter pupillae muscle* of the iris. In the normal patient, light shined in one eye will result in a pupillary reflex in that eye (*direct response*) and in the opposite eye (*consensual response*).

Example One: In the case of a lesion of the optic nerve and the light is shined in the eye on the lesioned side: this patient perceives no light in that eye, and both the direct and consensual papillary responses are absent; *the afferent limb is interrupted.* In this example, there is no input to either pretectal area.

Example Two: In the case of a lesion of one optic nerve and the light is shined in the eye opposite the side of the lesion: this patient perceives light, and there is both a direct and consensual response. In this example, the *afferent limb to both pretectal nuclei is intact* and there is a response in the blind eye because its efferent limb is intact.

Example Three: In the case of a lesion of the oculomotor nerve on one side, light shined in the eye on the lesioned side will be perceived and will result in a consensual response, but no direct response; *the efferent limb is interrupted.* If the light is shined in the eye on the side opposite the oculomotor root lesion, the light is perceived, and there is a direct response but no consensual response.

Table 8-1 Flow Diagrams of Additional Common Reflexes*

Sneezing

Receptors in nasal membranes → Cell bodies in trigeminal ganglion → Projection to spinal trigeminal nucleus → Trigeminal projection to nucleus ambiguus (NuAmb) and reticular formation (RetFor)

NuAmb and RetFor to phrenic nucleus and anterior horn cells → Phrenic nucleus to diaphragm and anterior horn cells to intercostal muscles → Patient sneezes

Vomiting

Receptors in the pharynx and gut, travel via the vagus and splanchnic → Cell bodies in inferior vagal and posterior root ganglia → Projection to solitary nucleus (SolNu), dorsal motor vagal nucleus (DVagNu)

SolNu and DVagNu project to RetFor and to intramural ganglia via DVagNu → Reticulospinal fibers to intermediolateral cell column (IMLCC), to phrenic nucleus, and anterior horn cells → IMLCC projects to sympathetic preganglionic cells, DVagNu to preganglionic parasympathetic cells, phrenic nucleus to diaphragm, and anterior horn cells to intercostal muscles

Smooth muscles of gut activated; intercostal muscles and diaphragm activated → Patient vomits (Note: Gag reflex may proceed to a vomiting reflex)

Swallowing

Receptors in larynx and pharynx → Cell bodies in inferior ganglia of CNs IX and X → Project to DVagNu and SolNu; SolNu projects to DVagNu

DVagNu projects to intramural ganglia in esophagus → Contraction along length of esophagus → Patient swallows

Baroreceptor

Receptors in carotid body and aortic arch → Cell bodies in inferior ganglia of CNs IX and X → Projects to SolNu; SolNu projects to DVagNu and to vasopressor neurons in medulla (VaPress)

VaPress projects to IMLCC via reticulospinal fibers (DVagNu activity is decreased, while sympathetic activity is increased) → IMLCC projects to postganglionic cells serving heart and peripheral vessels

Peripheral vascular tone and cardiac rate and output increased → Patient's blood pressure and cardiac output maintained upon rising from a recumbent position

Vagovagal

Vagal receptors may be in airway, thorax, and abdomen (may be mechanical stimulation) → Cell bodies in inferior ganglia of CN X → Projects to SolNu

SolNu projects to DVagNu → DVagNu projects to intramural ganglion in thoracic and abdominal viscera → Postganglionic parasympathetic fiber activation results in vagal cardioinhibition

Patient experiences bradycardia, hypotension, pallor, and light-headedness

* All of these reflexes are mediated through the brainstem. As is the case with brainstem reflexes, the pathways may involve several centers, or nuclei, within the brainstem; only the basic pathways are diagrammed here.

■ Blank Drawing for the Spinal Cord and Brainstem ■

8-35 Blank master drawings for spinal cord and cranial nerve/brainstem reflexes. These illustrations are provided for self-evaluation of the understanding of circuits related to reflexes, for the instructor to expand on reflexes not covered in this atlas, or for both activities. To provide for a wider variety of review possibilities, a cervical spinal cord level and brainstem diagram is provided here.

■ Spinocerebellar Tracts in Anatomical Orientation ■

8-36 The origin, course, and distribution pattern of fibers to the cerebellar cortex and nuclei from the spinal cord (posterior [dorsal] and anterior [ventral] spinocerebellar tracts, rostral spinocerebellar fibers) and from the accessory (lateral) cuneate nucleus (cuneocerebellar fibers). Also illustrated is the somatotopy of those fibers originating from the spinal cord. These fibers enter the cerebellum via the restiform body, the larger portion of the inferior cerebellar peduncle, or in relationship to the superior cerebellar peduncle. After these fibers enter the cerebellum, collaterals are given off to the cerebellar nuclei while the parent axons of spinocerebellar and cuneocerebellar fibers pass on to the cortex, where they end as mossy fibers in the granule cell layer. Although not shown here, there are important ascending spinal projections to the medial and dorsal accessory nuclei of the inferior olivary complex (spino-olivary fibers). The accessory olivary nuclei (as well as the principal olivary nucleus) project to the cerebellar cortex and send collaterals into the nuclei (see Figure 8-26 on p. 225).

Neurotransmitters

Glutamate (+) is found in some spinocerebellar fibers, in their mossy fiber terminals in the cerebellar cortex, and in their collateral branches that innervate the cerebellar nuclei.

Clinical Correlations

Lesions, or tumors, that selectively damage only spinocerebellar fibers are rarely, if ever, seen in humans. The *ataxia* one might expect to see in patients with a spinal cord hemisection (e.g., the *Brown-Séquard syndrome*) is masked by the *hemiplegia* resulting from the concomitant damage to lateral corticospinal (and other) fibers.

Friedreich ataxia (hereditary spinal ataxia) is an autosomal recessive disorder, the symptoms of which usually appear between 8 and 15 years of age. There is degeneration of anterior and posterior spinocerebellar tracts plus the posterior columns and corticospinal tracts. Degenerative changes are also seen in Purkinje cells in the cerebellum, in posterior root ganglion cells, in neurons of the Clarke column, and in some nuclei of the pons and medulla. These patients have *ataxia, dysarthria,* muscle weakness/paralysis (particularly in the LEs), and skeletal defects. The axial and appendicular *ataxia* seen in these patients correlates partially with the spinocerebellar degeneration and also partially with proprioceptive losses via the degeneration of posterior column fibers.

ABBREVIATIONS

ACNu	Accessory (lateral) cuneate nucleus	**PSNu**	Principal (chief) sensory nucleus of trigeminal nerve
ALS	Anterolateral system	**Py**	Pyramid
AMV	Anterior medullary velum	**RB**	Restiform body
ASCT	Anterior (ventral) spinocerebellar tract	**RSCF**	Rostral spinocerebellar fibers
Cbl	Cerebellum	**RuSp**	Rubrospinal tract
CblNu	Cerebellar nuclei	**S**	Sacral representation
CCblF	Cuneocerebellar fibers	**SBC**	Spinal border cells
DNuC	Dorsal nucleus of Clarke	**SCP**	Superior cerebellar peduncle
FNL	Flocculonodular lobe	**SpTNu**	Spinal trigeminal nucleus
IZ	Intermediate zone	**SpTTr**	Spinal trigeminal tract
L	Lumbar representation	**T**	Thoracic representation
MesNu	Mesencephalic nucleus	**TriMoNu**	Trigeminal motor nucleus
ML	Medial lemniscus	**VesNu**	Vestibular nuclei
PRG	Posterior (dorsal) root ganglion		
PSCT	Posterior (dorsal) spinocerebellar tract		

Review of Blood Supply to Spinal Cord Gray Matter, Spinocerebellar Tracts, RB, and SCP

Structures	Arteries
Spinal Cord Gray	Branches of central artery (see Figure 6-6)
PSCT and **ASCT** in Cord	Penetrating branches of arterial vasocorona (see Figure 6-6)
RB	Posterior inferior cerebellar (see Figure 6-14)
SCP	Long circumferential branches of basilar and superior cerebellar (see Figure 6-21)
Cerebellum	Posterior and anterior inferior cerebellar and superior cerebellar

■ 8-36 Spinocerebellar Tracts in Anatomical Orientation ■

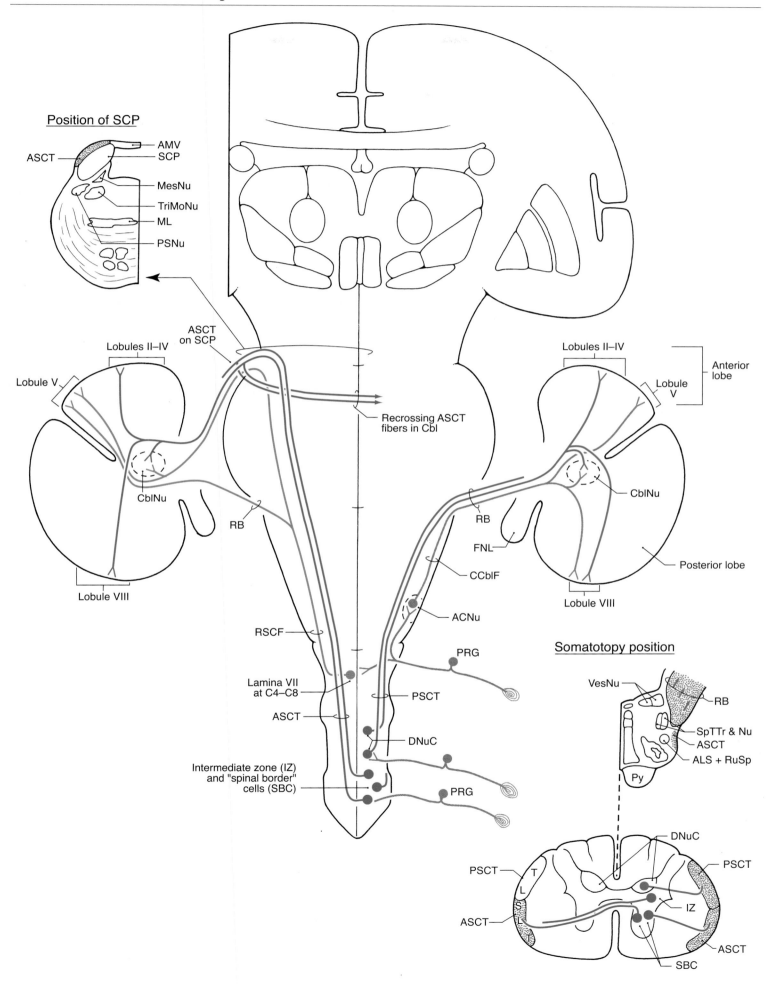

Position of SCP

ASCT — AMV
SCP
MesNu
TriMoNu
ML
PSNu

ASCT on SCP

Lobules II–IV
Lobule V
Recrossing ASCT fibers in Cbl
CblNu
RB
Lobule VIII

Lobules II–IV
Anterior lobe
Lobule V
CblNu
RB
FNL
Posterior lobe
CCblF
Lobule VIII

ACNu
PRG
RSCF
PSCT
Lamina VII at C4–C8
ASCT
DNuC
Intermediate zone (IZ) and "spinal border" cells (SBC)
PRG

Somatotopy position

VesNu
RB
SpTTr & Nu
ASCT
ALS + RuSp
Py

DNuC
PSCT
PSCT
T
L
S
L
T
IZ
ASCT
ASCT
SBC

■ Pontocerebellar, Reticulocerebellar, Olivocerebellar, Ceruleocerebellar, Hypothalamocerebellar, and Raphecerebellar Fibers in Anatomical Orientation ■

8-37 Afferent fibers to the cerebellum from selected brainstem areas and the organization of corticopontine fibers in the internal capsule and crus cerebri as shown here. Pontocerebellar axons are mainly crossed, reticulocerebellar fibers may be bilateral (from RetTegNu) or mainly uncrossed (from LRNu and PRNu), and olivocerebellar fibers (OCblF) are exclusively crossed. Raphecerebellar, hypothalamocerebellar, and ceruleocerebellar fibers are, to varying degrees, bilateral projections. Although all afferent fibers to the cerebellum give rise to collaterals to the cerebellar nuclei, those from pontocerebellar axons are relatively small, having comparatively small diameters. Olivocerebellar axons end as climbing fibers, reticulocerebellar and pontocerebellar fibers as mossy fibers, and hypothalamocerebellar and ceruleocerebellar axons end in all cortical layers. These latter fibers have been called multilayered fibers in the literature because they branch in all layers of the cerebellar cortex.

Neurotransmitters

Glutamate (+) is found in corticopontine projections and in most pontocerebellar fibers. Aspartate (+) and corticotropin (+)-releasing factor are present in many olivocerebellar fibers. Ceruleocerebellar fibers contain noradrenalin, histamine is found in hypothalamocerebellar fibers, and some reticulocerebellar fibers contain enkephalin. Serotonergic fibers to the cerebellum arise from neurons found in medial areas of the reticular formation (open gray cell in Figure 8-37 on the facing page) and, most likely, from some cells in the adjacent raphe nuclei.

Clinical Correlations

Common symptoms seen in patients with lesions involving nuclei and tracts that project to the cerebellum are *ataxia* (of trunk or limbs), an *ataxic gait, dysarthria, dysphagia,* and disorders of eye movement such as *nystagmus.* These deficits are seen in some hereditary diseases (e.g., *olivopontocerebellar degeneration, ataxia telangiectasia,* or *hereditary cerebellar ataxia*), in tumors (brainstem gliomas), in vascular diseases *(lateral pontine syndrome),* or in other conditions, such as *alcoholic cerebellar degeneration* or pontine hemorrhages (see Figures 8-38 and 8-40B on pp. 242 and 247 for more information on cerebellar lesions).

ABBREVIATIONS

AntLb	Anterior limb of internal capsule	PonNu	Pontine nuclei
CblNu	Cerebellar nuclei	PO	Principal olivary nucleus
CerCblF	Ceruleocerebellar fibers	PPon	Parietopontine fibers
CPonF	Cerebropontine fibers	PRNu	Paramedian reticular nuclei
CSp	Corticospinal fibers	Py	Pyramid
DAO	Dorsal accessory olivary nucleus	RB	Restiform body
FPon	Frontopontine fibers	RCblF	Reticulocerebellar fibers
Hyth	Hypothalamus	RetLenLb	Retrolenticular limb of internal capsule
HythCblF	Hypothalamocerebellar fibers	RNu	Red nucleus
IC	Internal capsule	RetTegNu	Reticulotegmental nucleus
IO	Inferior olive	SCP	Superior cerebellar peduncle
LoCer	Nucleus (locus) ceruleus	SubLenLb	Sublenticular limb of internal capsule
LRNu	Lateral reticular nucleus	SN	Substantia nigra
MAO	Medial accessory olivary nucleus	TPon	Temporopontine fibers
MCP	Middle cerebellar peduncle		
ML	Medial lemniscus		
NuRa	Raphe nuclei		**Number Key**
OCblF	Olivocerebellar fibers		
OPon	Occipitopontine fibers	1	Nucleus raphe, pontis
PCblF	Pontocerebellar fibers	2	Nucleus raphe, magnus
PostLb	Posterior limb of internal capsule	3	Raphecerebellar fibers

---

Review of Blood Supply to Precerebellar Relay Nuclei in Pons and Medulla, MCP, and RB	
Structures	**Arteries**
Pontine Tegmentum	Long circumferential branches of basilar plus some from superior cerebellar (see Figure 6-21)
Basilar Pons	Paramedian and short circumferential branches of basilar (see Figure 6-21)
Medulla **RetF** and **IO**	Branches of vertebral and posterior inferior cerebellar (see Figure 6-14)
MCP	Long circumferential branches of basilar and branches of anterior inferior and superior cerebellar (see Figure 6-21)
RB	Posterior inferior cerebellar (see Figure 6-14)

■ 8-37 Pontocerebellar, Reticulocerebellar, Olivocerebellar, Ceruleocerebellar, Hypothalamocerebellar, and Raphecerebellar Fibers in Anatomical Orientation ■

Position of associated tracts and nuclei

AntLb (FPon)
PostLb (PPon)
SubLenLb (TPon)
RetLenLb (OPon)
IC

ML
RNu
SN
PPon OPon TPon
FPon

NuRa
RetTegNu
MCP
ML
CPonF
CSp
PonNu

PRNu
OCblF
PO
Py
RB
LRNu

Hyth
CPonF
HythCblF   LoCer
RetTegNu   CerCblF
SCP
MCP
1
PonNu
PCblF
2   3
OCblF
DAO   CblNu
RB
RCblF
PO
MAO
LRNu
PRNu

OCblF
PCblF   CerCblF

■ Cerebellar Corticonuclear, Nucleocortical, and Corticovestibular Fibers in Anatomical Orientation ■

8-38 Cerebellar corticonuclear fibers arise from all regions of the cortex and terminate in an orderly (mediolateral and rostrocaudal) sequence in the ipsilateral cerebellar nuclei. For example, corticonuclear fibers from the vermal cortex terminate in the fastigial nucleus, those from the intermediate cortex terminate in the emboliform and globosus nuclei, and those from the lateral cortex terminate in the dentate nucleus. Also, cerebellar corticonuclear fibers from the anterior lobe typically terminate in more rostral regions of these nuclei whereas those from the posterior lobe terminate more caudally. Cerebellar corticovestibular fibers originate primarily from the vermis and flocculonodular lobe, exit the cerebellum via the juxtarestiform body, and end in the ipsilateral vestibular nuclei. Corticonuclear and corticovestibular fibers arise from Purkinje cells.

Nucleocortical processes originate from cerebellar nuclear neurons and pass to the overlying cortex in a pattern that basically reciprocates that of the corticonuclear projection; they end as mossy fibers. Some nucleocortical fibers are collaterals of cerebellar efferent axons. The cerebellar cortex may influence the activity of lower motor neurons through many combinations of circuits, for example, the cerebellovestibular–vestibulospinal route.

Neurotransmitters

γ-Aminobutyric acid (GABA) (−) is found in Purkinje cells and is the principal transmitter substance present in cerebellar corticonuclear and corticovestibular projections. However, taurine (−) and motilin (−) are also found in some Purkinje cells. GABA-ergic terminals are numerous in the cerebellar nuclei and vestibular complex. Some of the glutamate-containing mossy fibers in the cerebellar cortex represent the endings of nucleocortical fibers that originate from cells in the cerebellar nuclei.

Clinical Correlations

Numerous disease entities can result in cerebellar dysfunction, including viral infections *(echovirus)*, hereditary diseases (see Figure 8-37), trauma, tumors *(glioma, medulloblastoma)*, occlusion of cerebellar arteries (cerebellar stroke), *arteriovenous malformation* of cerebellar vessels, developmental errors (e.g., the *Dandy-Walker syndrome* or the *Arnold-Chiari deformity*), or the intake of toxins. Usually, damage to only the cortex results in transient deficits unless the lesion is quite large or causes an increase in intracranial pressure. However, lesions involving both the cortex and nuclei, or only the nuclei, will result in long-term deficits.

Lesions involving midline structures (vermal cortex, fastigial nuclei) and/or the flocculonodular lobe result in *truncal ataxia (titubation* or *tremor)*, *nystagmus*, and head tilting. These patients also may have a wide-based *(cerebellar) gait*, are unable to walk in tandem (heel to toe), and may be unable to walk on their heels or on their toes. Generally, midline lesions result in bilateral motor deficits affecting axial and proximal limb musculature.

Damage to the intermediate and lateral cortices and the globose, emboliform, and dentate nuclei results in various combinations of the following deficits: *dysarthria, dysmetria (hypometria, hypermetria), dysdiadochokinesia, tremor (static, kinetic, intention), rebound phenomenon*, unsteady and wide-based *(cerebellar) gait*, and *nystagmus*. One of the more commonly observed deficits in patients with cerebellar lesions is an *intention tremor*, which is best seen in the *finger-nose test*. The *finger-to-finger test* is also used to demonstrate an intention tremor and to assess cerebellar function. The *heel-to-shin test* will show *dysmetria* in the lower extremity. If the heel-to-shin test is normal in a patient with his or her eyes open, the cerebellum is intact. If this test is repeated in the same patient with eyes closed and is abnormal, this would suggest a lesion in the posterior column–medial lemniscus system.

Cerebellar damage in intermittent and lateral areas (nuclei or cortex plus nuclei) causes movement disorders on the side of the lesion with ataxia and gait problems on that side; the patient may tend to fall toward the side of the lesion. This is because the cerebellar nuclei project to the contralateral thalamus, which projects to the motor cortex on the same side, which projects to the contralateral side of the spinal cord via the corticospinal tract. Other circuits (cerebellorubral–rubrospinal) and feedback loops (cerebello-olivary–olivocerebellar) follow similar routes. Consequently, the motor expression of unilateral cerebellar damage is toward the lesioned side because of these doubly crossed pathways.

Lesions of cerebellar efferent fibers, after they cross the midline in the decussation of the superior cerebellar peduncle, will give rise to motor deficits on the side of the body (excluding the head) contralateral to the lesion. This is seen in midbrain lesions such as the *Claude syndrome*.

ABBREVIATIONS

CorNu	Corticonuclear fibers	MLF	Medial longitudinal fasciculus
CorVes	Corticovestibular fibers	MVesSp	Medial vestibulospinal tract
Flo	Flocculus	MVNu	Medial vestibular nucleus
IC	Intermediate cortex	NL, par	Lateral cerebellar nucleus, parvocellular region
InfVesNu	Inferior (spinal) vestibular nucleus	NM, par	Medial cerebellar nucleus, parvocellular region
JRB	Juxtarestiform body	NuCor	Nucleocortical fibers
LC	Lateral cortex	SVNu	Superior vestibular nucleus
LVesSp	Lateral vestibulospinal tract	VC	Vermal cortex
LVNu	Lateral vestibular nucleus		

Review of Blood Supply to Cerebellum and Vestibular Nuclei

Structures	Arteries
Cerebellar Cortex	Branches of posterior and anterior inferior cerebellar and superior cerebellar
Cerebellar Nuclei	Anterior inferior cerebellar and superior cerebellar
Vestibular Nuclei	Posterior inferior cerebellar in medulla, long circumferential branches of basilar in pons

■ 8-38 Cerebellar Corticonuclear, Nucleocortical, and Corticovestibular
Fibers in Anatomical Orientation ■

Cerebellar Nuclei
1= Medial (fastigial)
2= Posterior interposed (globose)
3= Anterior interposed (emboliform)
4= Lateral (dentate)

■ Cerebellar Efferent Fibers in Anatomical Orientation ■

8-39 The origin, course, topography, and general distribution of fibers arising in the cerebellar nuclei. Cerebellofugal fibers project to several thalamic areas (VL and VA), to intralaminar relay nuclei in addition to the centromedian, and a number of midbrain, pontine, and medullary targets. Most of the latter nuclei project back to the cerebellum (e.g., reticulocerebellar, pontocerebellar), some in a highly organized manner. For example, cerebello-olivary fibers from the dentate nucleus (DNu) project to the principal olivary nucleus (PO), and neurons of the PO send their axons back to the lateral cerebellar cortex, with collaterals going to the DNu.

The cerebellar nuclei can influence motor activity through, as examples, the following routes: 1) cerebellorubral-rubrospinal; 2) cerebelloreticular-reticulospinal; 3) cerebellothalamic-thalamocortical-corticospinal; and 4) others. In addition, some direct cerebellospinal fibers arise in the fastigial nucleus as well as in the interposed nuclei.

Neurotransmitters

Many cells in the cerebellar nuclei contain glutamate (+), aspartate (+), or γ-aminobutyric acid (−). Glutamate and aspartate are found in cerebellorubral and cerebellothalamic fibers, whereas some GABA-containing cells give rise to cerebellopontine and cerebello-olivary fibers. Some cerebelloreticular projections also may contain GABA.

Clinical Correlations

Lesions of the cerebellar nuclei result in a range of motor deficits depending on the location of the injury. Many of these are described in Figures 8-38 and 8-40B on pp. 242 and 247, respectively.

ABBREVIATIONS

ALS	Anterolateral system
AMV	Anterior medullary velum
BP	Basilar pons
CblOl	Cerebello-olivary fibers
CblTh	Cerebellothalamic fibers
CblRu	Cerebellorubral fibers
CC	Crus cerebri
CeGy	Central gray (periaqueductal gray)
CM	Centromedian nucleus of thalamus
CSp	Corticospinal fibers
DAO	Dorsal accessory olivary nucleus
DNu	Dentate nucleus (lateral cerebellar nucleus)
ENu	Emboliform nucleus (anterior interposed cerebellar nucleus)
EWpgNu	Edinger-Westphal preganglionic nucleus
FNu	Fastigial nucleus (medial cerebellar nucleus)
GNu	Globose nucleus (posterior interposed cerebellar nucleus)
IC	Inferior colliculus
InfVNu	Inferior (spinal) vestibular nucleus
INu	Interstitial nucleus
LRNu	Lateral reticular nucleus
LVNu	Lateral vestibular nucleus
MAO	Medial accessory olivary nucleus
ML	Medial lemniscus
MLF	Medial longitudinal fasciculus
MVNu	Medial vestibular nucleus
NuDark	Nucleus of Darkschewitsch

OcNu	Oculomotor nucleus
PO	Principal olivary nucleus
PonNu	Pontine nuclei
RetForm	Reticular formation
RNu	Red nucleus
RuSp	Rubrospinal tract
SC	Superior colliculus
SCP	Superior cerebellar peduncle
SCP,Dec	Superior cerebellar peduncle, decussation
SN	Substantia nigra
SVNu	Superior vestibular nucleus
ThCor	Thalamocortical fibers
ThFas	Thalamic fasciculus
TriMoNu	Trigeminal motor nucleus
VL	Ventral lateral nucleus of thalamus
VPL	Ventral posterolateral nucleus of thalamus
VSCT	Ventral spinocerebellar tract
ZI	Zona incerta

Number Key

1 Ascending projections to superior colliculus, and possibly ventral lateral and ventromedial thalamic nuclei
2 Descending crossed fibers from superior cerebellar peduncle
3 Uncinate fasciculus (of Russell)
4 Juxtarestiform body to vestibular nuclei
5 Reticular formation

Review of Blood Supply to Cerebellar Nuclei and Their Principal Efferent Pathways

Structures	Arteries
Cerebellar Nuclei	Anterior inferior cerebellar and superior cerebellar
SCP	Long circumferential branches of basilar and superior cerebellar (see Figure 6-21)
Midbrain Tegmentum (RNu, CblTh, CblRu, OcNu)	Paramedian branches of basilar bifurcation, short circumferential branches of posterior cerebral, branches of superior cerebellar (see Figure 6-27)
VPL, CM, VL, VA	Thalamogeniculate branches of posterior cerebral, thalamo-perforating branches of the posteromedial group of posterior cerebral (see Figure 6-38)
IC	Lateral striate branches of middle cerebral (see Figure 6-38)

■ 8-39 Cerebellar Efferent Fibers in Anatomical Orientation ■

Motor cortex

CSp

VL

ThCor

CM

VPL

ThFas
ZI

Position of SCP,
CblTh, and CblRu

NuDark, INu,
OcNu, EWpgNu

RNu

CeGy

SCP

1

CeGy   SC

ML

RNu   CblTh and
CblRu

SN
CC

2

RetForm

3

4

PonNu

DNu

FNu

SVNu

5

ENu
GNu

LVNu

InfVNu

MVNu

CblOl

5

LRNu

5

DAO

PO

MAO

Cerebellospinal
fibers

5

IC

MLF
ML

SN

SCP,Dec

VSCT   AMV

SCP

TriMoNu
ALS and RuSp
ML

BP

■ Cerebellar Efferent Fibers in Clinical Orientation ■

Body of caudate nucleus

Posterior limb of internal capsule

Red nucleus

Decussation of the superior cerebellar peduncle

Superior cerebellar peduncle

Reticular formation

Cerebellar efferent fibers forming the superior cerebellar peduncle

Dentate nucleus

Emboliform nucleus

Globose nucleus

Fastigial nucleus

Cerebral cortex (motor area)

Corticospinal fiber

Thalamocortical fiber

Ventral lateral nucleus (pars caudalis)

Thalamic fasciculus

Red nucleus

Corticospinal fiber in crus cerebri

Cerebellothalamic fibers (also cerebellorubral fibers)

Crossed descending cerebellar projections to pons and medulla

Juxtarestiform body (JRB)

Dentate nucleus

Emboliform nucleus

Globose nucleus

Fastigial nucleus

JRB

Principal oilvary nucleus

Dorsal accessory olivary nucleus

Medial accessory olivary nucleus

8-40A Efferent fibers of the cerebellar nuclei superimposed on MRI (brainstem and forebrain, T2-weighted images) showing their origin, location, and trajectory in a clinical orientation. The blue, gray, and green fibers are shown arising in the right cerebellar nuclei, crossing in the decussation of the superior cerebellar peduncle, and after decussating, they either descend or ascend to various brainstem and thalamic targets. The red fibers originating in the fastigial nucleus project bilaterally to various nuclei of the brainstem and, in much lesser numbers, to select thalamic nuclei. The blue, gray, green, and red fibers correlate with those of the same color in Figure 8-28.

■ Cerebellar Efferent Fibers in Clinical Orientation: Representative Lesions and Deficits ■

Body of caudate nucleus

Cerebral cortex (motor area)

Corticospinal fiber

Thalamocortical fiber

Ventral lateral nucleus (pars caudalis)

Midbrain lesion
-Involves red nucleus, root of third nerve, cerebellothalamic fibers (Claude syndrome)
-Right-sided oculomotor paralysis
-Hyperkinesia/tremor (red nucleus) and akinesia (substantia nigra) on left
-Left-sided cerebellar tremor
-Possible left-sided proprioceptive loss

Thalamic fasciculus

Red nucleus

Corticospinal fiber in crus cerebri

Superior cerebellar peduncle

Cerebellothalamic fibers (also cerebellorubral fibers)

Crossed descending cerebellar projections to pons and medulla)

Reticular formation

Cerebellar efferent fibers forming the superior cerebellar peduncle

JRB

Cortex + nuclei lesion
-Left-sided intention tremor (finger-nose test)
-Dyssynergia, ataxia, hypotonia, unsteady gait
-Dysdiadochokinesia
-Rebound phenomenon
-Dysmetria (heel-to-shin test) (also hypermetria/hypometria)
-Dysarthria, nystagmus, static tremor
-Lesion on left = deficits on left

Dentate nucleus

Emboliform nucleus

Globose nucleus

Cortex lesion only
-Ataxia, tremor (static/kinetic), unsteady gait, dysmetria
-Lesion on left = deficits on left
-Deficits usually transient, full recovery commonly seen

Midline lesion
-Lesion usually bilateral
-Truncal ataxia, wide-based stance
-Unable to walk-in-tandem or on heels or on toes
-Titubation, nystagmus

Principal oilvary nucleus

Dorsal accessory olivary nucleus

Medial accessory olivary nucleus

8-40B Representative lesions of the cerebellum and of cerebellothalamic fibers in the midbrain (and the adjacent red nucleus) and the deficits that correlate with each lesion. It is important to remember that the motor deficits seen in patients with cerebellar lesions are expressed through the corticospinal tract. Consequently, if a lesion is proximal to the decussation of the supe-rior cerebellar peduncle, the deficits are ipsilateral to the lesion; if a lesion is distal to the decussation, the deficits are on the contralat-eral side. Note that the laterality (R/L) of the deficits is determined by whether the lesion is on the left or right side of the MRI; this reinforces important clinical concepts. For additional information on deficits related to cerebellar lesions see Figure 8-38 on p. 242.

■ Blank Master Drawing for Efferent Cerebellar Connections ■

8-41 Blank master drawing for pathways projecting to the cerebellar cortex, and for efferent projections of cerebellar nuclei. This illustration is provided for self-evaluation of understanding of pathways to the cerebellar cortex and from the cerebellar nuclei, for the instructor to expand on cerebellar afferent/efferent pathways not covered in the atlas, or both.

NOTES

■ 8-41 Blank Master Drawing for Efferent Cerebellar Connections ■

■ Striatal Connections in Anatomical Orientation ■

8-42 The origin, course, and distribution of afferent fibers to, and efferent projections from, the neostriatum. These projections are extensive, complex, and, in large part, topographically organized; only their general patterns are summarized here. Afferents to the caudate and putamen originate from the cerebral cortex (corticostriate fibers), from several of the intralaminar thalamic nuclei (thalamostriate), from the substantia nigra-pars compacta (nigrostriate), and from some of the raphe nuclei. Neostriatal cells send axons into the globus pallidus (paleostriatum) as striopallidal fibers and into the substantia nigra pars reticulata as a strionigral projection.

Neurotransmitters

Glutamate (+) is found in corticostriate fibers, and serotonin is found in raphe striatal fibers from the nucleus raphe dorsalis. Four neuroactive substances are associated with striatal efferent fibers, these being γ-aminobutyric acid (GABA) (−), dynorphin, enkephalin (−), and substance P (+). Enkephalinergic and GABA-ergic striopallidal projections are numerous to the lateral pallidum (origin of pallidosubthalamic fibers), whereas GABA-ergic and dynorphin-containing terminals are more concentrated in its medial segment (source of pallidothalamic fibers). Enkephalin and GABA are also present in strionigral projections to the pars reticulata. Substance P and GABA are found in striopallidal *and* strionigral fibers. Dopamine is present in nigrostriatal projection neurons and in their terminals in the neostriatum.

Clinical Correlations

Degenerative changes and neuron loss in the caudate nucleus and putamen result in movement disorders. Examples are seen in *Sydenham chorea (rheumatic chorea)*, *Huntington disease* (a dominantly inherited disease), and *Wilson disease* (a genetic error in the patient's ability to metabolize copper). In *Parkinson disease*, there is a loss of the dopamine-containing cells in the pars compacta of the substantia nigra and of their terminals in the neostriatum.

Sydenham chorea is a disease usually seen in children between 5 and 15 years of age, resulting from infection with hemolytic streptococcus. The *choreiform movements* are brisk and flowing, irregular, and may involve muscles of the limbs, face, oral cavity, and trunk. *Dystonia* may be seen; muscle weakness is common. In most patients, the disease resolves after successful treatment of the infection.

Huntington disease is a progressive inherited disorder, the symptoms of which appear at 35 to 45 years of age. A feature of this disease is excessive CAG repeats on chromosome 4 (4p16.3); the greater the number of repeats, the earlier the onset, and more severe the disease. There is loss of GABA-ergic and enkephalinergic cells in the neostriatum (primarily the caudate) and cell loss in the cerebral cortex. Loss of neostriatal cell terminals in the lateral and medial segments of the globus pallidus correlates with the development of *choreiform movements* and later with *rigidity* and *dystonia*. Loss of cortical neurons correlates with personality changes and eventual *dementia*. Huntington chorea is rapid, unpredictable, and may affect muscles of the extremities, face, and trunk. Patients commonly attempt to mask the abnormal movement by trying to make it appear to be part of an intended movement (*parakinesia*).

Symptoms in *Wilson disease (hepatolenticular degeneration)* appear in persons between 10 and 25 years of age. Copper accumulates in the basal nuclei and the frontal cortex, with resultant spongy degeneration in the putamen. These patients may show *athetoid movements*, *rigidity* and *spasticity*, *dysarthria*, *dysphagia*, contractures, and *tremor*. A unique movement of the hand and/or upper extremity in these patients is called a *flapping tremor (asterixis)* sometimes described as a wing-beating tremor. Copper also can be seen in the cornea *(Kayser-Fleischer ring)* in these patients.

In *Parkinson disease* (onset at 50 to 60 years of age), there is a progressive loss of dopaminergic cells in the substantia nigra-pars compacta, their terminals in the caudate and putamen, and their dendrites that extend into the substantia nigra-pars reticulata. Patients with Parkinson disease characteristically show a *resting tremor* (pill-rolling), *rigidity (cogwheel* or *lead-pipe)*, and *bradykinesia* or *hypokinesia*. The slowness of movement also may be expressed in speech (*dysarthria*, *hypophonia*, *trachyphonia*) and writing (*micrographia*). These patients have a distinct stooped *flexed posture* and a *festinating gait*. Parkinson disease and Huntington disease are progressive neurodegenerative disorders.

Dystonia, a movement disorder seen in some patients with basal nuclei disease, is characterized by increased/sustained muscle contractions that cause twisting of the trunk or extremities resulting in abnormal posture. These patients also may have unusual and repetitive movements of the extremities or of the neck (*cervical dystonia or spasmodic torticollis*). Dystonia may be an inherited progressive disease or have other causes and may be seen in children or young adults. The symptoms may initially appear during movements or when talking, but in later stages may be present at rest.

ABBREVIATIONS

CaNu	Caudate nucleus	**RaSt**	Raphestriatal fibers
CorSt	Corticostriate fibers	**SNpc**	Substantia nigra, pars compacta
GPL	Globus pallidus, lateral segment	**SNpr**	Substantia nigra, pars reticulata
GPM	Globus pallidus, medial segment	**StNig**	Striatonigral fibers
IC	Internal capsule	**StPal**	Striatopallidal fibers
NigSt	Nigrostriatal fibers	**SThNu**	Subthalamic nucleus
Put	Putamen	**ThSt**	Thalamostriatal fibers
RaNu	Raphe nuclei	**ZI**	Zona incerta

Review of Blood Supply to Caudate, Putamen, SN, CC, and IC

Structures	Arteries
Caudate, Putamen, and IC	Medial striate artery for head of caudate and lateral striate branches of middle cerebral for Put and IC (see Figure 6-38)
SN and CC	Paramedian branches of basilar bifurcation, short circumferential branches of posterior cerebral and some from superior cerebellar (see Figure 6-27)

■ 8-42 Striatal Connections in Anatomical Orientation ■

Cerebral cortex

CorSt

CorSt

Ca,Nu

StPal

ThSt

Intralaminar nuclei

Put

StPal

NigSt

ZI

CorSt

SThNu

NigSt

GPL

StNig

GPM

SNpc

SNpr

RaSt

RaNu

■ Pallidal Efferents and Nigral Connections in Anatomical Orientation ■

8-43 The origin, course, and distribution of efferent projections of the globus pallidus (upper illustration), and connections of the substantia nigra (lower drawing) that were not shown in relation to the pallidum or in Figure 8-42 on p. 251 (see also Figure 8-44A on p. 254). The ansa lenticularis (dashed line) arches around the internal capsule and passes caudally to join in the formation of the thalamic fasciculus. Pallidosubthalamic fibers originate primarily from the lateral pallidal segment, but pallidothalamic projections, via the ansa lenticularis and lenticular fasciculus, arise mainly from its medial segment. The substantia nigra has extensive connections, the clinically most important being the dopaminergic nigrostriatal fibers. The globus pallidus influences motor activity by way of pallidothalamic-thalamocortical-corticospinal (and corticonuclear) pathways.

Neurotransmitters

γ-Aminobutyric acid (−)–containing cells in the globus pallidus give rise to pallidonigral projections, which end primarily in the substantia nigra-pars reticulata. Although GABA is also found in some subthalamopallidal axons, this latter projection contains many glutaminergic (+) fibers.

Dopamine-, GABA (−)-, and glycine (−)-containing cells are present in the substantia nigra. Of these, dopamine is found in pars compacta neurons, which give rise to nigrostriatal, nigroamygdaloid, and several other projections; GABA in pars reticulata cells, which give rise to nigrocollicular and nigrothalamic fibers; and glycine in some local circuit nigral neurons. Glutamate (+) is found in corticonigral fibers, and serotonin (−) is associated with raphenigral fibers; these latter fibers originate primarily from the nucleus raphe dorsalis.

The dopaminergic projections to the frontal cortex, shown here as arising only from SNpc, originate from this cell group as well as from the immediately adjacent ventral tegmental area. Excessive activity in neurons comprising this projection may play a partial role in *schizophrenia*.

Clinical Correlations

Movement disorders associated with lesions in the neostriatum and substantia nigra are reviewed in Figures 8-42 and 8-44B on pp. 250 and 255. Hemorrhage into, the occlusion of vessels serving or a tumor within, the subthalamic nucleus will result in violent flailing movements of the extremities, a condition called *hemiballismus*. Hemiballistic movements are seen contralateral to the lesion because the motor expression of this lesion is through the corticospinal tract. Lesions confined to the globus pallidus, as in hemorrhage of lenticulostriate arteries, may result in *hypokinesia* and *rigidity* without tremor.

ABBREVIATIONS

AmyNig	Amygdalonigral fibers	**PedPonNu**	Pedunculopontine nucleus
AmyNu	Amygdaloid nucleus (complex)	**Put**	Putamen
AnLent	Ansa lenticularis	**RaNu**	Raphe nuclei
CaNu	Caudate nucleus	**SC**	Superior colliculus
CM	Centromedian nucleus of thalamus	**SNpc**	Substantia nigra, pars compacta
CorNig	Corticonigral fibers	**SNpr**	Substantia nigra, pars reticulata
CSp	Corticospinal fibers	**SThFas**	Subthalamic fasciculus
GPL	Globus pallidus, lateral segment	**SThNig**	Subthalamonigral fibers
GPM	Globus pallidus, medial segment	**SThNu**	Subthalamic nucleus
LenFas	Lenticular fasciculus (H₂)	**ThCor**	Thalamocortical fibers
NigAmy	Nigroamygdaloid fibers	**ThFas**	Thalamic fasciculus (H₁)
NigCol	Nigrocollicular fibers	**VA**	Ventral anterior nucleus of thalamus
NigTec	Nigrotectal fibers	**VL**	Ventral lateral nucleus of thalamus
NigSTh	Nigrosubthalamic fibers	**VM**	Ventromedial nucleus of thalamus
NigTh	Nigrothalamic fibers	**ZI**	Zona incerta
PalNig	Pallidonigral fibers		

Review of Blood Supply to Pallidum, Subthalamic Area, and SN

Structures	Arteries
GPM/GPL	Lateral striate branches of middle cerebral and branches of anterior choroidal (see Figure 6-38)
SThNu	Posteromedial branches of posterior cerebral and posterior communicating (see Figure 6-38)
SN	Branches of basilar bifurcation, medial branches of posterior cerebral and posterior communicating, short circumferential branches of posterior cerebral (see Figure 6-27)

■ 8-43 Pallidal Efferents and Nigral Connections in Anatomical Orientation ■

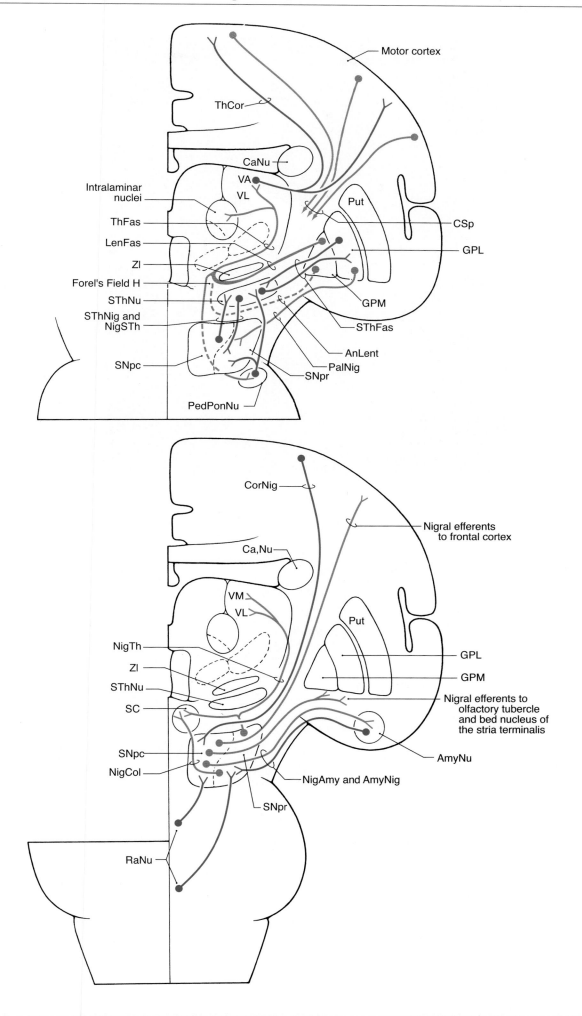

Motor cortex

ThCor

CaNu

VA

VL

Intralaminar
nuclei

Put

ThFas

CSp

LenFas

GPL

ZI

Forel's Field H

SThNu

GPM

SThNig and
NigSTh

SThFas

AnLent

SNpc

PalNig

SNpr

PedPonNu

CorNig

Nigral efferents
to frontal cortex

Ca,Nu

VM

VL

Put

NigTh

GPL

ZI

GPM

SThNu

SC

Nigral efferents to
olfactory tubercle
and bed nucleus of
the stria terminalis

SNpc

NigCol

AmyNu

NigAmy and AmyNig

SNpr

RaNu

■ Pallidal Efferents, Subthalamic, and Nigral Connections in Clinical Orientation ■

Cerebral cortex

Corticospinal fibers

Thalamocortical fibers

White matter

Corticostriate fibers

Corpus callosum

Body of fornix

Ventral lateral nucleus

Body of caudate nucleus

Insular cortex

Dorsal thalamus

Posterior limb, internal capsule

Putamen

Internal and external segments, globus pallidus

Nigrostriatial fibers

Subthalamic nucleus

Corticospinal fibers in crus cerebri

Substantia nigra

Crus cerebri

Corticospinal fibers in basilar pons

Basilar pons

Corticospinal fibers in pyramid

Pyramid of medulla

Corticospinal fiber
Corticostriate fiber (+)

Thalamocortical fiber (+)

Striatopallidal cell/fiber (−)

Ventral lateral nucleus of thalamus

Thalamic fasciculus

Pallidosubthalamic cell/fiber (−)
Striatopallidal cell/fiber (−)

Lenticular fasciculus

Pallidothalamic fiber (−)

Subthalamopallidal cell/fiber (+)

Corticospinal fiber

Nigrostriatal cell/fiber
(+ through direct pathway;
− through indirect pathway)

Direct pathway = Gray →Red → Blue →Gray
Indirect pathway = Gray →Green → Blue → Gray

8-44A The direct and indirect pathways through the basal nuclei, subthalamic nucleus, and substantia nigra superimposed on MRI (forebrain, T2-weighted MRI) shown in clinical orientation. The exploded view below the MRI illustrates the specific fiber types, by name, that comprise these two pathways and specifies whether the synaptic influences are excitatory (+) or inhibitory (−).

■ Pallidal Efferents, Subthalamic, and Nigral Connections in Clinical Orientation: Representative Lesions and Deficits ■

Corticospinal fibers

Thalamocortical fibers

Corticostriate fibers

Ventral lateral nucleus

Insular cortex

Nigrostriatial fibers

Corticospinal fibers in crus cerebri

Corticospinal fibers in basilar pons

Corticospinal fibers in pyramid

Huntington disease
- Inherited disorder (excessive CAG nucleotide repeats)
- Loss of medium-sized spiny neostriatial neurons
- Choreiform movements (fingers, wrist, extremities, face, tongue)
- Dysarthria, dysphagia
- Dystonia and/or myoclonus
- Forgetfulness, diminished attention, irritability, depression, memory loss
- Dementia
- Lesion/deficits usually bilateral

Wilson disease
- Inherited error of copper metabolism: copper accumulates in liver and lenticular nucleus
- Kayser-Fleischer ring
- Aminoaciduria
- Asterixis (wing-beating tremor)
- Tremor, rigidity, dysarthria, dysphagia
- Cognitive decline, personality change
- Lesion/deficits usually bilateral
- Treatable

Subthalamic lesion
- Usually vascular in origin
- Hemiballism/hemiballismus (one side of body involved: deficits contralateral to lesion)
- Ballism/ballismus (both sides of body involved)
- Rapid jerky, flinging movements: more common in UE

Parkinson disease
- Neurodegenerative disease of unknown etiology: progressive
- Loss of dopamine-containing cells in substantia nigra, pars compacta
- Resting/pill-rolling tremor
- Akinesia, bradykinesia, hypokinesia
- Rigidity (lead-pipe/cogwheel)
- Flexed posture, shuffling/festinating gait; unsteady posture
- Expressionless face
- Dysarthria, hypophonia, micrographia, dystonia
- Dementia in late stages

8-44B Representative lesions of the basal nuclei, subthalamic nucleus, and substantia nigra and the deficits that correlate with lesions at each of these locations. As was the case with the cerebellum, motor deficits resulting from lesions of the basal nuclei and related structures are expressed through the corticospinal tract. Note that the laterality (R/L) of the deficits is determined by whether the lesion is on the left or right side of the MRI; this reinforces important clinical concepts.

■ Blank Master Drawing for Connections of the Basal Nuclei ■

8-45 Blank master drawing for connections of the basal nuclei. This illustration is provided for self-evaluation of under- standing of basal nuclei connections, for the instructor to expand on basal nuclei pathways not covered in this atlas, or both.

NOTES

■ **8-45 Blank Master Drawing for Connections of the Basal Nuclei** ■

■ Pupillary Pathways ■

8-46 The origin, course, and distribution of fibers involved in the pathway for the pupillary light reflex. In addition, the pathway for sympathetic innervation of the dilator muscle of the iris is also depicted. The intermediolateral cell column of the spinal cord receives input predominately from the paraventricular nucleus and also from cells in the lateral hypothalamic zone and posterior hypothalamus. This projection may be supplemented, in a minor way, by descending fibers through the reticular formation of the brainstem. Postganglionic sympathetic fibers to the head originate from the superior cervical ganglion. Although not shown, descending projections to the intermediolateral cell column also originate from various hypothalamic areas and nuclei (hypothalamospinal fibers), some of which receive retinal input.

Neurotransmitters

Acetylcholine is the transmitter found in the preganglionic and postganglionic autonomic fibers shown in this illustration. In addition, N-acetyl-aspartyl-glutamate is present in some retinal ganglion cells (retinogeniculate projections).

Clinical Correlations

Total or partial blindness in one or both eyes may result from a variety of causes (e.g., *gliomas, meningiomas, strokes, aneurysms,* infections, and demyelinating diseases); lesions may occur at any locus along the visual pathway. A complete lesion (i.e., a transection) of the optic nerve will result in *blindness* and loss of the *pupillary light reflex* (direct response) in the eye on the injured side and a loss of the *pupillary light reflex* (consensual response) in the opposite eye *when shining a light in the blind eye.* On the other hand, shining a light in the normal eye will result in a *pupillary light reflex* (direct response) in that eye *and* a consensual response in the blind eye. See

also Figure 8-34 on p. 235. A *pituitary adenoma* may damage the crossing fibers in the optic chiasm (producing a *bitemporal hemianopia*) or damage the uncrossed fibers in the right (or left) side of the optic chiasm. These lateral lesions produce a *right* (or *left*) *nasal hemianopia.*

Optic (geniculocalcarine) radiations (see Figures 8-47 and 8-49 on pp. 260 and 262) may pass directly caudal to the upper lip (cuneus) of the calcarine sulcus or follow an arching route (the *Meyer,* or *Meyer-Archambault loop*) through the temporal lobe to the lower bank (lingual gyrus) of the calcarine sulcus. Temporal lobe lesions involving the Meyer-Archambault loop, or involving fibers entering the lingual gyrus, can produce a *homonymous superior quadrantanopia.* A *homonymous inferior quadrantanopia* is seen in patients with damage to upper (parietal) parts of the geniculocalcarine radiations or to these fibers as they enter the cuneus. See Figure 8-49B on p. 263 for additional lesions of the visual pathways and the corresponding visual field deficits.

Damage to the visual cortex adjacent to the calcarine sulcus (distal posterior cerebral artery occlusion) results in a *right* (or *left*) *homonymous hemianopia.* With the exception of macular sparing, this deficit is the same as that seen in optic tract lesions. See Figure 8-49B on p. 263 for additional lesions of the optic radiations and visual cortex and the corresponding visual field deficits.

Vascular lesions (e.g., the *lateral medullary syndrome*), tumors (e.g., *brainstem gliomas*), or *syringobulbia* may interrupt the descending projections from hypothalamus (hypothalamospinal fibers) and midbrain to the intermediolateral cell column at upper thoracic levels. This may result in a *Horner syndrome* (*ptosis, miosis,* and *anhidrosis*) on the ipsilateral side. The *enophthalmos* (a slight sinking of the eyeball into the orbit) frequently mentioned in relation to *Horner syndrome* is not really very apparent in afflicted patients.

ABBREVIATIONS

CC	Crus cerebri		PoCom	Posterior commissur
CilGang	Ciliary ganglion		PrTecNu	Pretectal nucleus
EWpgNu	Edinger-Westphal preganglionic nucleus		PulNu	Pulvinar nuclear complex
ILCC	Intermediolateral cell column		RetF	Reticular formation
LGNu	Lateral geniculate nucleus		RNu	Red nucleus
MGNu	Medial geniculate nucleus		SC	Superior colliculus
ML	Medial lemniscus		SC,Br	Superior colliculus, brachium
OcNr	Oculomotor nerve		SCerGang	Superior cervical ganglion
OpCh	Optic chiasm		SN	Substantia nigra
OpNr	Optic nerve		WRCom	White ramus communicans
OpTr	Optic tract			

Review of Blood Supply to OpTr, MGNu, LGNu, SC, and Midbrain Tegmentum, Including PrTecNu

Structures	Arteries
OpTr	Anterior choroidal (see Figure 6-38)
MGNu, LGNu	Thalamogeniculate branches of posterior cerebral (see Figure 6-38)
SC and PrTecNu	Long circumferential branches (quadrigeminal) of posterior cerebral, posterior choroidal, and some from superior cerebellar (to SC) (see Figures 6-27 and 6-38)
Midbrain Tegmentum	Paramedian branches of basilar bifurcation, medial branches of posterior cerebral and posterior communicating, short circumferential branches of posterior cerebral (see Figure 6-27)

■ 8-46 Pupillary Pathways ■

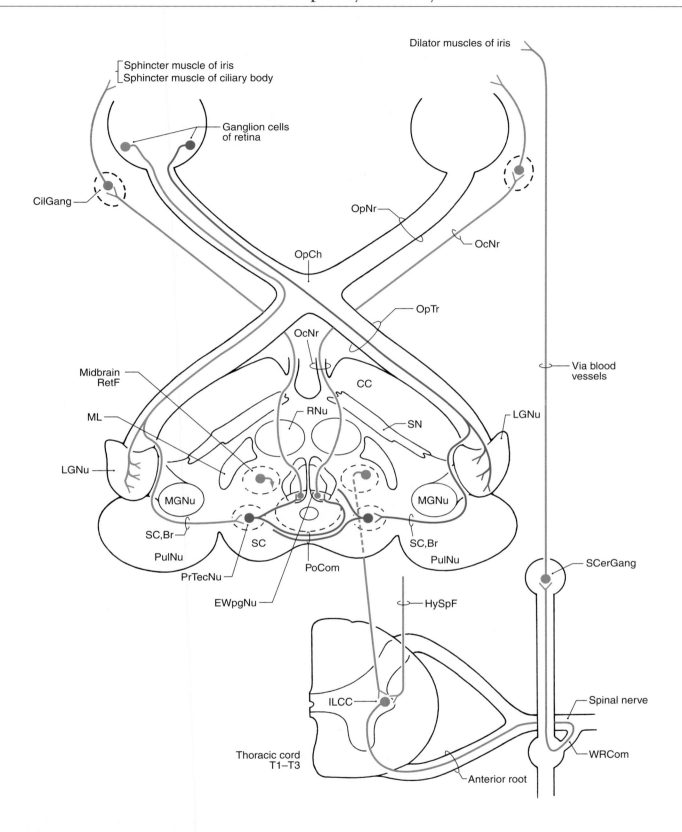

Dilator muscles of iris

Sphincter muscle of iris
Sphincter muscle of ciliary body

Ganglion cells
of retina

CilGang

OpNr

OcNr

OpCh

OpTr

OcNr

Via blood
vessels

Midbrain
RetF

CC

RNu

SN

LGNu

ML

LGNu

MGNu

MGNu

SC,Br

SC

SC,Br

PulNu

PulNu

SCerGang

PrTecNu

PoCom

EWpgNu

HySpF

ILCC

Spinal nerve

Thoracic cord
T1–T3

WRCom

Anterior root

■ Visual Pathways ■

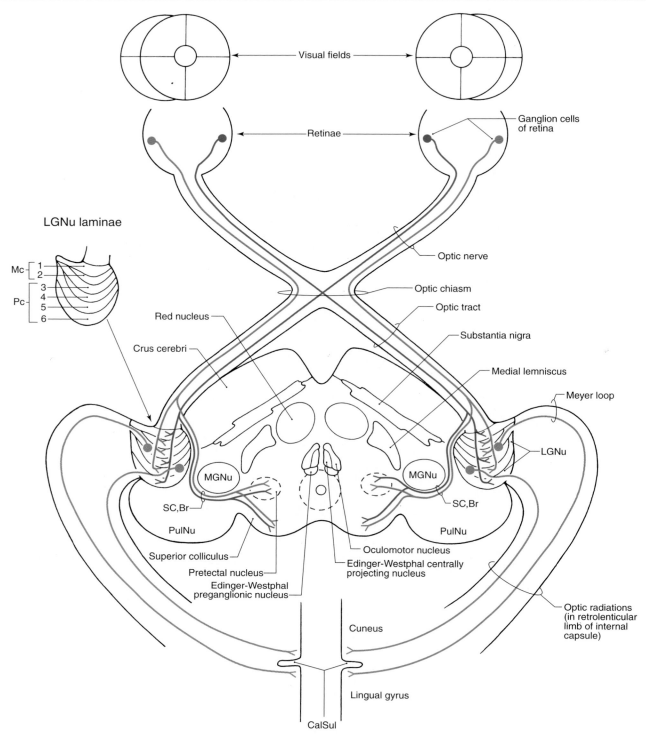

8-47 The origin, course, and distribution of the visual pathway are shown. Uncrossed retinogeniculate fibers terminate in laminae 2, 3, and 5, whereas crossed fibers end in laminae 1, 4, and 6. Geniculocalcarine fibers arise from laminae 3 through 6. Retinogeniculate and geniculocalcarine pathways are retinotopically organized (see facing page).

Neurotransmitters

Cholecystokinin (+) is present in some geniculocalcarine fibers. N-acetyl-aspartyl-glutamate is found in some retinogeniculate fibers, and in some lateral geniculate and visual cortex neurons.

Clinical Correlations

Deficits seen following lesions of various parts of visual pathways are described in Figures 8-46 and 8-49B on pp. 258 and 263.

ABBREVIATIONS	
CalSul	Calcarine sulcus
LGNu	Lateral geniculate nucleus
Mc	Magnocellular
Pc	Parvocellular
MGNu	Medial geniculate nucleus
PulNu	Pulvinar nuclear complex
SC,Br	Superior colliculus, brachium

■ Visual Pathways ■

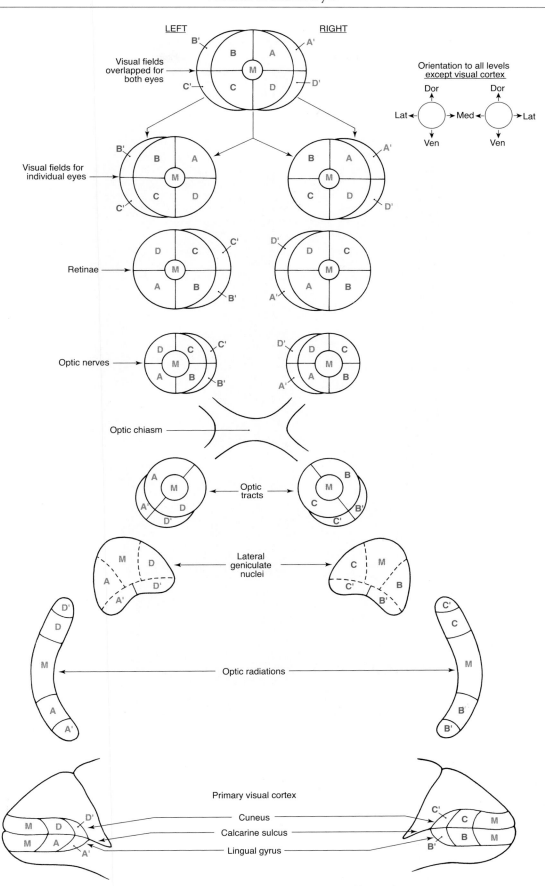

8-48 Semi-diagrammatic representation of the retinographic arrangement of visual and retinal fields, and the subsequent topography of these projections throughout the visual system. Upper case letters identify the binocular visual fields (A, B, C, D), the macula (M), and the monocular visual fields (A', B', C', D').

Clinical Correlations

Deficits seen following lesions of various parts of the visual pathway are described in Figures 8-46 and 8-49B on pp. 258 and 263.

■ Visual Pathways in Clinical Orientation ■

Ganglion cell of retina

Optic nerve

Optic nerve

Optic chiasm

Optic tract

Lateral geniculate nucleus

Meyer loop

Medial geniculate nucleus

Brachium of superior colliculus

Pulvinar

Pretectal nucleus

Optic radiations

Cuneus

Lingual gyrus

Optic nerve

Optic chiasm

Crus cerebri

Lateral geniculate nucleus

Medial geniculate nucleus

Pulvinar

Optic radiations

Cuneus

Calcarine sulcus

Optic radiations

Lingual gyrus

Cuneus

Calcarine sulcus

Lingual gyrus

8-49A The visual pathway from retina to primary visual cortex superimposed on MRI in clinical orientation. The upper T1-weighted image is in the axial plane and the lower T1-weighted image is in the coronal plane. The red, blue, and gray fibers in the upper image correlate with those of the same color in Figure 8-48.

8-49B Representative lesions at 13 different locations in the visual pathway and the patterns of visual field deficits that correlate with each lesion. As indicated by the letters (A–G), some lesions, especially those caudal to the optic chiasm, may result in comparable visual field deficits even though the lesions may be at different locations within the pathway.

International clinical convention dictates that *Visual Field Deficits* are illustrated *as the patient sees the environment*. In this respect *the patient's right eye and visual field are on the right and the patient's left eye and visual field are on the left*. Axial and coronal MRI and CT images are viewed as if the observer is standing at the patient's feet looking toward the head (axial) or looking at the

■ Visual Pathways in Clinical Orientation: Representative Lesions and Deficits ■

Ganglion cell of retina

Optic nerve

Optic nerve

Optic tract

Lateral geniculate nucleus

Meyer loop

Medial geniculate nucleus

Brachium of superior colliculus

Pulvinar

Pretectal nucleus

Optic radiations

Cuneus

Lingual gyrus

Retinal disorders/trauma
- Visual field defects of various patterns
- Scotoma   A

Optic nerve lesion
- Blind in left eye
- Loss of pupillary light reflex in both eyes when light shined in left eye   B

Midline optic chiasm lesion
- Bitemporal hemianopia
- May have relative afferent pupillary defect (RAPD)   C

Lateral optic chiasm lesion
- Binasal hemianopia
- May have RAPD   D

Optic tract lesion
- Right homonymous hemianopia
- May have RAPD   E

- Right superior homonymous quadrantanopia   F

- Right inferior homonymous quadrantanopia   G

Total optic radiation lesion
- Right homonymous hemianopia   E

Cuneus lesion
- Right inferior homonymous quadrantanopia   G

Cuneus

Calcarine sulcus

Lingual gyrus

Lingual gyrus lesion
- Right superior homonymous quadrantanopia   F

- Right inferior homonymous quadrantanopia   G

Total optic radiation lesion
- Right homonymous hemianopia (also seen in lesion of total primary visual cortex)   E

- Right superior homonymous quadrantanopia   F

Visual Field Deficits

Lesion Left Right   Left Right   Left Right

A   B   C   D   E   F   G

patient's face (coronal). In this case, when looking at MRI/CT *the observer's right is the patient's left and the observer's left is the patient's right.* Understanding the reality of how these images are used and viewed in the clinical environment is absolutely essential to the diagnosis of the patient with visual system lesions and the corresponding visual field deficits.

■ Blank Master Drawing for Visual Pathways ■

8-50 Blank master drawing for visual pathways. This illustration is provided for self-evaluation of visual pathway understanding, for the instructor to expand on aspects of the visual pathways not covered in the atlas, or both.

NOTES

■ 8-50 Blank Master Drawing for Visual Pathways ■

■ 8-50 Blank Master Drawing for Visual Pathways ■

■ Auditory Pathways in Anatomical Orientation ■

8-51 The origin, course, and distribution of the fibers collectively composing the auditory pathway. Central to the cochlear nerve and dorsal and ventral cochlear nuclei, this system is, largely, bilateral and multisynaptic, as input is relayed to the auditory cortex. Synapse and crossing (or re-crossing) of information can occur at several levels in the neuraxis. Consequently, central lesions rarely result in a total unilateral hearing loss. The medial geniculate body is the thalamic station for the relay of auditory information to the temporal cortex.

Neurotransmitters

Glutamate (+) and aspartate (+) are found in some spiral ganglion cells and in their central terminations in the cochlear nuclei. Dynorphin-containing and histamine-containing fibers are also present in the cochlear nuclei; the latter arises from the hypothalamus. A noradrenergic projection to the cochlear nuclei and the inferior colliculus originates from the nucleus locus ceruleus. Cells in the superior olive that contain cholecystokinin and cells in the nuclei of the lateral lemniscus that contain dynorphin project to the inferior colliculus. Although the olivocochlear bundle is not shown, it is noteworthy that enkephalin is found in some of the cells that contribute to this projection.

Clinical Correlations—Categories of Deafness

Conductive deafness is caused by problems of the external ear (obstruction of the canal, wax build-up) or disorders of the middle ear *(otitis media, otosclerosis). Nerve deafness (sensorineural hearing loss)* results from diseases involving the cochlea or the cochlear portion of the vestibulocochlear nerve. *Central deafness* results from damage to the cochlear nuclei or their central connections.

Hearing loss may result from trauma (e.g., fracture of the petrous bone), demyelinating diseases, tumors, certain medications (*streptomycin*), or occlusion of the labyrinthine artery. Damage to the cochlear part of the eighth nerve (e.g., *vestibular schwannoma*) results in *tinnitus* and/or *deafness* (partial or total) in the ipsilateral ear. High-frequency hearing losses (*presbyacusis*), such as a woman's voice or discrimination between sounds, are more commonly seen in older patients.

The *Weber test* and *Rinne test* are used to differentiate between neural hearing loss and conduction hearing loss, and to lateralize the deficit. In the *Weber test*, a tuning fork (512 Hz) is applied to the midline of the forehead or apex of the skull. In the normal patient, the sound (conducted through the skull bones) is heard the same in each ear. In the case of *nerve deafness* (cochlea or cochlear nerve lesions), the sound is best heard in the normal ear, whereas in *conductive deafness*, the sound is best heard in the abnormal ear. In the *Rinne test*, a tuning fork (512 Hz) is placed against the mastoid process. When the sound is no longer perceived, the prongs are moved close to the external acoustic meatus, where the sound is again heard; this is the situation in a normal individual (positive Rinne test). In middle ear disease, the sound is not heard at the external meatus after it has disappeared from touching the mastoid bone (abnormal or negative Rinne test). Therefore, a negative Rinne test signifies conductive hearing loss in the ear tested. In mild nerve deafness (cochlea or cochlear nerve lesions), the sound is heard by application of the tuning fork to the mastoid and movement to the ear (the Rinne test is positive). In severe nerve deafness, the sound may not be heard at either position.

In addition to hearing loss and tinnitus, large vestibular schwannomas may result in nausea, vomiting, ataxia/unsteady gait (vestibular root involvement), facial muscle weakness (facial root), altered facial sensations, and a diminished corneal reflex (trigeminal root). There also may be general signs associated with increased intracranial pressure (lethargy, headache, and vomiting).

Central lesions (e.g., gliomas or vascular occlusions) rarely produce unilateral or bilateral hearing losses that can be detected, the possible exception being pontine lesions, which damage the trapezoid body and nuclei. Injury to central auditory pathways and/or primary auditory cortex may diminish auditory acuity, decrease the ability to hear certain tones, or make it difficult to precisely localize sounds in space. Patients with damage to the secondary auditory cortex in the temporal lobe experience difficulty in understanding and/or interpreting sounds *(auditory agnosia).*

ABBREVIATIONS

AbdNu	Abducens nucleus	**MLF**	Medial longitudinal fasciculus
ACNu	Anterior (ventral) cochlear nucleus	**PCNu**	Posterior (dorsal) cochlear nucleus
ALS	Anterolateral system	**PulNu**	Pulvinar nuclear complex
CC	Crus cerebri	**RB**	Restiform body
FacNu	Facial nucleus	**RetF**	Reticular formation
IC	Inferior colliculus	**SC**	Superior colliculus
IC,Br	Inferior colliculus, brachium	**SCP,Dec**	Superior cerebellar peduncle, decussation
IC,Com	Inferior colliculus, commissure	**SO**	Superior olive
IC,SL	Internal capsule, sublenticular limb	**SpGang**	Spiral ganglion
LGNu	Lateral geniculate nucleus	**SpTTr**	Spinal trigeminal tract
LL	Lateral lemniscus	**TrapB**	Trapezoid body
LL,Nu	Lateral lemniscus, nucleus	**TrapNu**	Trapezoid nucleus
MGNu	Medial geniculate nucleus	**TTGy**	Transverse temporal gyrus
ML	Medial lemniscus		

Review of Blood Supply to Cochlear Nuclei, LL (and Associated Structures), Pontine Tegmentum, IC, and MGNu

Structures	Arteries
Cochlear Nuclei	Anterior inferior cerebellar (see Figure 6-14)
LL, SO in Pons	Long circumferential branches of basilar (see Figure 6-21)
IC	Long circumferential branches (quadrigeminal branches) of basilar, superior cerebellar (see Figure 6-27)
MGNu	Thalamogeniculate branches of posterior cerebral (see Figure 6-38)

■ 8-51 Auditory Pathways in Anatomical Orientation ■

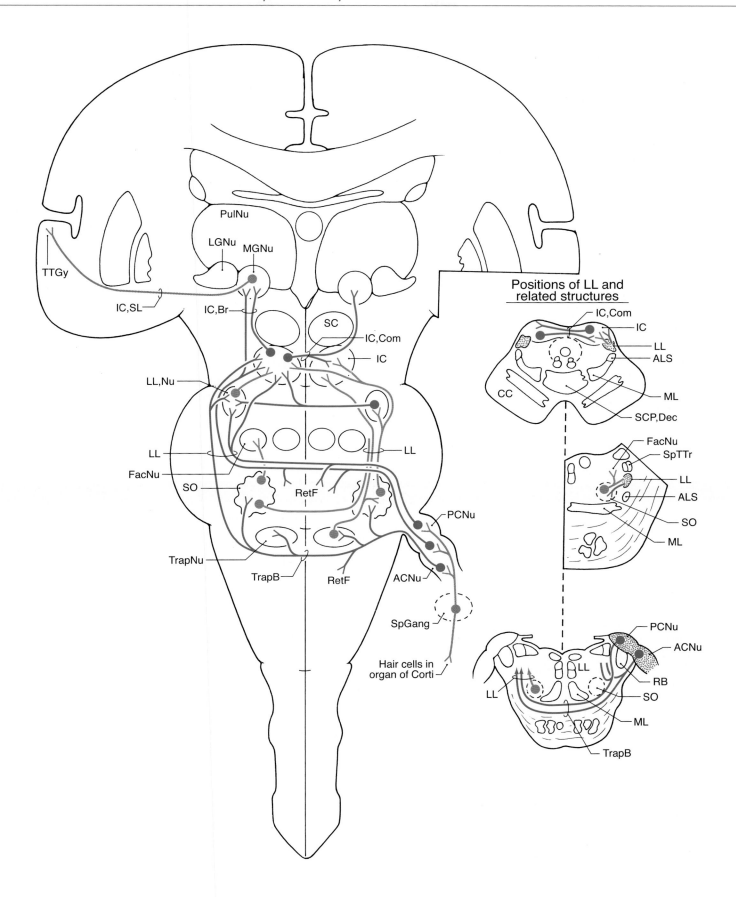

Positions of LL and
related structures

■ Vestibular Pathways in Anatomical Orientation ■

8-52 The origin, course, and distribution of the main afferent and efferent connections of the vestibular nuclei (see also Figures 8-18, 8-38, and 8-39 on pp. 217, 243, and 245). Primary vestibular afferent fibers may end in the vestibular nuclei or pass to cerebellar structures via the juxtarestiform body. Secondary vestibulocerebellar axons originate from the vestibular nuclei and follow a similar path to the cerebellum. Efferent projections from the vestibular nuclei also course to the spinal cord through vestibulospinal tracts (see Figures 8-18, 8-38, and 8-39), as well as to the motor nuclei of the oculomotor, trochlear, and abducens nerves via the MLF. Cerebellar structures most extensively interconnected with the vestibular nuclei include the lateral regions of the vermal cortex of anterior and posterior lobes, the flocculonodular lobe, and the fastigial (medial) cerebellar nucleus.

Neurotransmitters

γ-Aminobutyric acid (−) is the transmitter associated with many cerebellar corticovestibular fibers and their terminals in the vestibular complex; this substance is also seen in cerebellar corticonuclear axons. The medial vestibular nucleus also has fibers that are dynorphin-positive and histamine-positive; the latter arise from cells in the hypothalamus.

Clinical Correlations

The vestibular part of the eighth nerve can be damaged by many of the same insults that affect the cochlear nerve (see Figure 8-40).

Damage to vestibular receptors of the vestibular nerve commonly results in *vertigo*. The patient may feel that his or her body is moving (*subjective vertigo*) or that objects in the environment are moving (*objective vertigo*). They have equilibrium problems, an *unsteady (ataxic) gait*, and a tendency to fall to the lesioned side. Deficits seen in nerve lesions, or in brainstem lesions involving the vestibular nuclei, include *nystagmus, nausea*, and vomiting, along with *vertigo* and gait problems. *Vestibular schwannoma* is a relatively common lesion (about 8%–10% of CNS tumors), commonly results in hearing loss (95+%), is frequently characterized by disequilibrium and tinnitus (65%–70%), and is sometimes related to headache and facial numbness (about 30%); the latter indicates that the lesion is large and has encroached on the trigeminal nerve root. Facial weakness (*facial palsy*) occurs in about 10% of cases. These vestibular deficits, along with partial or complete deafness, are seen in *Ménière disease*.

Lesions of those parts of the cerebellum with which the vestibular nerve and nuclei are most intimately connected (flocculonodular lobe and fastigial nucleus) result in *nystagmus, truncal ataxia, ataxic gait*, and a propensity to fall to the injured side. The nystagmus seen in patients with vestibular lesions and the *internuclear ophthalmoplegia* seen in some patients with *multiple sclerosis* are signs that correlate with the interruption of vestibular projections to the motor nuclei of III, IV, and VI via the MLF.

ABBREVIATIONS			
AbdNu	Abducens nucleus	**OcNu**	Oculomotor nucleus
ALS	Anterolateral system	**PAG**	Periaqueductal gray
Cbl	Cerebellar	**Py**	Pyramid
Cbl-CoVes	Cerebellar corticovestibular fibers	**RB**	Restiform body
CblNu	Cerebellar nuclei	**RNu**	Red nucleus
HyNu	Hypoglossal nucleus	**SC**	Superior colliculus
IC	Inferior colliculus	**SCP,Dec**	Superior cerebellar peduncle, decussation
InfVNu	Inferior (spinal) vestibular nucleus	**SN**	Substantia nigra
JRB	Juxtarestiform body	**SolNu**	Solitary nucleus
LVesSp	Lateral vestibulospinal tract	**SolTr**	Solitary tract
LVNu	Lateral vestibular nucleus	**SpTTr**	Spinal trigeminal tract
MesNu	Mesencephalic nucleus	**SVNu**	Superior vestibular nucleus
ML	Medial lemniscus	**TroNu**	Trochlear nucleus
MLF	Medial longitudinal fasciculus	**VesGang**	Vestibular ganglion
MVesSp	Medial vestibulospinal tract	**VesCbl,Prim**	Vestibulocerebellar fibers, primary
MVNu	Medial vestibular nucleus	**VesCbl,Sec**	Vestibulocerebellar fibers, secondary

Review of Blood Supply to Vestibular Nuclei, TroNu, and OcNu	
Structures	**Arteries**
Vestibular Nuclei	Posterior inferior cerebellar in medulla (see Figure 6-14), long circumferential branches of basilar in pons (see Figure 6-21)
TroNu and OcNu	Paramedian branches of basilar bifurcation, medial branches of posterior cerebral and posterior communicating, short circumferential branches of posterior cerebral (see Figure 6-27)

■ 8-52 Vestibular Pathways in Anatomical Orientation ■

Position of vestibular nuclei, MLF, and related structures

SC
PAG
OcNu
MesNu
ML
RNu
SN

IC
TroNu
ALS
MLF
ML
SCP,Dec

LVNu
JRB
AbdNu
SVNu
MLF
SpTTr
ALS
ML

HyNu
MVNu and InfVNu
MLF
RB
SpTTr
ML
SolTr and Nu
Py

OcNu
TroNu
MLF
AbdNu
SVNu
CblNu
Cbl-CoVes
JRB
LVNu
VesCbl, Sec
Cbl cortex
VesCbl, Prim
VesGang
Crista ampullaris
Macula utriculi
Macula sacculi
MVNu
InfVNu
MVesSp in MLF
LVesSp

■ Blank Master Drawing for Auditory or Vestibular Pathways ■

8-53 Blank master drawing for auditory or vestibular pathway. This illustration is provided for self-evaluation of auditory or vestibular pathway understanding, for the instructor to expand on aspects of these pathways not covered in the atlas, or both.

NOTES

■ 8-53 Blank Master Drawing for Auditory or Vestibular Pathways ■

■ The Internal Capsule: Relationships and Contents ■

8-54 The internal capsule, its relationship to the basal nuclei and thalamus, and its major constituent fiber bundles in the axial plane. Pathways conveying sensory information (with the exception of olfaction) from the entire body and pathways influencing motor activity of cranial nerves and the extremities all traverse some part of the internal capsule.

The *internal capsule* is divided into five parts, called *limbs*, which are most easily recognized in the axial plane (see facing page). Each limb has a characteristic relationship to adjacent structures and contains particular fiber groups.

Anterior limb: The *anterior limb* is located between the head of the caudate nucleus and the lenticular nucleus. The major fiber populations found in the anterior limb are frontopontine fibers, the anterior thalamic radiations (medial and anterior thalamic projections to the frontal and cingulate cortex), and, adjacent to the genu, small fascicles of descending fibers from the frontal eye fields.

Genu: The positions of the column of the fornix, the interventricular foramen, and the anterior tubercle of the thalamus indicate the location of the *genu of the internal capsule*. The most clinically significant fiber bundles in the genu are corticonuclear fibers projecting to the motor nuclei of cranial nerves (see also Figures 8-15 and 8-16 on pp. 210–213).

Posterior limb: The *posterior limb* is the largest part of the internal capsule, is located between the thalamus and the lenticular nucleus, and contains a number of important fiber populations. These larger bundles include corticospinal fibers, superior thalamic radiations (ventral anterior, ventral lateral, ventral posteromedial, and posterolateral projections to motor and sensory cortices), and, in its more caudal region, parietopontine fibers. Smaller bundles of fibers including corticorubral, corticoreticular, corticonigral, corticosubthalamic, the general category of corticotegmental fibers, and pallidothalamic fibers that arise in the medial segment of the globus pallidus, traverse the posterior limb.

Sublenticular limb: The *sublenticular limb* is difficult to identify, although its trajectory and contents are well known. It extends between the medial geniculate nucleus and the temporal lobe, particularly the auditory cortex, and contains auditory radiations (geniculotemporal radiations), temporopontine fibers, and corticotectal fibers.

Retrolenticular limb: The *retrolenticular limb* is that large mass of fibers located immediately caudal the lenticular nucleus; hence its name, retrolenticular. The larger fiber bundles within this limb are visual radiations (geniculocalcarine or optic radiations) and occipitopontine fibers; the smaller bundles comprise corticotectal, corticotegmental, and some corticorubral fibers.

Recall that the optic radiations are composed of fibers that arise in the lateral geniculate nucleus and pass caudally directly to the primary visual cortex, and of fibers that arise in the lateral geniculate nucleus, arch forward into the temporal lobe, turn sharply caudal (as the Meyer loop), and then proceed to the primary visual cortex. These two portions of the optic radiations are conveying information from different parts of the visual fields; lesions of these parts result in specific visual deficits (see Figures 8-46 through 8-49 on pp. 258–263).

General note: Most of the limbs of the internal capsule also contain thalamocortical projections (other than those mentioned above), corticothalamic fibers (from all cortical areas to their respective thalamic nuclei), and corticostriate fibers.

Neurotransmitters

There are no nuclei within the internal capsule, only fibers of passage conveying a variety of motor and sensory information, and fibers that are integrative in nature. The major transmitters associated with fibers within the internal capsule are *glutamate* (most cortical efferent fibers, thalamocortical fibers) and *GABA* (pallidothalamic fibers), and smaller populations of *cholinergic, dopaminergic, serotoninergic, histaminergic,* and *GABA-ergic* fibers.

Clinical Correlations

Lesions of the internal capsule are usually expressed as movement disorders related to involvement of corticospinal or corticonuclear fibers (depending on the general location of the lesion) and somatosensory losses related to damage to thalamocortical projections. A general characteristic of forebrain lesions is motor and sensory deficits that are all on the same side (the side of the body opposite the location of the lesion). Cranial nerve deficits are lacking unless the damage involves the genu of the internal capsule.

A lesion in the genu of the internal capsule results in deficits that generally reflect damage to corticonuclear fibers to the facial and hypoglossal nuclei, and to the nucleus ambiguus. The facial muscles are weak on the lower half of the face opposite the lesion (a *central seven* as opposed to a *Bell palsy*), the tongue deviates to the opposite side on attempted protrusion, and the uvula deviates toward the lesioned side when the patient makes an "ah" sound. In addition, the patient may not be able to elevate the ipsilateral shoulder against resistance (trapezius weakness) or to rotate the head to the contralateral side against resistance (sternocleidomastoid weakness) assuming injury to fibers of the accessory nucleus. This combination of deficits is unique to genu lesions and is clearly different from cranial nerve deficits resulting from brainstem lesions.

Damage to the posterior limb of the internal capsule may result in a frank contralateral *hemiplegia* or *hemiparesis* (-*plegia* refers to paralysis and -*paresis* refers to weakness or incomplete paralysis) affecting upper and lower extremities and a *hemianesthesia* on the same side as the weakness. This sensory loss may affect the body only or the body plus the head.

The *anterior choroidal artery syndrome* (also called *von Monakow syndrome*) is characterized by a *hemiplegia* and a *homonymous hemianopia*, both contralateral to the side of the lesion. If this lesion (which is in the lower portion of the posterior limb) extends upward, it may also involve thalamocortical fibers from sensory relay nuclei, producing a *hemianesthesia* on the same side as the other deficits. This vessel serves portions of the genu, and corticonuclear deficits may sometimes be seen.

ABBREVIATIONS	
f.	Fibers
rad.	Radiations

Review of Blood Supply to the Internal Capsule	
Structures	**Arteries**
Anterior Limb	Lateral striate branches of middle cerebral; medial striate branches of anterior cerebral (see Figure 6-38)
Genu	Lateral striate branches of middle cerebral; anterior choroidal artery (see Figure 6-38)
Posterior Limb	Lateral striate branches of middle cerebral; anterior choroidal artery (see Figure 6-38)
Sublenticular Limb	Penetrating branches of middle cerebral (temporal, angular branches)
Retrolenticular Limb	Posterior cerebral; small branches from anterior choroidal

■ 8-54 The Internal Capsule: Relationships and Contents ■

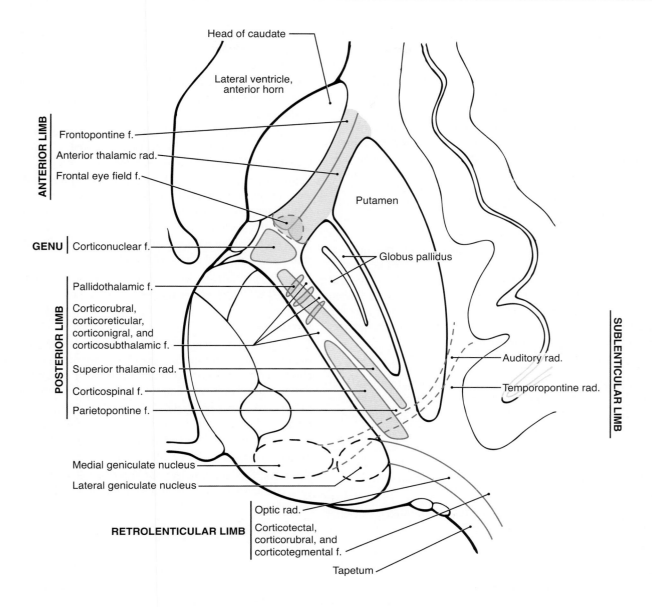

Head of caudate

Lateral ventricle, anterior horn

ANTERIOR LIMB

Frontopontine f.

Anterior thalamic rad.

Frontal eye field f.

Putamen

GENU Corticonuclear f.

Globus pallidus

POSTERIOR LIMB

Pallidothalamic f.

Corticorubral, corticoreticular, corticonigral, and corticosubthalamic f.

Superior thalamic rad.

Corticospinal f.

Parietopontine f.

Auditory rad.

Temporopontine rad.

SUBLENTICULAR LIMB

Medial geniculate nucleus

Lateral geniculate nucleus

Optic rad.

RETROLENTICULAR LIMB Corticotectal, corticorubral, and corticotegmental f.

Tapetum

■ The Topography of Thalamocortical Connections ■

8-55 The major nuclei of the dorsal thalamus, commonly called the thalamus, and their major cortical targets. The thalamic nuclei may generally be divided into *association nuclei, relay nuclei*, and *intralaminar nuclei*. Association nuclei project to multiple cortical regions and receive input from similar diverse regions (e.g., pulvinar, centromedian). Relay nuclei are those which receive a specific type of information (discriminative touch, vision) and send this information on to a precise cortical target (primary somatosensory cortex, primary visual cortex); examples are: the ventral posterolateral nucleus and the lateral geniculate nucleus. Intralaminar nuclei are located within the internal medullary lamina; the most obvious is the centromedian nucleus; smaller intralaminar nuclei include the central lateral, central medial, and the parafascicular nuclei. The *thalamic reticular nucleus* is a group of neurons forming a shell around the thalamus, separated from it by the internal medullary lamina, and located medial to the internal capsule.

The thalamic nuclei receive information from many sources and project to the cerebral cortex. The more important thalamic nuclei, their afferents, and the cortical areas/gyri to which they project are summarized below and illustrated in Figure 8-55 on the facing page. Some generalizations are made for clarity.

Association nuclei:

Dorsomedial nucleus: *afferents*—amygdala, pallidum, temporal and orbitofrontal cortex, olfactory system, basal forebrain; *efferents*—orbital cortex, medial and lateral frontal lobe (excluding the motor cortex)

Pulvinar: *afferents*—superior colliculus, visual cortex (areas 17, 18, 19), temporal and occipital cortex; *efferents*—superior colliculus, visual cortex (areas 17, 18, 19), temporal and occipital cortex

Relay nuclei:

Anterior thalamic nuclei: *afferents*—medial mammillary nucleus, hippocampal formation; *efferents*—cingulate gyrus, small amount to limbic and orbitofrontal cortex

Ventral anterior nucleus: *afferents*—globus pallidus, substantia nigra, cortical areas 6 and 8; *efferents*—frontal cortex (excluding area 4), orbital cortex

Ventral lateral nucleus: *afferents*—globus pallidus, cerebellar nuclei, motor cortex (area 4); *efferents*—motor cortex (area 4), supplemental motor cortex

Ventral posterolateral nucleus: *afferents*—posterior column–medial lemniscus system, anterolateral system; *efferents*—primary somatosensory cortex (areas 3, 1, 2)

Ventral posteromedial nucleus: *afferents*—spinal and principal sensory nuclei, solitary nucleus (taste); *efferents*—face area of primary somatosensory cortex (areas 3, 1, 2), frontal operculum and adjacent insular cortex (taste areas)

Medial geniculate nucleus: *afferent*—inferior colliculus; *efferents*—transverse temporal gyrus (of Heschl)

Lateral geniculate nucleus: *afferents*—portions of both retina, visual area 17; *efferents*—primary visual cortex (area 17, some to 18 and 19)

Intralaminar nuclei:

Centromedian nucleus: *afferents*—frontal, limbic and motor cortex, pallidum, cerebellar nuclei, reticular formation, spinal cord, sensory cortex; *efferents*—corpus striatum (putamen, globus pallidus, caudate), subthalamic nucleus, substantia nigra, frontal lobe

Other intralaminar nuclei: *afferents*—cerebral cortex, brainstem reticular formation, nucleus accumbens, olfactory tubercle; *efferents*—similar to centromedian, cingulate gyrus

Other:

Thalamic reticular nucleus: *afferents*—collaterals of thalamocortical, corticothalamic, thalamostriate, and pallidothalamic fibers; *efferents*—thalamic nuclei

Review of Blood Supply to the Dorsal Thalamus	
Structures	**Arteries**
Anterior Thalamic Areas	Thalamoperforating branches of P_1 (see Figure 6-38)
Posterior Thalamic Areas	Thalamogeniculate branches of P_2 (see Figure 6-38)
Caudomedial Thalamic Area	Medial posterior choroidal artery, P_2 branch (see Figure 6-38)

■ 8-55 The Topography of Thalamocortical Connections ■

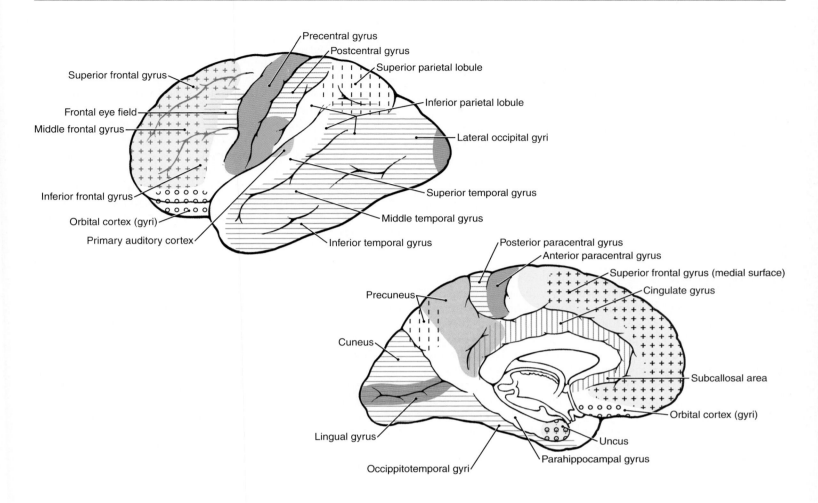

Precentral gyrus
Postcentral gyrus
Superior parietal lobule
Superior frontal gyrus
Inferior parietal lobule
Frontal eye field
Lateral occipital gyri
Middle frontal gyrus
Superior temporal gyrus
Inferior frontal gyrus
Middle temporal gyrus
Orbital cortex (gyri)
Primary auditory cortex
Inferior temporal gyrus

Posterior paracentral gyrus
Anterior paracentral gyrus
Superior frontal gyrus (medial surface)
Cingulate gyrus
Precuneus
Cuneus
Subcallosal area
Orbital cortex (gyri)
Lingual gyrus
Uncus
Parahippocampal gyrus
Occippitotemporal gyri

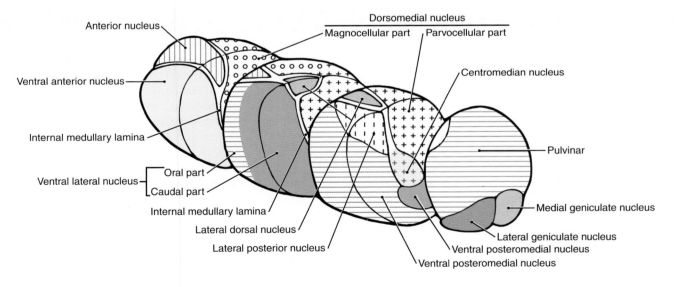

Dorsomedial nucleus
Anterior nucleus
Magnocellular part   Parvocellular part
Centromedian nucleus
Ventral anterior nucleus
Internal medullary lamina
Pulvinar
Ventral lateral nucleus
Oral part
Caudal part
Medial geniculate nucleus
Internal medullary lamina
Lateral dorsal nucleus
Lateral geniculate nucleus
Lateral posterior nucleus
Ventral posteromedial nucleus
Ventral posteromedial nucleus

■ Hippocampal Connections in Anatomical Orientation ■

8-56 Selected afferent and efferent connections of the hippocampus (upper) and the mammillary body (lower) with emphasis on the circuit of Papez. The hippocampus receives input from, and projects to, diencephalic nuclei (especially the mammillary body via the postcommissural fornix), the septal region, and amygdala. The hippocampus receives cortical input from the superior and middle frontal gyri, superior temporal and cingulate gyri, precuneus, lateral occipital cortex, occipitotemporal gyri, and subcallosal cortical areas. The mammillary body is connected with the dorsal and ventral tegmental nuclei, anterior thalamic nucleus (via the mammillothalamic tract), septal nuclei, and through the mammillotegmental tract, to the tegmental pontine and reticulotegmental nuclei.

Neurotransmitters

Glutamate (+)-containing cells in the subiculum and Ammon's horn project to the mammillary body, other hypothalamic centers, and the lateral septal nucleus through the fornix. Cholecystokinin (+) and somatostatin (−) are also found in hippocampal cells that project to septal nuclei and hypothalamic structures. The septal nuclei and the nucleus of the diagonal band give rise to cholinergic afferents to the hippocampus that travel in the fornix. In addition, a γ-aminobutyric acid (−) septohippocampal projection originates from the medial septal nucleus. Enkephalin and glutamate containing hippocampal afferent fibers arise from the adjacent entorhinal cortex; the locus ceruleus gives origin to noradrenergic fibers to the dentate gyrus, Ammon horn, and subiculum; and serotoninergic fibers arise from the rostral raphe nuclei.

Clinical Correlations

Dysfunction associated with damage to the hippocampus is seen in patients with trauma to the temporal lobe, as a sequel to alcoholism, and as a result of neurodegenerative changes seen in the dementing diseases (e.g., *Alzheimer disease* and *Pick disease*). Bilateral injury to the hippocampus results in loss of recent memory (remote memory is unaffected), impaired ability to remember recent (new) events, and difficulty in turning a new experience (something just done or experienced) into a longer-term memory that can be retrieved at a later time. Also, memory that depends on visual, tactile, or auditory discrimination is noticeably affected. These represent *visual agnosia, tactile agnosia,* and *auditory agnosia,* respectively.

In the *Korsakoff syndrome (amnestic confabulatory syndrome)* there is memory loss, dementia, amnesia, and a tendency to give confabulated responses. This type of response is fluent (the patient's response is immediate, smooth, and in appropriate cadence), but consists of a string of unrelated, or even made up, "memories" that never actually occurred or make no sense (hence, the confabulation). This may lead to an incorrect conclusion that the patient is suffering from *dementia*. In addition to lesions in the hippocampus in these patients, the mammillary bodies and dorsomedial nucleus of the thalamus are noticeably affected. The Korsakoff syndrome (see also the *Wernicke-Korsakoff* syndrome) as seen in chronic alcoholics is largely owing to thiamin deficiency and can be treated with therapeutic doses of this vitamin.

ABBREVIATIONS

AC	Anterior commissure		**LT**	Lamina terminalis
AmHrn	Ammon horn		**MB**	Mammillary body
Amy	Amygdaloid nucleus (complex)		**MedFCtx**	Medial frontal cortex
AntNu	Anterior nucleus of thalamus		**MedTh**	Medial thalamus
CC,G	Corpus callosum, genu		**MTegTr**	Mammillotegmental tract
CC,Spl	Corpus callosum, splenium		**MtTr**	Mammillothalamic tract
Cing	Cingulum		**NuAcc**	Nucleus accumbens
CingGy	Cingulate gyrus		**OpCh**	Optic chiasm
CorHip	Corticohippocampal fibers		**Pi**	Pineal
DenGy	Dentate gyrus		**RSplCtx**	Retrosplenial cortex
EnCtx	Entorhinal cortex		**SepNu**	Septal nuclei
For	Fornix		**SMNu**	Supramammillary nucleus
GyRec	Gyrus rectus		**Sub**	Subiculum
Hip	Hippocampus		**TegNu**	Tegmental nuclei
Hyth	Hypothalamus		**VmNu**	Ventromedial hypothalamic nucleus
IC,G	Internal capsule, genu			

Review of Blood Supply to Hip, MB, Hyth, and CingGy	
Structures	**Arteries**
Hip	Anterior choroidal (see Figure 6-38)
MB, Hyth	Branches of circle of Willis (see Figure 2–21)
AntNu	Thalamoperforating (see Figure 6-38)
CingGy	Branches of anterior cerebral

■ 8-56 Hippocampal Connections in Anatomical Orientation ■

■ Amygdaloid Connections in Anatomical Orientation ■

8-57 The origin, course, and distribution of selected afferent and efferent connections of the amygdaloid nuclear complex in sagittal (upper) and coronal (lower) planes. The amygdala receives input from, and projects to, brainstem and forebrain centers via the stria terminalis and the ventral amygdalofugal pathway. Corticoamygdaloid and amygdalocortical fibers interconnect the basal and lateral amygdaloid nuclei with select cortical areas.

Neurotransmitters

Cells in the amygdaloid complex contain vasoactive intestinal polypeptide (VIP, +), neurotensin (NT), somatostatin (SOM, −), enkephalin (ENK, −), and substance P (SP, +). These neurons project, via the stria terminalis or the ventral amygdalofugal path, to the septal nuclei (VIP, NT), the bed nucleus of the stria terminalis (NT, ENK, SP), the hypothalamus (VIP, SOM, SP), the nucleus accumbens septi, and the caudate and putamen (NT). Serotonergic amygdaloid fibers originate from the nucleus raphe dorsalis and the superior central nucleus, dopaminergic axons from the ventral tegmental area and the substantia nigra–pars compacta, and noradrenalin-containing fibers from the locus ceruleus. Glutamate (+) is found in olfactory projections to the prepiriform cortex and the amygdaloid complex. Acetylcholine is present in afferents to the amygdala from the substantia innominata, as well as from the septal area. In patients with Alzheimer disease and the associated dementia, there is a marked loss of acetylcholine-containing neurons in the basal nucleus of the substantia innominata, the cortex, and the hippocampus.

Clinical Correlations

Dysfunctions related to damage to the amygdaloid complex are seen in patients with trauma to the temporal lobes, *herpes simplex encephalitis*, bilateral temporal lobe surgery to treat intractable epileptic activity, and in some CNS degenerative disorders (e.g., *Alzheimer disease* and *Pick disease*). The behavioral changes seen in individuals with what are usually bilateral amygdala lesions collectively form the *Klüver-Bucy syndrome*. In humans these changes/deficits are: 1) *hyperorality*; 2) *visual, tactile,* and *auditory agnosia*; 3) *placidity*; 4) *hyperphagia* or other dietary manifestations; 5) an intense desire to explore the immediate environment (*hypermetamorphosis*); and 6) what is commonly called *hypersexuality*. These changes in sexual attitudes are usually in the form of comments, suggestions, and attempts to make a sexual contact (e.g., touching) rather than in actual intercourse or masturbation. These patients also may show *aphasia, dementia,* and *amnesia.*

ABBREVIATIONS

AC	Anterior commissure	NuRa,d	Nucleus raphe, dorsalis
Amy	Amygdaloid nuclear complex	NuRa,m	Nucleus raphe, magnus
AmyCor	Amygdalocortical fibers	NuRa,o	Nucleus raphe, obscurus
AmyFugPath	Amygdalofugal pathway	NuRa,p	Nucleus raphe, pallidus
AntHyth	Anterior hypothalamus	NuStTer	Nucleus of the stria terminalis
Ba-LatNu	Basal and lateral nuclei	OlfB	Olfactory bulb
CaNu	Caudate nucleus	OpCh	Optic chiasm
Cen-MedNu	Central, cortical and medial nuclei	PAG	Periaqueductal (central) gray
CorAmy	Corticoamygdaloid fibers	PbrNu	Parabrachial nuclei
DVagNu	Dorsal motor vagal nucleus	PfNu	Parafascicular nucleus
EnCtx	Entorhinal cortex	Pi	Pineal
For	Fornix	POpNu	Preoptic nucleus
GP	Globus pallidus	PPriCtx	Prepiriform cortex
Hyth	Hypothalamus	Put	Putamen
LT	Lamina terminalis	SepNu	Septal nuclei
LHAr	Lateral hypothalamic area	SNpc	Substantia nigra, pars compacta
MedThNu	Medial thalamic nuclei	SolNu	Solitary nucleus
MGNu	Medial geniculate nucleus	StTer	Stria terminalis
MidTh	Midline thalamic nuclei	Sub	Subiculum
NuAcc	Nucleus accumbens	SubLn	Substantia innominata
NuCen,s	Nucleus centralis, superior	VenTegAr	Ventral tegmental area
NuCer	Nucleus ceruleus	VmNu	Ventromedial hypothalamic nucleus

---

Review of Blood Supply to Amy and Related Centers	
Structures	**Arteries**
Amy	Anterior choroidal (see Figure 6-38)
Hyth	Branches of circle of Willis (see Figure 6-38)
Brainstem	(see Figures 6-14, 6-21, and 6-27)
Thalamus	Thalamoperforating, thalamogeniculate (see Figure 6-38)

■ 8-57 Amygdaloid Connections in Anatomical Orientation ■

■ Hippocampal and Amygdaloid Efferents in Clinical Orientation ■

Amygdalofugal pathway: To septal nuclei, medial thalamic nuclei, pre-optic nucleus, hypothalamus, substantia innominata, and brainstem nuclei

Middle cerebral artery

Amygdaloid complex

Temporal horn, lateral ventricle

Stria terminalis: To hypothalamus, nucleus accumbens, preoptic nucleus, putamen, and caudate nucleus

Hippocampus

Crus cerebri

Interpeduncular fossa

Midbrain tegmentum

Fornix: To anterior thalamic nucleus, medial mammillary nucleus and hypothalamus, septal nuclei, gyrus rectus and medial frontal cortex, and nucleus accumbens

Anterior lobe of cerebellum

Middle cerebral artery

Uncus

Amygdaloid complex

Temporal horn, lateral ventricle

Hippocampus

Crus cerebri

Stria terminalis

Fornix

Inferior colliculus

Superior (quadrigeminal) cistern

8-58A The principal efferent projections of the amygdaloid nucleus and the hippocampal formation superimposed on MRI in clinical orientation. This axial image is a T2-weighted MRI. The arrowheads on the efferent fibers, and the targets indicated for these fibers, indicate that these pathways have extensive and widespread connections.

■ Hippocampal and Amygdaloid Efferents in Clinical Orientation:
Representative Lesions and Deficits ■

Amygdalofugal pathway: to septal nuclei, medial thalamic nuclei, pre-optic nucleus, hypothalamus, substantia innominata, brainstem nuclei

Middle cerebral artery

Amygdaloid complex

Temporal horn, lateral ventricle

Stria terminalis: to hypothalamus, nucleus accumbens, preoptic nucleus, putamen, caudate nucleus

Hippocampus

Crus cerebri

Interpeduncular fossa

Midbrain tegmentum

Fornix: to anterior thalamic nucleus, hypothalamus, septal nuclei, gyrus rectus + medial frontal cortex, nucleus accumbens

Anterior lobe of cerebellum

Middle cerebral artery

Amygdaloid lesion(s)
-Klüver-Bucy syndrome consisting of hyperorality, hyperphagia, agnosia (visual, tactile, auditory), placidity, hypersexuality, hypermetamorphosis: seen only in bilateral lesions
-Aphasia, amnesia, dementia
-Stimulation = emotional outbursts
-Bilateral lesions more common and correlated with more severe deficits

Hippocampal lesion(s)
-Severe/long-lasting memory deficits in bilateral lesions
-Loss of short-term and immediate memory, unable to turn these into long-term memory; much of long-term (remote) memory is intact
-Other related conditions: Korsakoff and Wernicke-Korsakoff syndromes, Alzheimer disease
-Confabulation, amnesia

Inferior colliculus

Superior (quadrigeminal) cistern

8-58B Representative lesions of the amygdaloid nucleus and hippocampal formation and the deficits that correlate with each lesion. Damage to these regions of the rostral and medial temporal lobes is most frequently bilateral; motor vehicle collisions are common causes. Although there may be damage to only one side, as in stroke, deficits are most severe in situations of bilateral damage.

■ Blank Master Drawing for Limbic Pathways ■

8-59 Blank master drawing for limbic pathways. This illustration is provided for self-evaluation of limbic pathways or connections, for the instructor to expand on aspects of these pathways not covered in the atlas, or both.

NOTES

■ 8-59 Blank Master Drawing for Limbic Pathways ■

■ Hypothalamic Structures and Connections: Stained Sections ■

8-60 The structure of the hypothalamus in three representative coronal sections showing the general arrangement of the nuclei at these levels and the relationships of immediately adjacent fiber bundles and nuclei. The various hypothalamic nuclei that are labeled are generally representative of that level; for a more detailed representation in the axial plane, see Figure 8-61 on p. 286.

The hypothalamus is organized into three rostrocaudally oriented zones. The comparatively narrow *periventricular zone* is located in the ventricular wall, is of an irregular thickness, and contains a number of small nuclei. Neurons within the *periventricular zone* function in the synthesis of releasing hormones that are conveyed to the pituitary via the *tuberoinfundibular tract*. The *medial zone* is located immediately lateral to the periventricular zone and is divided into three regions: a *supraoptic region* (located internal to the optic chiasm), a *tuberal region* (located internal to the location of the tuber cinereum), and a *mammillary region* (located internal to the mammillary body). For the large part, the medial zone is arranged into a number of named nuclei. The *lateral zone* is an area of diffusely arranged neurons commonly called the *lateral hypothalamic area* that contains relatively few named nuclei, but does contain the *medial forebrain bundle*. The positions of the *column of the fornix* and the *mammillothalamic tract* indicate the border between the medial and lateral zones. See Figure 8-61 on p. 286 for additional information on hypothalamic zones and nuclei.

Neurotransmitters

The entire diencephalon constitutes only about 2.0% of the entire CNS by weight and the hypothalamus, a small part of the diencephalon, represents well under 0.2% of the CNS. In spite of its minuscule size, the hypothalamus has a widespread and powerful influence over the CNS, and, indeed, the entire body. This is at least partially reflected by the fact that numerous neurotransmitter substances are found in the cells of the hypothalamus or in terminals ending in these nuclei that arise in other locations. The following is not intended to be an all-inclusive list of transmitters associated with the hypothalamus, but serves as a representative example.

Monoamines: The monoamines *histamine* (cells in the dorsomedial nucleus, posterior hypothalamic area, tuberal nuclei), *dopamine* (cells in the caudal hypothalamus A11 cell group, periventricular area), and *serotonin* (fibers in the dorsomedial, ventromedial, preoptic, suprachiasmatic, and infundibular nuclei) are found in the hypothalamus. Some of these cells may project to other of the hypothalamic nuclei.

Peptides: These are sometimes referred to as gut-brain peptides because they were initially isolated from brain and gut tissue. The principal peptides found in the hypothalamus are *neurotensin* (cells in rostral periventricular zone, the preoptic, paraventricular, and infundibular nuclei and lateral hypothalamic area; fibers in these nuclei and the median eminence), *cholecystokinin* (cells in the paraventricular, medial preoptic, supraoptic, and dorsomedial nuclei; fibers in the ventromedial nucleus), *vasoactive intestinal polypeptide* (cells in the suprachiasmatic nucleus; fibers in the dorsomedial, ventromedial, paraventricular, anterior nucleus, and preoptic regions); and *substance P* (cells and fibers in the supraoptic, paraventricular, dorsomedial, ventromedial, arcuate, preoptic nuclei,

and the lateral hypothalamic area). *Angiotensin II* is in a family of peptides that exhibits vasoconstrictive activity; these cells are found in the paraventricular and supraoptic nuclei (and project to the posterior pituitary), and fibers are found in the dorsomedial nucleus.

Releasing factors (RFs) and releasing hormones (RHs): Many of these substances are associated with projection systems that originate in the hypothalamus and travel to the pituitary. The main releasing factors and releasing hormones are *corticotrophin RF* (cells in the medial preoptic and paraventricular nuclei and the lateral hypothalamic area); *luteinizing RH* (cells in supraoptic, medial preoptic, and infundibular nuclei [the latter projects to the posterior pituitary lobe]); *somatostatin* (cells in infundibular, suprachiasmatic, medial preoptic, and paraventricular nuclei [these cells project to other hypothalamic nuclei]), and *thyrotropin RH* (cells in the median eminence; ventromedial, dorsomedial, preoptic, and suprachiasmatic nuclei; and the periventricular zone).

Dynorphin and enkephalin: These substances are found at many locations in the CNS; one of their functions is related to pain modulation. *Dynorphin* (cells in the supraoptic, suprachiasmatic, ventromedial, dorsomedial, and paraventricular nuclei [all of these nuclei plus the anterior nucleus and medial preoptic area also contain fibers]) and *enkephalin* (cells in the supraoptic and paraventricular nuclei and the preoptic region) are also found in cells located in many areas of the forebrain, brainstem, and spinal cord.

Clinical Correlations

Due to its compact nature and location, deficits related to lesions involving the hypothalamus are frequently complicated by endocrine disorders, visual field defects, and behavioral disorders. Only representative deficits are mentioned here that would relate to lesions within the hypothalamus.

The medial mammillary nucleus receives extensive connections from the hippocampus via the postcommissural part of the fornix. Lesions of the mammillary nuclei result in an inability to process short-term events into long-term memory. This may be seen in vascular lesions or in the *Korsakoff syndrome*.

The suprachiasmatic nucleus receives input from the retina and is involved in the establishment and maintenance of circadian rhythms; these are cycles consisting of a light phase and a dark phase collectively forming about 24 hours. Damage to this area may modify, or abolish, these rhythms.

The supraoptic and paraventricular nuclei synthesize oxytocin and vasopressin and transmit these substances to the posterior lobe of the pituitary via the supraopticohypophyseal tract. Damage to these nuclei, or to this tract, as in a *traumatic brain injury*, may result in *diabetes insipidus*; this condition is characterized by increased water intake (*polydipsia*) and increased urination (*polyuria*).

Damage to the nuclei of the lateral hypothalamic area results in a decrease in feeding behavior with a resultant weight loss, whereas injury to the ventromedial nucleus (commonly called a satiety center) will cause excessive eating and abnormal weight gain. The dorsomedial nucleus, which is dorsally adjacent to the ventromedial nucleus, is a behavioral center; stimulation causes sham rage; destruction results in a decrease in aggression and feeding.

Review of Blood Supply to the Hypothalamus	
Structures	**Arteries**
Anterior Hypothalamus	Anteromedial group from A_1 and ACom (see Figure 2-21)
Mid/Caudal Hypothalamus	Posteromedial group from PCom and P_1 (see Figure 2-21)

■ 8-60 Hypothalamic Structures and Connections: Stained Sections ■

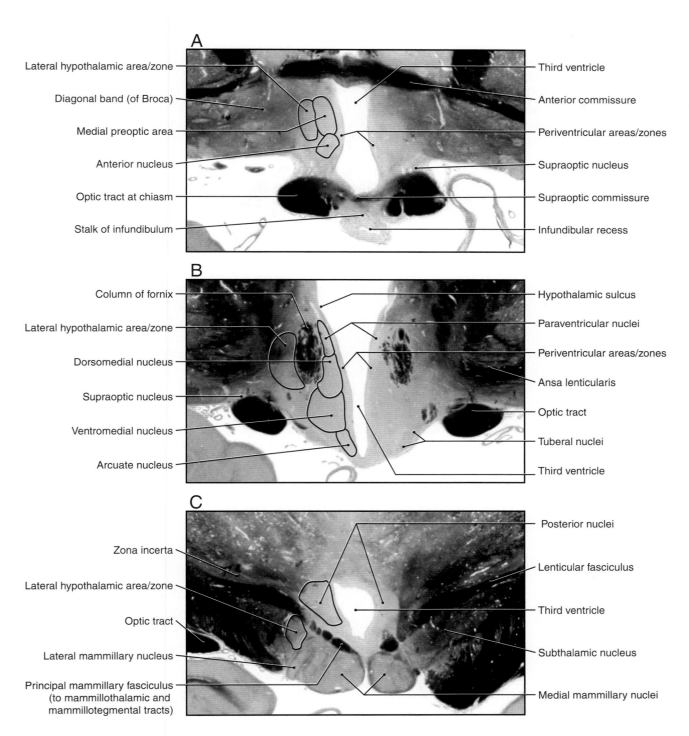

A

Lateral hypothalamic area/zone — Third ventricle

Diagonal band (of Broca) — Anterior commissure

Medial preoptic area — Periventricular areas/zones

Anterior nucleus — Supraoptic nucleus

Optic tract at chiasm — Supraoptic commissure

Stalk of infundibulum — Infundibular recess

B

Column of fornix — Hypothalamic sulcus

Lateral hypothalamic area/zone — Paraventricular nuclei

Dorsomedial nucleus — Periventricular areas/zones

— Ansa lenticularis

Supraoptic nucleus — Optic tract

Ventromedial nucleus — Tuberal nuclei

Arcuate nucleus — Third ventricle

C

— Posterior nuclei

Zona incerta — Lenticular fasciculus

Lateral hypothalamic area/zone — Third ventricle

Optic tract —

Lateral mammillary nucleus — Subthalamic nucleus

Principal mammillary fasciculus (to mammillothalamic and mammillotegmental tracts) — Medial mammillary nuclei

■ Hypothalamic Structures and Connections: Projections ■

8-61 The structure of the hypothalamus represented in the axial plane showing the three zones, the regions and nuclei of the medial zone, and the major afferent and efferent connections of the hypothalamus. The connections of the hypothalamus are complex and widespread within the central nervous system. In addition, many of these connections are reciprocal: structures that project to the hypothalamus frequently receive a return projection from the hypothalamus. An effort is made here to illustrate the hypothalamus in axial plane, its principal nuclei, and its major afferent and efferent pathways, all in a diagrammatic format. Hypothalamic afferents are shown in red (on right), efferents in blue (on left).

Zones: The *lateral zone* (shaded blue) contains diffuse cell groups, the tuberal nuclei, and the fibers of the medial forebrain bundle. The *medial zone* is organized into the *supraoptic region* (shaded green), the *tuberal region* (shaded red), and the *mammillary region* (shaded gray); each region is composed of several named nuclei. The *periventricular zone* (unshaded) is a thin sheet of cells in the wall of the hypothalamic portion of the third ventricle. See also Figure 8-58.

Retinohypothalamic fibers: Axons arising from ganglion cells of the retina project bilaterally to the suprachiasmatic nucleus via the optic nerve and tract. These projections are essential to the *maintenance of circadian rhythms*.

Amygdalohypothalamic fibers: The amydgala projects to the hypothalamus via the *ventral amygdalofugal pathway* (VAF) and the *stria terminalis* (ST). VAF fibers arise in the basolateral amygdala, course medially and inferior to the lenticular nucleus, to end in the septal area, lateral zone, and preoptic areas. Fibers forming the ST arise in the corticomedial amygdala, form a small bundle medial to the caudate and accompanied by the thalamostriate vein, and distribute to the septal area and nuclei of the supraoptic and tuberal regions.

Hippocampohypothalamic fibers: Cells of the hippocampal formation coalesce to form the *fornix*. The *precommissural fornix* distributes to septal, preoptic, and anterior hypothalamic nuclei, whereas the primary target of the *postcommissural fornix* is the medial mammillary nucleus with lesser projections to the dorsomedial nucleus and lateral hypothalamic zone.

Brainstem-hypothalamic fibers: Afferents to the hypothalamus that arise within the brainstem and ascend mainly in the *mammillary peduncle* and *posterior (dorsal) longitudinal fasciculus*, with fewer fibers traversing the *medial forebrain bundle*. These projections arise in the tegmental and raphe nuclei of the midbrain, the locus coeruleus, and the lateral parabrachial nucleus and terminate in the lateral zone and in many of the nuclei of the medial and paraventricular zones. Serotinergic fibers arise from the raphe nuclei, and monoaminergic projections originate from the locus coeruleus.

Other afferent fibers: The hypothalamus also receives spinohypothalamic fibers via the anterolateral system and corticohypothalamic fibers from widespread areas of the cerebral cortex including occipital, frontal, and parietal, and from the cortices of the limbic lobe.

Efferent hypothalamic connections: The double-headed arrows on the left signify the fact that the amygdaloid nuclear complex and the hippocampal formation receive input from the hypothalamic nuclei to which they project. This also applies to the fact that many of the cortical areas that give rise to a corticohypothalamic projection also receive hypothalamocortical fibers.

The *posterior (dorsal) longitudinal fasciculus* contains fibers arising in various nuclei of the periventricular and medial zones and projects to the midbrain tegmentum, tectum, and the central gray of the brainstem; some of these fibers target visceral motor nuclei.

The *principal mammillary fasciculus* is the bundle that passes out of the mammillary nuclei, then immediately divides into *the mammillothalamic tract* and the *mammillotegmental tract*. The former projects to the anterior thalamic nucleus, and the latter projects mainly to the midbrain tegmental nuclei.

Descending fibers that arise in the paraventricular and posterior hypothalamic nuclei (emphasis on the paraventricular) and in the lateral hypothalamic zone, influence brainstem visceral motor and sensory nuclei, parts of the nucleus ambiguus, the ventrolateral medullary regions, and the spinal cord (specifically the interomediolateral cell column). Through these descending fibers to visceral nuclei of the brainstem, the hypothalamus influences a wide range of essential activities controlled by these brainstem regions. Damage to these hypothalamospinal fibers results in a *Horner syndrome (ptosis, myosis, anhydrosis* on the ipsilateral side) along with other deficits characteristic of the lesion be it in the midbrain, lateral pontine tegmentum, lateral medulla, or cervical spinal cord.

The *medial forebrain bundle* is diffusely arranged and contains fibers arising in the lateral zone and ascending to hypothalamic, olfactory, and other basal forebrain areas and of some descending fibers to the brainstem.

Clinical Correlations

In addition to the clinical comments made above, a number of further clinical examples of hypothalamic lesions are described in Figure 8-60 on p. 284. It is important to recall that hypothalamic lesions may initially present with the patient complaining of various visual deficits; a thorough examination and evaluation will reveal the hypothalamic source of the primary lesion.

ABBREVIATIONS

n.	nucleus
tr.	tract

Review of Blood Supply to the Hypothalamus	
Structures	**Arteries**
Anterior Hypothalamus	Anteromedial group from A_1 and ACom (see Figure 2-21)
Mid/Caudal Hypothalamus	Posteromedial group from PCom and P_1 (see Figure 2-21)

■ 8-61 Hypothalamic Structures and Connections: Projections ■

Retina

Amygdalofugal pathway

Stria terminalis

Basolateral amygdala

Anterior commissure

Septal nuclei

Corticomedial amygdala

Hippocampal formation

Precommissural fornix

Postcommisural fornix

To preoptic, supraoptic, and suprachiasmatic nuclei

To anterior thalamic nucleus via mammillothalamic tract

To brainstem tegmentum; tegmental, superior central, dorsal motor vagal, and solitary nuclei; nucleus ambiguus; ventrolateral medulla; and intermediolateral cell column

Third ventricle

From tegmental, raphe, superior central, and parabrachial nuclei; locus coeruleus; central gray; midbrain and pontine tegmentum; and reticular formation

Key for nuclei

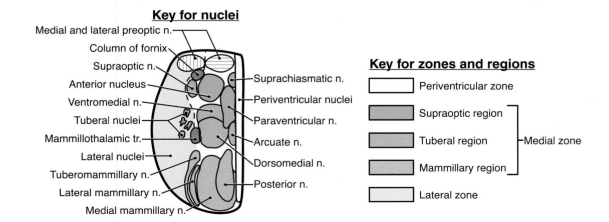

Medial and lateral preoptic n.

Column of fornix

Supraoptic n.

Anterior nucleus

Ventromedial n.

Tuberal nuclei

Mammillothalamic tr.

Lateral nuclei

Tuberomammillary n.

Lateral mammillary n.

Medial mammillary n.

Suprachiasmatic n.

Periventricular nuclei

Paraventricular n.

Arcuate n.

Dorsomedial n.

Posterior n.

Key for zones and regions

☐	Periventricular zone
▨	Supraoptic region
▨	Tuberal region
▨	Mammillary region
☐	Lateral zone

Medial zone

■ Blank Master Drawing for Hypothalamic Structures and Connections ■

8-62 Hypothalamic structures and connections are complex. This illustration is provided in the recognition that the instructor may wish to provide a less detailed, or a more detailed, treatment of the structure and connections of the hypothalamus than is covered in this atlas.

NOTES

■ 8-62 Blank Master Drawing for Hypothalamic Structures and Connections ■

■ The Pituitary Gland ■

8-63 The structure, relationships, and major pathways of the pituitary gland in the sagittal plane. The *pituitary gland*, also called the *hypophysis*, consists of two parts: one that arises from the developing oral cavity (adenohypophysis, anterior lobe) and the other that arises from the developing neural tube (neurohypophysis, posterior lobe).

The *adenohypophysis*, commonly called the anterior lobe of the pituitary, consists of a larger portion called the pars distalis (or pars anterior), a small portion, the pars intermedia, and the pars tuberalis, which is a small extension of the anterior lobe that wraps around the infundibular stalk. The *neurohypophysis*, also called the posterior lobe of the pituitary, consists of a neural lobe, the pars nervosa, and the infundibulum, or infundibular stalk, which joins the neural lobe with the hypothalamus.

The pituitary gland sits in the sella turcica of the sphenoid bone; the diaphragma sellae, a small extension of the dura, forms a donut-shaped structure through which the infundibular stalk passes. The anterior and posterior intercavernous sinuses pass across the midline (and between the cavernous sinuses) at the attachment of the diaphragma sellae to the sphenoid bone.

Hormones

There are numerous hormones and neuroactive substances associated with the hypothalamus and pituitary (see Figure 8-58). Of particular importance to the pituitary gland are those substances found in the *supraopticohypophyseal* and the *tuberoinfundibular* (or *tuberohypophyseal*) tracts.

The peptides *oxytocin* and *vasopressin* (*antidiuretic hormone*) are synthesized in the paraventricular and supraoptic nuclei and transported to the posterior lobe via the supraopticohypophyseal tract. Oxytocin is released during coitus, parturition, suckling, and regression of the uterus after birth. Vasopressin (ADH) is involved in the regulation of fluid homeostasis within the body and may either increase or reduce the production of urine.

A variety of *releasing hormones* are synthesized in the periventricular zone and in the arcuate nucleus, with further contributions coming from the paraventricular, medial preoptic, tuberal, and suprachiasmatic nuclei. These hormones are transported to the hypophyseal portal system and to the anterior lobe where they enter the vascular system.

Clinical Correlations

Due to its location, lesions of the pituitary may present as endocrine disorders, visual deficits (bitemporal hemianopia is most common), features of increased intracranial pressure, diplopia, and headache related to activation of nerves of the diaphragma sellae. In addition, lesions of the pituitary may be classified according to size: microadenomas (less than or equal to 1.0 cm in size) or macroadenomas (greater than 1.0 cm), or as secreting (excess hormone production) or nonsecreting (no hormone secretion). Hypersecreting tumors are those commonly seen in the clinical setting.

Excessive production of *growth hormone* may produce either *gigantism* or *acromegaly*. In the former, excessive hormone is produced before the growth plates have closed; the patient is abnormally tall and has large, but weak, muscles. In the latter, excessive hormone is produced after the growth plates have closed; the patient has large facial features, a large nose and thick lips, large hands and feet, and cardiac problems (hypertension, failure).

Excessive production of *corticotropin* results in *Cushing disease*. The patient has truncal obesity, a rounded ("moonlike") face, *hypertension, acne, osteoporosis,* violet stretch marks, and *diabetes mellitus.* Excessive production of *luteinizing hormone* may result in *hypogonadism* in males (testes may be present, but may not function normally) or disruption of the ovarian cycle in females.

Excessive production of *prolactin* in females results in *gallactorrhea* (milk production when not pregnant) and *amenorrhea* (absent menstrual cycles). *Hyperprolactinemia* in men may be signaled by infertility, decreased libido, or a combination of these signs and symptoms.

Excessive production of *vasopressin* (*antidiuretic hormone*) produces *hyponatremia* (low blood sodium levels and decreased urine excretion) and *natriuresis* (enhanced excretion of sodium in the urine). These patients may have hypotension, dehydration, headache, or may have more serious problems, such as *coma* and *seizures.*

Review of Blood Supply to the Pituitary Gland

The arterial blood supply to the pituitary comes from the *inferior hypophyseal arteries* (branches of the cavernous part of the internal carotid) and from the *superior hypophyseal arteries* (branches of the cerebral part of the internal carotid, A_1, and P_1). The venous drainage is via the hypophyseal portal system and inferior hypophyseal veins into locally adjacent dural sinuses.

▪ 8-63 The Pituitary Gland ▪

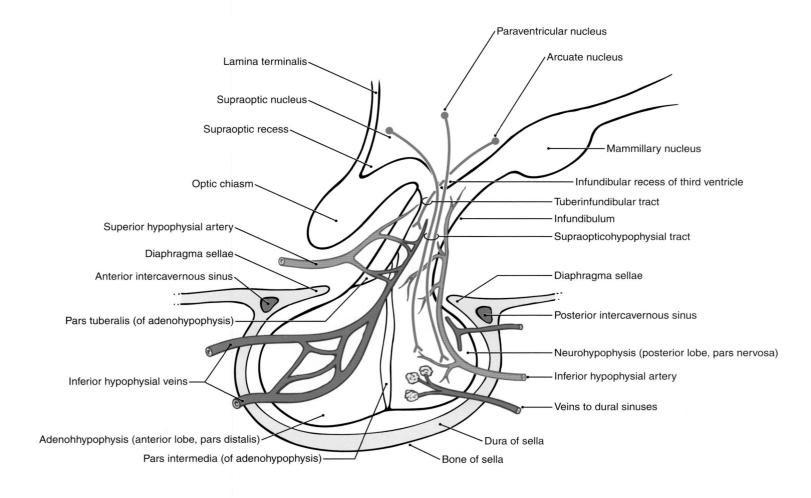

Paraventricular nucleus

Arcuate nucleus

Lamina terminalis

Supraoptic nucleus

Supraoptic recess

Mammillary nucleus

Optic chiasm

Infundibular recess of third ventricle

Tuberinfundibular tract

Superior hypophysial artery

Infundibulum

Supraopticohypophysial tract

Diaphragma sellae

Anterior intercavernous sinus

Diaphragma sellae

Pars tuberalis (of adenohypophysis)

Posterior intercavernous sinus

Neurohypophysis (posterior lobe, pars nervosa)

Inferior hypophysial veins

Inferior hypophysial artery

Veins to dural sinuses

Adenohypophysis (anterior lobe, pars distalis)

Dura of sella

Pars intermedia (of adenohypophysis)

Bone of sella

NOTES

9

Anatomical–Clinical Correlations: Cerebral Angiogram, MRA, and MRV

A

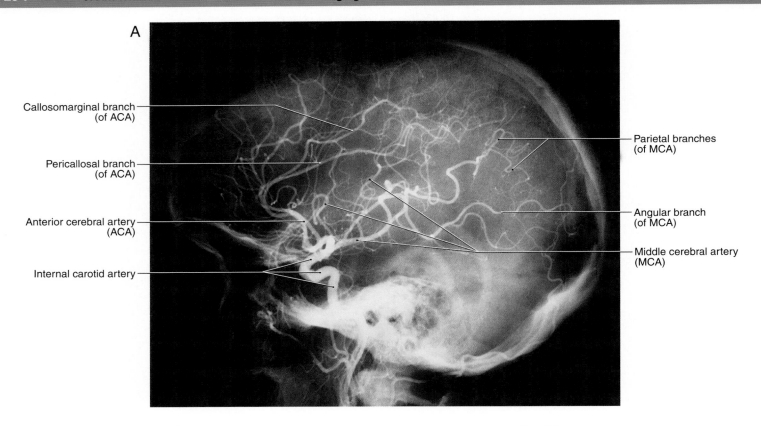

Callosomarginal branch
(of ACA)

Pericallosal branch
(of ACA)

Anterior cerebral artery
(ACA)

Internal carotid artery

Parietal branches
(of MCA)

Angular branch
(of MCA)

Middle cerebral artery
(MCA)

B

Ophthalmic artery

Internal carotid artery
(cavernous part)

Internal carotid artery
(petrous part)

Internal carotid artery
(cerebral part)

9-1 Internal carotid angiogram (left lateral projection, arterial phase) showing the general patterns of the internal carotid, middle, and anterior cerebral arteries (**A, B**) and an image with especially good filling of the ophthalmic artery (**B**). The ophthalmic artery leaves the cerebral part of the internal carotid and enters the orbit via the optic canal. This vessel gives rise to the central artery of the retina, which is an important source of blood supply to the retina. Occlusion of the ophthalmic artery may result in blindness in the eye on that side. The terminal branches of the ophthalmic artery anastomose with superficial vessels around the orbit. The venous drainage of the orbit generally mirrors that of the arteries serving the orbit. Orbital veins receive tributaries from the face and coalesce to form the ophthalmic vein, which ends in the cavernous sinus. This is a potential route through which infections of the face around the orbit, or within the orbit, may access the central nervous system. Compare with Figures 2-12 (p. 19), 2-21 (p. 25), 2-25 (p. 27), and 3-2 (p. 45).

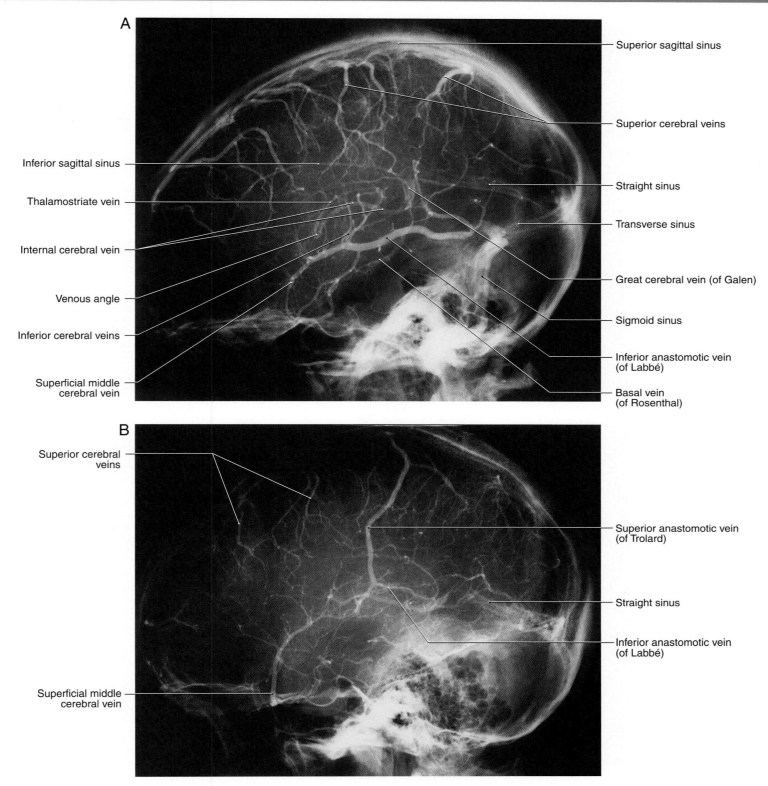

A

Superior sagittal sinus

Superior cerebral veins

Inferior sagittal sinus

Thalamostriate vein

Internal cerebral vein

Venous angle

Inferior cerebral veins

Superficial middle cerebral vein

Straight sinus

Transverse sinus

Great cerebral vein (of Galen)

Sigmoid sinus

Inferior anastomotic vein (of Labbé)

Basal vein (of Rosenthal)

B

Superior cerebral veins

Superior anastomotic vein (of Trolard)

Straight sinus

Inferior anastomotic vein (of Labbé)

Superficial middle cerebral vein

9-2 Two internal carotid angiograms (left lateral projection, venous phase). Superficial and deep venous structures are clear in (**A**), but (**B**) shows a particularly obvious vein of Trolard. The thalamostriate vein (**A**) at this location also can be called the superior thalamostriate vein. The junction of the superior thalamostriate vein with the internal cerebral vein is called the venous angle (**A**). The interventricular foramen is located immediately rostral to this point; small tumors at this location (such as a *colloid cyst*, or a small *choroid plexus papilloma*) may block the flow of cerebrospinal fluid from one or both lateral ventricles and result in *hydrocephalus*. Compare these images with the drawings of veins and sinuses in Figures 2-13 (p. 19), 2-19 (p. 23), and 2-28 (p. 29).

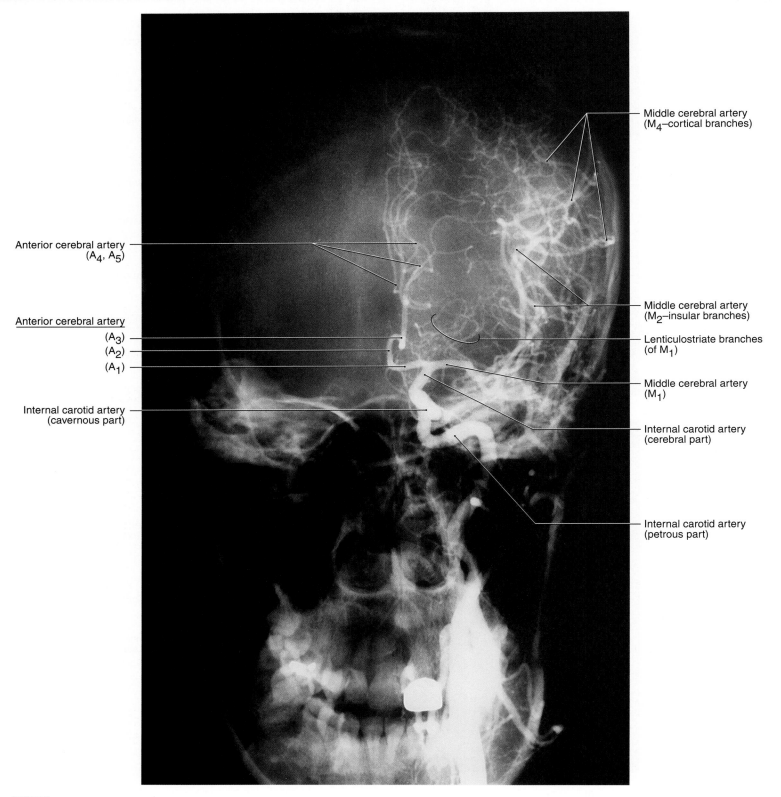

Anterior cerebral artery
(A₄, A₅)

Anterior cerebral artery
(A₃)
(A₂)
(A₁)

Internal carotid artery
(cavernous part)

Middle cerebral artery
(M₄–cortical branches)

Middle cerebral artery
(M₂–insular branches)

Lenticulostriate branches
(of M₁)

Middle cerebral artery
(M₁)

Internal carotid artery
(cerebral part)

Internal carotid artery
(petrous part)

9-3 Internal carotid angiogram (anterior–posterior projection, arterial phase). Note general distribution patterns of anterior and middle cerebral arteries and the location of lenticulostriate branches. The A_1 segment of the anterior cerebral artery is located between the internal carotid bifurcation and the anterior communicating artery. The distal portion of the anterior cerebral artery (ACA) immediately rostral to the anterior communicating artery and inferior to the rostrum of the corpus callosum is the A_2 segment (infracallosal). The portion of the ACA arching around the genu of the corpus callosum is the A_3 segment (precallosal) and the A_4

(supracallosal) and A_5 (postcallosal) segments are located superior (above), and caudal, to the corpus callosum.

The M_1 segment of the middle cerebral artery is located between the internal carotid bifurcation and the point at which this vessel branches into superior and inferior trunks on the insular cortex. As branches of the middle cerebral artery pass over the insular cortex, they are designated as M_2, as M_3 when these branches are located on the inner surface of the frontal, parietal, and temporal opercula, and as M_4 where they exit the lateral sulcus and fan out over the lateral aspect of the cerebral hemisphere. Compare with Figure 2-21 on p. 25.

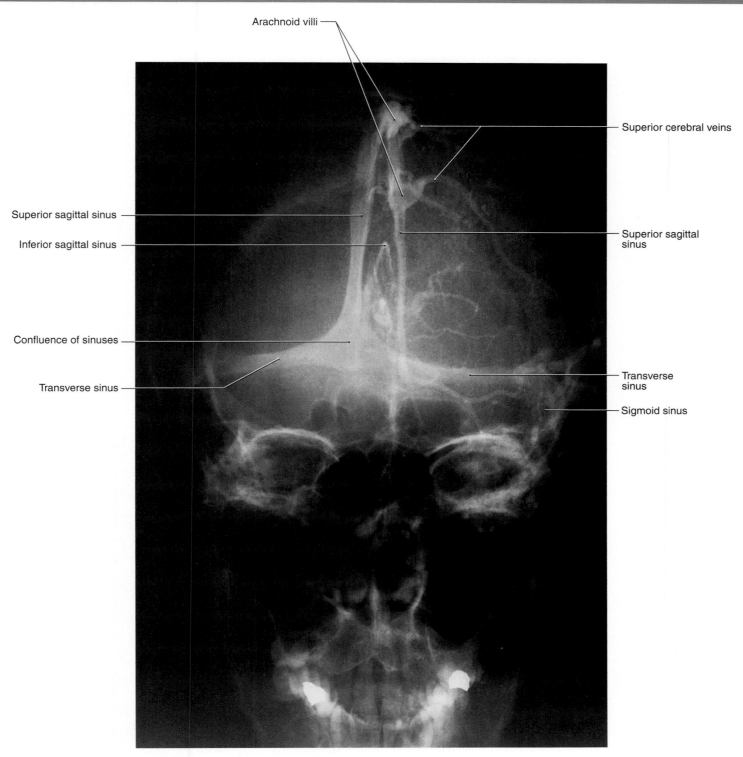

Arachnoid villi

Superior cerebral veins

Superior sagittal sinus

Superior sagittal sinus

Inferior sagittal sinus

Confluence of sinuses

Transverse sinus

Transverse sinus

Sigmoid sinus

9-4 Internal carotid angiogram (anterior–posterior projection, venous phase). The patient's head is tilted slightly; this shows the arching shapes of the superior and inferior sagittal sinuses to full advantage. In many individuals, the superior sagittal sinus turns predominately to the right at the confluence to form the right transverse sinus (see Figure 9-6 on p. 299), and the straight sinus turns mainly to the left to form the left transverse sinus. In some individuals, there is a true confluence of sinuses where both transverse sinuses and the superior sagittal and the straight sinuses meet. Note the other venous structures in this image and compare with the arterial phase shown in Figure 9-3 on p. 296 and the images in Figures 9-5 and 9-6 on pp. 298 and 299. Also compare with Figure 2-28 on p. 29.

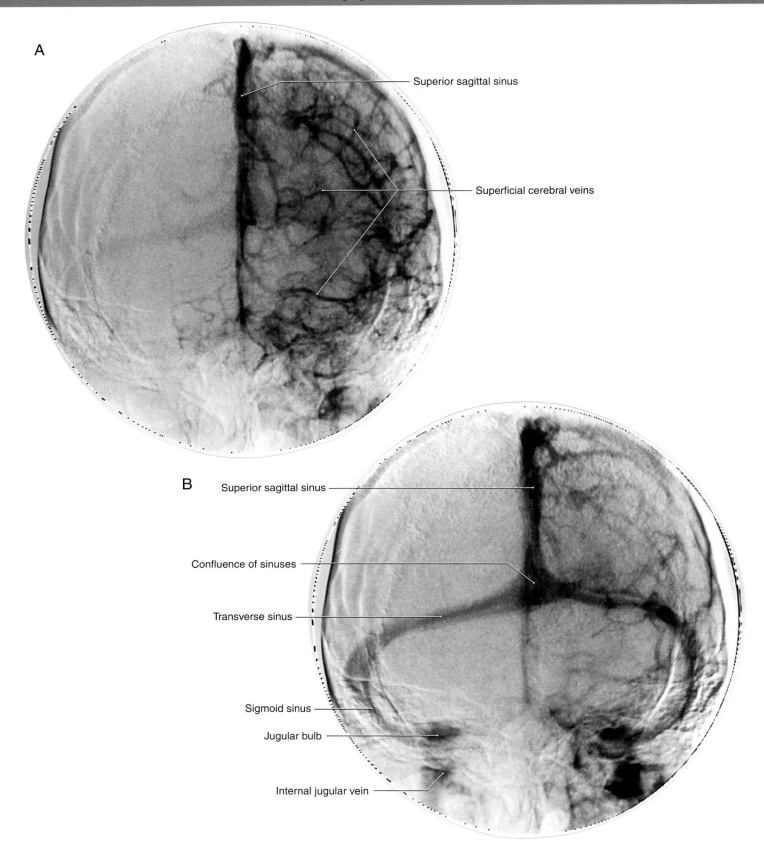

A

Superior sagittal sinus

Superficial cerebral veins

B

Superior sagittal sinus

Confluence of sinuses

Transverse sinus

Sigmoid sinus

Jugular bulb

Internal jugular vein

9-5 Digital subtraction image of an internal carotid angiogram (anterior–posterior projection, venous phase). Image (**A**) is early in the venous phase (greater filling of cortical veins), whereas image (**B**) is later in the venous phase (greater filling of the sinuses and jugular vein). Both images are of the same patient.

The jugular bulb is a dilated portion of internal jugular vein (IJV) in the jugular fossa at the point where the sigmoid sinus is continuous with the IJV; this continuity is through the jugular foramen. The jugular foramen also contains the roots of cranial nerves IX, X, and XI, the continuation of inferior petrosal sinus with the IJV and several small arteries. There are several syndromes that signify damage to the contents of the jugular foramen (such as the *Vernet syndrome*), or damage to these structures plus the hypoglossal root (*Collet-Sicard syndrome*). Recall that the jugular foramen and the hypoglossal canal are immediately adjacent, one to the other, in the posterior fossa. Compare with Figures 2-16 (p. 21) and 2-19 (p. 23).

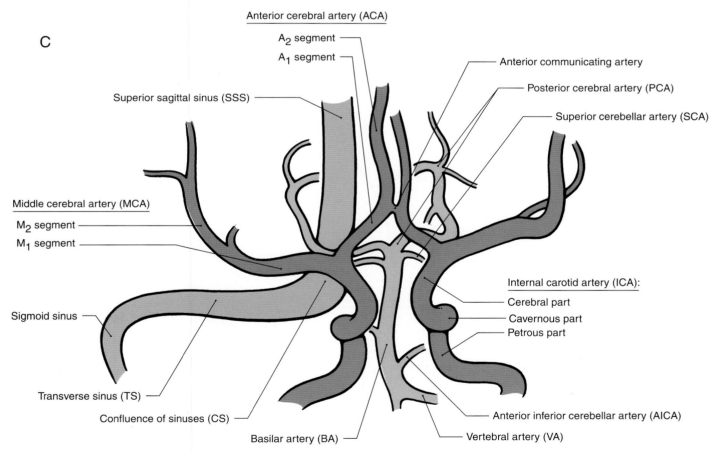

C

Anterior cerebral artery (ACA)

A₂ segment

A₁ segment

Superior sagittal sinus (SSS)

Anterior communicating artery

Posterior cerebral artery (PCA)

Superior cerebellar artery (SCA)

Middle cerebral artery (MCA)

M₂ segment

M₁ segment

Internal carotid artery (ICA):

Cerebral part

Sigmoid sinus

Cavernous part

Petrous part

Transverse sinus (TS)

Confluence of sinuses (CS)

Anterior inferior cerebellar artery (AICA)

Basilar artery (BA)

Vertebral artery (VA)

9-6 Magnetic resonance angiography (MRA) is a noninvasive method for imaging cerebral arteries, veins, and sinuses simultaneously. A three-dimensional phase contrast MRA (**A**) and an inverted video image window (**B**) of the same view show major vessels and sinuses from anterior to posterior. **C** shows the relative position of the major vessels and dural sinuses as imaged in (**A**) and (**B**). The superior sagittal sinus, as seen in (**A**) and (**B**), is usually continuous with the right transverse sinus at the confluence of sinuses.

A

Parieto-occipital branches (of PCA)

Thalamogeniculate arteries

Posterior choroidal arteries

Posterior cerebral arteries (PCA)

Thalamoperforating arteries

Basilar bifurcation

Posterior communicating artery

Superior cerebellar artery (SCA)

Basilar artery (BA)

Calcarine branch (of PCA)

Posterior inferior cerebellar artery (PICA)

Vertebral artery (VA)

B

Parieto-occipital branches

Calcarine branch

PCA

Basilar bifurcation

SCA

BA

Anterior inferior cerebellar artery

PICA

VA

9-7 A vertebral artery angiogram (left lateral projection, arterial phase) is shown in (**A**), and the same view, but in a different patient, is shown in (**B**), using digital subtraction methods. Note the characteristic orientation of the major vessels, particularly the loop of PICA around the medulla and through the cisterna magna. Compare with Figures 2-21 (p. 25) and 2-24 (p. 27).

A

PCA, Cortical branches

PCA

SCA

AICA

Thalamoperforating arteries

Basilar artery (BA)

Vertebral artery (VA)

B

Posterior cerebral arteries (PCA)

Superior cerebellar artery (SCA)

BA

AICA

PICA

Posterior cerebral artery, Cortical branches

Thalamoperforating arteries (of the basilar bifurcation)

SCA

Anterior inferior cerebellar artery (AICA)

Posterior inferior cerebellar artery (PICA)

VA

9-8 A vertebral artery angiogram (anterior–posterior projection, arterial phase) is shown in (**A**); the same view, but in a different patient, is shown in (**B**), using digital subtraction methods. Even though the injection is into the left vertebral, there is bilateral filling of the vertebral arteries and branches of the basilar artery. The thalamoperforating arteries are important branches of P_1 that generally serve rostral portions of the diencephalon.

The root of the oculomotor (third) nerve, after exiting the infe-

rior aspect of the midbrain, characteristically passes through the interpeduncular cistern and between the superior cerebellar and posterior cerebral arteries en route to its exit from the skull through the superior orbital fissure. In this position the third nerve may be damaged by large aneurysms of the rostral end of the basilar artery (called the basilar tip, or basilar head) that impinge on the nerve root. Compare with Figures 2-21 (p. 25), 3-2B (p. 45) and 3-3C (p. 46).

A

Anterior cerebral artery:
A₃ segment
A₂ segment
A₁ segment

Basilar artery (BA)

PCA, Temporal branch

Lateral ventricular vein

Transverse sinus (TS)

Middle cerebral artery (MCA):
M₁ segment
M₂ segment

MCA, Insular branches

Posterior cerebral artery (PCA)

MCA, Cortical branches (M₄ segment)

Internal cerebral vein
Superior petrosal sinus

Great cerebral vein (of Galen)

Straight sinus (SS)

TS

B

Anterior cerebral artery:
(A₃)
(A₂)
MCA, M₂ segment

Internal carotid artery

Posterior communicating artery   BA   PCA   TS

Superior cerebellar artery

Superior sagittal sinus

Great cerebral vein

SS

9-9 MRA images arteries, veins, and sinuses simultaneously, based on the movement of fluid in these structures. These are inverted video images of three-dimensional phase contrast MRA images as viewed in the axial plane (**A**) and from the lateral aspect, a sagittal view (**B**). The portion of the anterior cerebral artery (ACA) located between the internal carotid artery and the anterior communicating artery is the A₁ segment (precommunicating). The part of the ACA immediately rostral to the anterior communicating artery and inferior to the rostrum of the corpus callosum is the A₂ segment (infracallosal). The portion of the ACA arching around the genu of the corpus callosum is the A₃ segment (precallosal) and the A₄ (supracallosal) and A₅ (postcallosal) segments are located superior to (above), and caudal to, the corpus callosum. Compare these images with arteries and veins as depicted in Figures 2-18 and 2-19 (p. 23), 2-21 (p. 25), and 2-23 (p. 26).

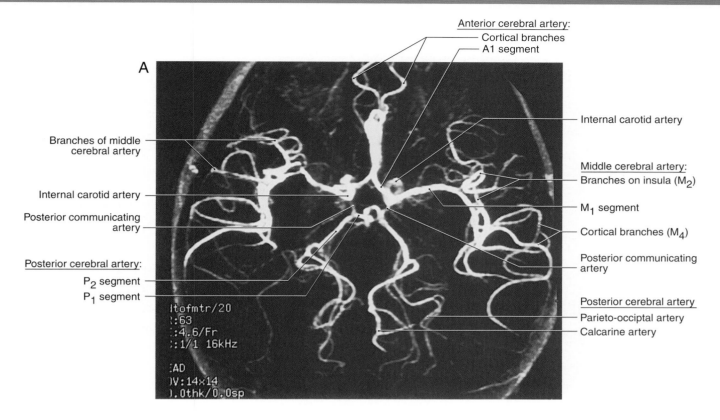

A

Anterior cerebral artery:
— Cortical branches
— A1 segment

Internal carotid artery

Middle cerebral artery:
— Branches on insula (M₂)

Branches of middle cerebral artery

Internal carotid artery

Posterior communicating artery

Posterior cerebral artery:
P₂ segment
P₁ segment

M₁ segment

Cortical branches (M₄)

Posterior communicating artery

Posterior cerebral artery
Parieto-occiptal artery
Calcarine artery

B

Anterior communicating artery

Anterior cerebral artery (A₁ segment)

Middle cerebral artery (branches on insula)

Middle cerebral artery (M₁ segment)

Posterior communicating artery

Basilar artery

Posterior cerebral artery

Orbit

Ophthalmic artery

Cavernosus sinus (containing internal carotid artery)

Petrosal segment of internal carotid artery

Superior cerebellar artery

Tumor (vestibular schwannoma)

Posterior cerebral artery

Calcarine artery

Vertebral arteries

9-10 MRA images, in the axial plane, of the vessels at the base of the brain forming much of the cerebral arterial circle (of Willis) (**A,B**). Note the anterior, middle, and posterior cerebral arteries as they extend outward from the circle. The upper image is from a normal individual, and the lower image is from a patient with a *vestibular schwannoma*. These tumors are generally slow growing, usually present (95%+ of the time) with hearing deficits (difficulty discriminating sounds, hearing loss), and, if especially large (generally, >2.5 cm in size), may involve the trigeminal root with a corresponding sensory loss on the face. Additional deficits include tinnitus, dysequilibrium, headache, facial numbness (about 30% of cases), and facial weakness (interestingly enough, only about 10%–14% of cases). Descriptions of the segments of the anterior, middle, and posterior cerebral arteries are found on pp. 21, 25, 29, 39, and 296.

Superior sagittal sinus

A

Callosomarginal branch of ACA

Pericallosal branch of ACA

Anterior cerebral artery (ACA)

Middle cerebral artery

Ophthalmic artery or vein

Carotid artery (cavernous portions)

Basal vein (of Rosenthal)

Basilar artery

Internal jugular vein

Superficial cerebral veins

Internal cerebral vein

Great cerebral vein (of Galen)

Straight sinus

Vein of Labbé

Transverse sinus

Confluence of sinuses

Sigmoid sinus

B

Superficial cerebral veins

Superior sagittal sinus

Superficial cerebral veins

Middle cerebral artery on insular cortex

Transverse sinus

Sigmoid sinus

Inferior petrosal sinus

Internal jugular vein

Superficial cerebral vein

Confluence of sinuses

Basilar artery

Internal carotid artery

Vertebral artery

9-11 Magnetic resonance venography (MRV) primarily demonstrates veins and venous sinuses, although arteries (seen in **A** and **B**) will also sometimes be visualized. Many veins and venous sinuses can be seen in this lateral, or sagittal, view (**A**) and in the anterior–posterior, or coronal, view (**B**). Note that the continuation of the superior sagittal sinus is most prominent into the right transverse sinus (**B**, compare with Figure 9-6 on p. 299). Compare with Figures 2-13 (p. 19), 2-16 (p. 21), 2-19 (p. 23), and 2-28 (p. 29).

A

Anterior cerebral artery
A₂
A₁

Internal carotid artery
Cerebral part
Cavernous part
Petrosal part
Cervical part

Posterior inferior
cerebellar artery

Maxillary artery
(branch of external
carotid artery)

Middle cerebral artery
M₂
M₁

Basilar artery
Anterior inferior
cerebellar artery

Vertebral artery

Internal carotid artery

Vertebral artery

External carotid artery

Common carotid artery

B

Posterior cerebral artery
Superior cerebellar artery

Basilar artery

Anterior inferior
cerebellar artery

Position of
oculomotor nerve

Anterior inferior
cerebellar artery

Vertebral artery
(intracranial portion)

Vertebral artery
(passing caudally and
medially around the lateral
mass of the atlas)

Vertebral artery
(passing through transverse
foramen of the atlas)

9-12   Overview (**A**) of the arteries in the neck that serve the brain (internal carotid and vertebral) and of their main terminal branches (anterior cerebral artery and middle cerebral artery, vertebrobasilar system) as seen in an MRA (anterior–posterior view). In approximately 40%–45% of individuals, the left vertebral artery is larger, as seen here, and in about 5%–10% of individuals, one or the other of the vertebral arteries may be hypoplastic as seen here on the patient's right. The MRI in (**B**) is a detailed view of the vertebrobasilar system from the point where the vertebral arteries exit the transverse foramen to where the basilar artery bifurcates into the posterior cerebral arteries. Compare this image with Figure 2-21 on p. 25.

The vertebral artery (VA) is generally described as being composed of four segments sometimes designated as V_1 to V_4. The first segment (V_1) is between the VA origin from the subclavian artery and the entrance of VA into the first transverse foramen (usually C6); the second segment (V_2) is that part of VA ascending through the transverse foramen of C6 to C2; the third segment (V_3) is between the exit of VA from the transverse foramen of the axis and the dura at the foramen magnum (this includes the loop of the VA that passes through the transverse foramen of C1/the atlas); the fourth segment (V_4) pierces the dura and joins its counterpart to form the basilar artery.

NOTES

10

Q&As: A Sampling of Study and Review Questions, Many in the USMLE Style, All With Explained Answers

There are two essential goals of a student studying human neurobiology, or, for that matter, the student of any of the medical sciences. The *first* is to gain the knowledge base and diagnostic skills to become a competent health care professional. Addressing the medical needs of the patient with insight, skill, and compassion is paramount. The *second* is to successfully negotiate whatever examination procedures are used in a given setting. These may be standard class examinations, Subject National Board Examination (now used/required in many courses), the USMLE Step 1 Examination (required of all U. S. medical students), or simply the desire, on the part of the student, for self-assessment.

The questions in this chapter are prepared in two general styles. First, there are *study* or *review* questions that test general knowledge concerning the structure of the central nervous system. Many of these have a functional flavor. Second, there are single one-best-answer questions in the *USMLE Style* that use a patient vignette approach in the stem. These questions have been carefully reviewed for clinical accuracy and relevance as used in these examples. At the end of each explained answer, page numbers appear in parentheses that specify where the *correct answer*, be it in a figure or the text, may be found. In order to make this a fruitful learning exercise, some answers may contain additional relevant information to extend the educational process.

In general, the questions are organized by individual chapters, although Chapters 1 and 2 are combined. Reference to the page (or pages) containing the correct answer are usually to the chapter(s) from which the question originated. However, recognizing that neuroscience is dynamic and three-dimensional, some answers contain references to chapters other than that from which the question originated. This provides a greater level of integration by bringing a wider range of information to bear on a single question. Correct diagnosis of the neurologically compromised patient may also require inclusion of concepts gained in other basic science courses. In this regard, a few questions, and their answers, may include such additional basic concepts.

This is not an all-inclusive list of questions, but rather a sampling that covers a wide variety of neuroanatomical and clinically relevant points. There is certainly a much larger variety of questions that can be developed from the topics covered in this atlas. It is hoped that this sample will give the user a good idea of how basic neuroscience information correlates with a range of clinically relevant topics and how questions on these topics may be developed.

▪ Print and On-Line Q&As ▪

The following is a sampling of Questions and Answers that are random and not divided according to chapters. This sample of 60 Q&As plus an additional 225 (for a total of 285) are all available online as one of the several Bonus Materials available for this atlas. This entire set of 285 online Q&As is organized according to chapter and follows the other general guidelines described above.

1. A 69-year-old woman is brought to the Emergency Department. The daughter reports that her mother suddenly seemed to be unable to speak. The examination reveals that the woman has a nonfluent (Broca) aphasia. A sagittal MRI shows a lesion in which of the following gyri?
   (A) Angular
   (B) Inferior frontal
   (C) Lingual
   (D) Middle frontal
   (E) Supramarginal

2. A 71-year-old morbidly obese man is brought to the Emergency Department by his son. The son reports that the man complained of a sudden excruciating headache and then became stuporous. Suspecting a ruptured aneurysm, the physician orders a CT. Which of the following describes the appearance of acute blood in the subarachnoid space in this patient?
   (A) Black (hypodense)
   (B) Black to gray
   (C) Light gray
   (D) Medium gray
   (E) White (hyperdense)

3. Which of the following venous structures is found deep in the lateral sulcus on the surface of the insular cortex?
   (A) Anterior cerebral vein
   (B) Basal vein of Rosenthal
   (C) Deep middle cerebral vein
   (D) Superficial middle cerebral vein
   (E) Vein of Labbé

4. A 47-year-old man presents with an intense pain on his face arising from stimulation at the corner of his mouth. This is characteristic of trigeminal neuralgia (tic douloureux). MRI shows a vessel compressing the root of the trigeminal nerve. Aberrant branches of which of the following vessels would most likely be involved?

(A) Anterior inferior cerebellar artery

(B) Basilar artery

(C) Posterior cerebral artery

(D) Posterior inferior cerebellar artery

(E) Superior cerebellar artery

5. A 22-year-old man is brought to the Emergency Department from the site of a motor vehicle collision. The examination reveals facial lacerations, a dilated right pupil, and loss of most eye movement on the right. He has no other motor or sensory difficulties. CT reveals fractures of the face and orbit. A fracture that traverses which of the following, and damages its contents, would most likely explain this man's deficits?

(A) Foramen ovale

(B) Foramen rotundum

(C) Inferior orbital fissure

(D) Superior orbital fissure

(E) Stylomastoid foramen

6. A 71-year-old woman is diagnosed with a one-and-a-half syndrome resultant to a lesion on the right side of the pons. Movement of which of the following muscles is preserved in this patient?

(A) Left laternal rectus

(B) Left medial rectus

(C) Left superior rectus

(D) Right lateral rectus

(E) Right medial rectus

7. Bacterial meningitis is an inflammation of the meninges that generally is found in which of the following locations?

(A) Epidural space

(B) Subarachnoid space

(C) Subdural space

(D) Subpial space

(E) Ventricular space

8. An 85-year-old woman is brought to the Emergency Department by her family because she suddenly became confused and lethargic. CT shows a hemorrhage into the medial and lateral geniculate bodies. Which of the following structures would also likely be involved in this vascular lesion?

(A) Anterior thalamic nucleus

(B) Rostral dorsomedial nucleus

(C) Globus pallidus

(D) Pulvinar nucleus(i)

(E) Subthalamic nucleus

9. A 16-year-old boy is brought to the Emergency Department following a diving accident at a local quarry. The examination reveals a bilateral loss of motor and sensory function in the trunk and lower extremities. At 36 hours after the accident the boy is able to dorsi-

flex his toes, barely move his right lower extremity at the knee, and is able to perceive pinprick stimulation of the perianal skin (sacral sparing). Which of the following most specifically describes the spinal cord lesion in this patient?

(A) Central cord

(B) Complete

(C) Hemisection

(D) Incomplete

(E) Large syringomyelia

10. A 71-year-old man is brought to the Emergency Department by his wife. She explains that he suddenly became weak in his left lower extremity. She immediately rushed him to the hospital, a trip of about 20 minutes. The examination reveals an alert man who is obese and hypertensive. He has no cranial nerve deficits, is slightly weak on his left side, and has no sensory deficits. Within 2 hours the weakness has disappeared. An MRI obtained the following day shows no lesions. Which of the following most specifically describes this man's medical experience?

(A) Central cord syndrome

(B) Small embolic stroke

(C) Small hemorrhagic stroke

(D) Syringobulbia

(E) Transient ischemic attack

11. An 81-year-old woman is brought to the Emergency Department by her adult grandson. He explains that during dinner she slumped off of her chair, did not lose consciousness, but had trouble speaking. The examination reveals weakness of the upper and lower extremities on the left and deviation of the tongue to the right on protrusion. Which of the following most specifically describes this deficit in this elderly patient?

(A) Alternating hemianesthesia

(B) Hemihypesthesia

(C) Inferior alternating hemiplegia

(D) Middle alternating hemiplegia

(E) Superior alternating hemiplegia

12. Which of the following structures is located immediately internal to the crus cerebri and appears as a dark shade of gray (hypointense) in a sagittal T1-weighted MRI?

(A) Brachium of the inferior colliculus

(B) Periaqueductal gray

(C) Pretectal area

(D) Red nucleus

(E) Substantia nigra

13. A 15-year-old boy is brought to the Emergency Department after an accident on his father's farm. The examination reveals weakness of the left lower extremity, but no frank paralysis. There is a loss of pinprick sensation on the right side beginning at the T8 dermatome (about half way between the nipple and umbilicus), and dorsiflexion of the great toe in response to plantar stimulation. Based on this examination, which of the following represents the most likely approximate location of this lesion?

(A) T6 on the left side

(B) T6 on the right side

(C) T8 on the left side

(D) T8 on the right side

(E) T10 on the left side

14. The physician is conducting a routine neurological examination of a 16-year-old boy in preparation for summer football camp. As part of this examination, he taps the patellar tendon and elicits a knee-jerk reflex. The functional integrity of which of the following spinal levels is tested by this reflex?

    (A) C5–C6

    (B) C7–C8

    (C) T8–T10

    (D) L2–L4

    (E) L5–S1

15. During a busy day in the Emergency Department, the neurology resident sees three patients with brainstem lesions. The first is an 83-year-old woman with a lesion in the territory of the midbrain served by the quadrigeminal and lateral posterior choroidal arteries. The second is a 68-year-old man with a posterior inferior cerebellar artery (lateral medullary or Wallenberg) syndrome. The third is a 47-year-old woman with a presumptive glioblastoma multiforme invading the mid to lateral portions of the pontine tegmentum and adjacent portions of the middle cerebellar peduncle. Which of the following would most likely be seen in all three patients assuming a thorough neurological examination?

    (A) Claude syndrome

    (B) Contralateral hemiplegia

    (C) Facial hemiplegia

    (D) Horner syndrome

    (E) Medial medullary syndrome

16. Somato-visceral reflexes are those in which the afferent limb arises from some type of cutaneous receptor (a somatic afferent), and the efferent limb is mediated through visceromotor fibers. A grain of sand blown into the eye results in increased secretions of the lacrimal gland in an effort to flush the offending object. In the tearing (or lacrimal) reflex, which of the following represents the location of the postganglionic cell bodies that innervate the lacrimal gland?

    (A) Dorsal motor vagal nucleus

    (B) Geniculate ganglion

    (C) Otic ganglion

    (D) Pterygopalatine ganglion

    (E) Superior salivatory nucleus

17. A 23-year-old man is brought to the Emergency Department from an accident at a construction site. CT shows a fracture of the left mastoid bone with total disruption of the stylomastoid foramen. Which of the following deficits would most likely be seen in this man?

    (A) Alternating hemianesthesia

    (B) Alternating hemiplegia

    (C) Central seven

    (D) Facial hemiplegia

    (E) Hemifacial spasm

18. A 59-year-old man, who is a family physician, confides in a neurology colleague that he believes he has early-stage Parkinson disease.

The neurological examination reveals a slight resting tremor of the left hand, slow gait, and lack of the normal range of facial expression. Which of the following is the most likely location of the degenerative changes at this stage of the physician's disease?

    (A) Bilateral substantia nigra

    (B) Left globus pallidus

    (C) Left substantia nigra

    (D) Right globus pallidus

    (E) Right substantia nigra

19. An inherited (autosomal recessive) disorder may appear early in the teenage years. These patients have degenerative changes in the spinocerebellar tracts, posterior columns, corticospinal fibers, cerebellar cortex, and at select places in the brainstem. The symptoms of these patients may include ataxia, paralysis, dysarthria, and other clinical manifestations. This constellation of deficits is most characteristically seen in which of the following?

    (A) Friedreich ataxia

    (B) Huntington disease

    (C) Olivopontocerebellar degeneration (atrophy)

    (D) Parkinson disease

    (E) Wallenberg syndrome

20. A 20-year-old man is brought to the Emergency Department from the site of a motorcycle accident. The examination reveals multiple head injuries and a broken humerus. Cranial CT shows a basal skull fracture extending through the jugular foramen. Assuming that the nerve or nerves that traverse this opening are damaged, which of the following deficits would most likely be seen in this man?

    (A) Deviation of the tongue to the injured side on protrusion

    (B) Diplopia and ptosis

    (C) Drooping and difficulty elevating the shoulder

    (D) Drooping of the face on the ipsilateral side

    (E) Loss of the efferent limb of the corneal reflex

21. Which of the following represents a relay nucleus of the thalamus?

    (A) Centromedian

    (B) Dorsomedial

    (C) Medial geniculate

    (D) Pulvinar

    (E) Thalamic reticular

22. A 39-year-old woman presents with sustained and oscillating muscle contractions that have twisted her trunk and extremities into unusual and abnormal postures. This woman is most likely suffering from which of the following?

    (A) Dysarthria

    (B) Dysmetria

    (C) Dysphagia

    (D) Dyspnea

    (E) Dystonia

23. The mother of a 16-year-old girl brings her to the family physician. The girl explains that she occasionally has drops of a white fluid coming from her breasts. Further examination confirms that the girl is not sexually active and not pregnant. An MRI reveals a small

tumor in the area of the pituitary and hypothalamus. Based on this girl's signs and symptoms, she is most likely suffering from which of the following?

(A) Excessive corticotrophin production

(B) Excessive growth hormone production

(C) Excessive luteinizing hormone production

(D) Excessive prolactin production

(E) Excessive vasopressin production

24. The physician sees three patients in the Emergency Department. The first is a 61-year-old woman with a superior alternating hemiplegia, the second a 12-year-old boy with an ependymoma of the fourth ventricle that is impinging on the facial colliculus, and the third a 72-year-old man with a vascular infarct in the territory of the paramedian branches of the basilar artery in the caudal pons. Which of the following do these patients have in common?

(A) Aphasia

(B) Agnosia

(C) Diplopia

(D) Dysarthria

(E) Dysphagia

25. A 44-year-old woman presents to her family physician with intermittent headache and the complaint that she cannot see with her left eye. The examination reveals that the woman is blind in her left eye. When a light is shined into her left eye there is no direct or consensual pupillary light reflex. Magnetic resonance angiography (MRA) shows a large aneurysm at the origin of the ophthalmic artery. Which of the following represents the usual point of origin of this vessel?

(A) Cavernous part of the internal carotid artery

(B) Cerebral part of the internal carotid artery

(C) First segment (A_1) of the anterior cerebral artery

(D) First segment (M_1) of the middle cerebral artery

(E) Petrous part of the internal carotid artery

Questions 26 and 27 are based on the following patient.
A 59-year-old woman complains of a sudden severe headache that did not seen to respond to OTC medications, but cleared after several hours. Upon questioning her physician discovers that she has recently had prior similar episodes and he orders an MRI. This series of images reveals a large fusiform aneurysm of the P_3 segment.

26. Based on its location, which of the following gyri would most likely be impinged upon by this aneurysm?

(A) Cuneus

(B) Lingual

(C) Orbital

(D) Parahippocampal

(E) Superior temporal

27. Assuming the neurosurgeon decides that this is a serious lesion that requires clipping, which of the following deficits might this patient experience?

(A) Blindness in one eye

(B) Partial bilateral hearing loss

(C) Partial bilateral visual loss

(D) Somatomotor loss on the body

(E) Somatosensory loss on the body

Questions 28 and 29 are based on the following patient.
A 63-year-old man has hearing loss, tinnitus (ringing or buzzing sounds in the ear), vertigo, and unsteady gait; all of these have developed over several years. MRI reveals a large tumor (3 cm in diameter) at the cerebellopontine angle, most likely a vestibular schwannoma (sometimes incorrectly called an acoustic neuroma).

28. What additional deficit could this patient also have?

(A) Anosmia

(B) Hemianopsia

(C) Numbness on the face

(D) Visual field deficits

(E) Weakness of the tongue

29. In addition to the vestibulocochlear nerve, which of the following structures would most likely also be affected by the tumor in this man?

(A) Anterior inferior cerebellar artery

(B) Facial nerve

(C) Glossopharyngeal nerve

(D) Posterior inferior cerebellar artery

(E) Vagus nerve

Questions 30 and 31 are based on the following patient.
A 23-year-old man is brought to the Emergency Department from the site of an automobile collision. The neurological examination reveals weakness of the right lower extremity and a loss of pain and thermal sensations on the left side beginning at the level of the umbilicus. CT shows a fracture of the vertebral column with displacement of bone fragments into the vertebral canal.

30. Damage to which of the following tracts would correlate with weakness of the lower extremity in this man?

(A) Left lateral corticospinal tract

(B) Reticulospinal fibers on the right

(C) Right lateral corticospinal tract

(D) Right rubrospinal tract

(E) Vestibulospinal fibers on the right

31. Which of the following represents the most likely level of damage to the spinal cord resulting from the fracture to the vertebral column in this man?

(A) T6 on the left

(B) T8 on the left

(C) T8 on the right

(D) T10 on the left

(E) T10 on the right

Questions 32 and 33 are based on the following patient.
A 71-year-old woman presents to her family physician with the complaint that "food dribbles out of my mouth when I eat." The examination reveals a unilateral weakness of muscles around the eye (palpebral fissure) and the opening of the mouth (oral fissure). She also has a loss of pain and thermal sensations on the opposite side of the body excluding the head. CT shows an infarcted area in the lateral portion of the pontine tegmentum.

32. Damage to which of the following nuclei would most likely explain the muscle weakness experienced by this woman?

(A) Abducens

(B) Arcuate

(C) Facial motor

(D) Hypoglossal

(E) Trigeminal motor

33. The loss of pain and thermal sensations experienced by this woman would most likely correlate with a lesion involving which of the following structures?

(A) Anterior (ventral) trigeminothalamic tract

(B) Anterolateral system

(C) Lateral lemniscus

(D) Medial lemniscus

(E) Spinal trigeminal tract

Questions 34 and 35 are based on the following patient.
A 41-year-old man is brought to the Emergency Department after an accident at a construction site. The examination reveals a weakness (hemiplegia) and a loss of vibratory sensation and discriminative touch all on the left lower extremity, and a loss of pain and thermal sensations on the right lower extremity. CT shows a fracture of the vertebral column adjacent to the T8 level of the spinal cord.

34. Damage to which of the following fiber bundles or tracts would most likely explain the loss of vibratory sensation in this man?

(A) Anterolateral system on the right

(B) Cuneate fasciculus on the left

(C) Cuneate fasciculus on the right

(D) Gracile fasciculus on the left

(E) Gracile fasciculus on the right

35. The loss of pain and thermal sensation in this man reflects damage to which of the following fiber bundles or tracts?

(A) Anterolateral system on the left

(B) Anterolateral system on the right

(C) Cuneate fasciculus on the left

(D) Gracile fasciculus on the left

(E) Posterior spinocerebellar tract on the left

Questions 36 through 38 are based on the following patient.
An 88-year-old man is brought to the Emergency Department by his daughter. She indicates that he complained of weakness of his "arm" and "leg" (upper and lower extremities) on the right side and of "seeing two of everything" (double vision—diplopia). CT shows an infarcted area in the medial area of the pons at the pons-medulla junction. The infarcted area is consistent with the vascular territory served by paramedian branches of the basilar artery.

36. Weakness of the extremities on the right can be explained by damage to which of the following structures?

(A) Corticospinal fibers on the left

(B) Corticospinal fibers on the right

(C) Middle cerebellar peduncle on the left

(D) Rubrospinal fibers on the left

(E) Rubrospinal fibers on the right

37. The diplopia (double vision) this man is having is most likely the result of damage to which of the following structures?

(A) Abducens nerve root

(B) Facial nerve root

(C) Oculomotor nerve root

(D) Optic nerve

(E) Trochlear nerve or root

38. Recognizing that this patient's lesion involves the territory served by paramedian branches of the basilar artery, which of the following structures is also most likely included in the area of infarction?

(A) Anterolateral system

(B) Facial motor nucleus

(C) Hypoglossal nucleus

(D) Medial lemniscus

(E) Spinal trigeminal tract

Questions 39 through 42 are based on the following patient.
A 69-year-old man is brought to the Emergency Department with the complaint of a sudden loss of sensation. The history reveals that the man is overweight, hypertensive, and does not regularly take medication. When the man speaks his voice is gravelly and hoarse. The examination further reveals a loss of pain and thermal sensations on the right side of his body and on the left side of his face. CT shows an infarcted area in the medulla.

39. Damage to which of the following structures would most likely explain the man's hoarse, gravelly voice?

(A) Facial nucleus

(B) Gracile nucleus

(C) Hypoglossal nucleus

(D) Nucleus ambiguus

(E) Spinal trigeminal nucleus

40. Injury to which of the following structures in this man is most specifically related to the loss of pain and thermal sensations on the body below the neck?

(A) Anterolateral system

(B) Cuneate fasciculus

(C) Gracile fasciculus

(D) Medial lemniscus

(E) Spinal trigeminal tract

41. Damage to which of the following structures would most specifically explain the loss of pain and thermal sensations on the man's face?

(A) Anterolateral system

(B) Medial lemniscus

(C) Medial longitudinal fasciculus

(D) Solitary tract

(E) Spinal trigeminal tract

42. The CT shows an infarcted area in the medulla in this man. Based on the deficits described, and the corresponding structures involved, which of the following vessels is most likely occluded?

(A) Anterior spinal artery

(B) Posterior spinal artery

(C) Posterior inferior cerebellar artery

(D) Anterior inferior cerebellar artery

(E) Penetrating branches of the vertebral artery

Questions 43 through 45 are based on the following patient.
A 73-year-old man is brought to the Emergency Department after losing consciousness at his home. CT shows a hemorrhage into the right hemisphere. The man regains consciousness, but is not fully alert. After 3 to 4 days the man begins to rapidly deteriorate. His pupils are large (dilated) and respond slowly to light, eye movement becomes restricted, there is weakness in the extremities on the left side, and the man becomes comatose. Repeat CT shows an uncal herniation.

43. Based on its location, which of the following parts of the brainstem is most likely to be directly affected by uncal herniation, especially in the early stages?

    (A) Diencephalon/thalamus

    (B) Mesencephalon/midbrain

    (C) Myelencephalon/medulla

    (D) Pons and cerebellum

    (E) Pons only

44. Damage to corticospinal fibers in which of the following locations would most likely explain the weakness in his extremities?

    (A) Left basilar pons

    (B) Left crus cerebri

    (C) Right basilar pons

    (D) Right crus cerebri

    (E) Right posterior limb of the internal capsule

45. The dilated, and slowly responsive, pupils in this man are most likely explained by damage to fibers in which of the following?

    (A) Abducens nerve

    (B) Corticonuclear fibers in the crus

    (C) Oculomotor nerve

    (D) Optic nerve

    (E) Sympathetic fibers on cerebral vessels

46. A newborn girl baby is unable to suckle. The examination reveals that muscles around the oral cavity and of the cheek are poorly developed or absent. A failure in proper development of which of the following structures would most likely contribute to this problem for this baby?
    (A) Head mesoderm

    (B) Pharyngeal arch 1

    (C) Pharyngeal arch 2

    (D) Pharyngeal arch 3

    (E) Pharyngeal arch 4

Questions 47 through 48 are based on the following patient.
A 62-year-old woman presents with tremor and ataxia on the right side of the body excluding the head, and with a loss of most eye movement on the left; the woman's eye is rotated slightly down and out at rest. The left pupil is dilated. There are no sensory losses on her face or body.

47. Based on the deficits seen in this woman, which of the following represents the most likely location of the causative lesion?

    (A) Cerebellum on the left

    (B) Cerebellum on the right

    (C) Midbrain on the left

    (D) Midbrain on the right

    (E) Rostral pons on the right

48. The dilated pupil in this woman is most likely a result of which of the following?

    (A) Intact parasympathetic fibers on the left

    (B) Intact parasympathetic fibers on the right

    (C) Intact sympathetic fibers on the left

    (D) Intact sympathetic fibers on the right

    (E) Interrupted hypothalamospinal fibers on the left

Questions 49 through 50 are based on the following patient.
A 69-year-old man is diagnosed with dysarthria. The history reveals that the man has had this problem for several weeks. MRI shows an infarcted area in the brainstem on the right side.

49. Damage to which of the following structures would most likely explain this deficit in this man?

    (A) Cuneate nucleus

    (B) Nucleus ambiguus

    (C) Solitary tract and nuclei

    (D) Spinal trigeminal tract

    (E) Vestibular nuclei

50. Assuming that the infarcted area in the brain of this man is the result of a vascular occlusion, which of the following arteries is most likely involved?

    (A) Anterior inferior cerebellar

    (B) Labyrinthine

    (C) Posterior inferior cerebellar

    (D) Posterior spinal

    (E) Superior cerebellar

Questions 51 through 53 are based on the following patient.
An 80-year-old woman is brought to the Emergency Department from an assisted care facility. The woman, who is in a wheelchair, complains of not feeling well, numbness on her face, and being hoarse, although she claims not to have a cold. The examination reveals a loss of pain and thermal sensations on the right side of her face and the left side of her body. CT shows an infarcted area in the lateral portion of the medulla.

51. A lesion of which of the following structures in this woman would explain the loss of pain and thermal sensations on her body excluding the head?

    (A) Anterolateral system on the left

    (B) Anterolateral system on the right

    (C) Medial lemniscus on the left

    (D) Spinal trigeminal nucleus on the left

    (E) Spinal trigeminal tract on the left

52. The hoarseness in this woman is most likely due to which of the following?

    (A) Lesion of the facial nucleus

    (B) Lesion of the hypoglossal nucleus/nerve

    (C) Lesion of the nucleus ambiguus

    (D) Lesion of the spinal trigeminal tract

    (E) Lesion of the trigeminal nucleus

53. Assuming this woman suffered a vascular occlusion, which of the following vessels is most likely involved?

    (A) Anterior inferior cerebellar artery

    (B) Anterior spinal artery

    (C) Posterior inferior cerebellar artery

    (D) Posterior spinal artery

    (E) Superior cerebellar artery

Questions 54 and 55 are based on the following patient.
A 37-year-old-man is brought to the Emergency Department from the site of an automobile collision. He was unrestrained and, as a result, has extensive injuries to his face and head. CT shows numerous fractures of the facial bones and skull and blood in the rostral areas of the frontal lobes and in the rostral 3–4 cm of the temporal lobes, bilaterally. After several weeks of recovery the man is moved to a long-term care facility. His behavior is characterized by: (1) difficulty recognizing sounds such as music or words; (2) a propensity to place inappropriate objects in his mouth; (3) a tendency to eat excessively or to eat non-food items such as the leaves on the plant in his room; and (4) a tendency to touch his genitalia.

54. Which of the following most specifically describes the tendency of this man to eat excessively?

    (A) Aphagia

    (B) Dysphagia

    (C) Dyspnea

    (D) Hyperorality

    (E) Hyperphagia

55. Based on the totality of this man's deficits he is most likely suffering from which of the following?

    (A) Klüver-Bucy syndrome

    (B) Korsakoff syndrome

    (C) Senile dementia

    (D) Wallenberg syndrome

    (E) Wernicke aphasia

Questions 56 and 57 are based on the following patient.
A 23-year-old man is brought to the Emergency Department from the site of an automobile collision. CT shows fractures of the facial bones and evidence of bilateral trauma to the temporal lobes (blood in the substance of the brain).

56. As this man recovers, which of the following deficits is most likely to be the most obvious?

    (A) A bilateral sensory loss in the lower body

    (B) A loss of immediate and short-term memory

    (C) A loss of long-term (remote) memory

    (D) Dementia

    (E) Dysphagia and dysarthria

57. Assuming that this man also has sustained bilateral injury to the Meyer-Archambault loop, which of the following deficits would he also most likely have?

    (A) Bitemporal hemianopsia

    (B) Bilateral inferior quadrantanopia

    (C) Bilateral superior quadrantanopia

    (D) Left superior quadrantanopia

    (E) Right superior quadrantanopia

Questions 58 through 60 are based on the following patient.
A 67-year-old man is brought to the Emergency Department by his wife. She explains that he fell suddenly, could not get out of his bed, and complained of feeling sick. The examination revealed a left-sided weakness of the upper and lower extremities, a lack of most movement of the right eye, and a dilated pupil on the right. MRI shows an infarcted area in the brainstem.

58. The weakness of this man's extremities is explained by damage to the axons of cell bodies that are located in which of the following regions of the brain?

    (A) Left somatomotor cortex

    (B) Right anterior paracentral gyrus

    (C) Right crus cerebri

    (D) Right precentral gyrus

    (E) Right somatomotor cortex

59. This man's dilated pupil is due to damage to which of the following fiber populations?

    (A) Preganglionic fibers from the Edinger-Westphal nucleus

    (B) Preganglionic fibers from the inferior salivatory nucleus

    (C) Postganglionic fibers from the ciliary ganglion

    (D) Postganglionic fibers from the geniculate ganglion

    (E) Postganglionic fibers from the superior cervical ganglion

60. Which of the following descriptive phrases best describes the constellation of signs and symptoms seen in this man?

    (A) Alternating hemianesthesia

    (B) Brown-Séquard syndrome

    (C) Inferior alternating hemiplegia

    (D) Middle alternating hemiplegia

    (E) Superior alternating hemiplegia

■ Answers ■

1. **Answer B:** The inferior frontal gyrus consists of the pars orbitalis (Brodmann area 47), pars triangularis (area 45), and pars opercularis (area 44). A lesion located primarily in areas 44 and 45 in the dominant hemisphere will result in a nonfluent (Broca) aphasia. The supramarginal (area 40) and angular (area 39) gyri represent what is called the Wernicke area, and the middle frontal gyrus contains areas 6 and 8. The lingual gyrus is located below the calcarine sulcus; the superior quadrant of the opposite visual fields is represented in this gyrus. (pp. 14, 18)

2. **Answer E:** Patients who experience rupture of an intracranial aneurysm frequently complain of an intense, sudden headache ("the most horrible headache I have ever had"). Acute blood in the subarachnoid space will appear white to very white on CT; this blood is hyperdense. This will contrast with the medium gray of the brain and the black of cerebrospinal fluid (CSF) in the ventricles. The degree of white may vary somewhat, based on the relative concentration of blood, from very white (concentrated blood) to white (mostly blood, some CSF), to very light gray (mixture of blood and CSF). (pp. 2–4)

3. Answer C: The deep middle cerebral vein is located on the insular cortex and, by joining with the anterior cerebral vein, forms the basal vein of Rosenthal. The superficial middle cerebral vein is located on the lateral aspect of the hemisphere in the vicinity of the lateral sulcus, arches around the temporal lobe, and joins the cavernous sinus. The vein of Labbé drains the lateral aspect of the hemisphere into the transverse sinus. (pp. 19, 21, 39)

4. Answer E: Branches of the superior cerebellar artery are most frequently involved in cases of trigeminal neuralgia that are presumably of vascular origin. The posterior cerebral artery and its larger branches serve the midbrain–diencephalic junction or join the medial surface of the hemisphere. The basilar artery serves the basilar pons and the anterior inferior cerebellar artery serves the caudal midbrain, inner ear, and the inferior surface of the cerebellar surface. The basal vein drains the medial portions of the hemisphere and passes through the ambient cistern to enter the great cerebral vein (of Galen). (p. 47)

5. Answer D: This man's deficits, loss of most (but not all) eye movement and dilation of the pupil on that side. These losses, with no other deficits, indicate damage to the oculomotor nerve; this nerve exits the cranial cavity via the superior orbital fissure. This fissure also transmits the ophthalmic nerve. The foramen ovale transmits the mandibular nerve (plus fibers to the masticatory muscles) and the foramen rotundum transmits the maxillary nerve. After the maxillary nerve passes through the rotundum, it shifts course and enters the orbit via the inferior orbital fissure. The facial nerve passes through the stylomastoid foramen. (pp. 42, 43)

6. Answer A: In this patient the pontine lesion is on the right side. This results in a paralysis of the right lateral rectus (abducens lower motor neurons) and the right and left medial recti (damage to the axons of interneurons in the medial longitudinal fasciculus on both sides). The surviving muscle is the left lateral rectus. (pp. 51, 52)

7. Answer B: The inflammation in meningitis generally occupies the subarachnoid space and its minute extensions into the sulci; the infection may extend into cisterns. The commonly used clinical terms leptomeningitis (signifying arachnoid + pia) or pia-arachnitis reflect the fact that this infection is frequently sequestered within the subarachnoid space. Meningitis may involve the dura (pachymeningitis) and, by extension, invade the minute spaces between the pia and brain surface (subpial space). However, these are not the main locations of this disease process. Epidural and subdural spaces are the result of trauma or some pathologic process and, around the brain, are not naturally occurring spaces. (pp. 56–59)

8. Answer D: The geniculate bodies are tucked-up under the caudal and inferior aspect of the pulvinar. The groove between the medial geniculate body and pulvinar contains the brachium of the superior colliculus. The geniculate bodies and the pulvinar have a common blood supply from the thalamogeniculate artery, a branch of P_2. None of the other choices have a close apposition with the geniculate bodies. The anterior thalamic, rostral dorsomedial, and subthalamic nuclei do not share a common blood supply with the pulvinar. (pp. 80, 87)

9. Answer D: Although this patient initially presented with complete motor and sensory losses, some function had returned by 36 hours; in this case, the lesion is classified as an incomplete lesion of the spinal cord. Patients with no return of function at 24+ hours and no sacral sparing have suffered a lesion classified as complete and it is unlikely that they will recover useful neurological function. In

a central cord and a large syringomyelia, there is sparing of posterior column sensations and in a hemisection the loss of motor function is unilateral. (pp. 104–105)

10. Answer E: The short-term loss of function, frequently involving a specific part of the body, is characteristic of a transient ischemic attack (commonly called a TIA). The follow-up MRI shows no lesion because there has been no permanent damage. TIAs are caused by a brief period of inadequate perfusion of a localized region of the nervous system; recovery is usually rapid and complete. However, TIAs, especially if repeated, may be indicative of an impending stroke. Hemorrhagic strokes frequently result in some type of permanent deficit, and the central cord syndrome has bilateral deficits. A small embolic stroke would be visible on the follow-up MRI and, in this patient, would have resulted in a persistent deficit. Syringobulbia may include long tract signs as well as cranial nerve signs. (pp. 160, 168–169)

11. Answer C: Weakness of the extremities accompanied by paralysis of muscles on the contralateral side of the tongue (seen as a deviation of the tongue to that side on protrusion) indicates a lesion in the medulla involving the corticospinal fibers in the pyramid and the exiting hypoglossal roots. This is an inferior alternating hemiplegia. Middle alternating hemiplegia refers to a lesion of the pontine corticospinal fibers and the root of the abducens nerve, and superior alternating hemiplegia specifies damage to the oculomotor root and crus cerebri. Alternating (alternate) hemianesthesia and hemihypesthesia are sensory losses. (pp. 120–121)

12. Answer E: The substantia nigra is located internal to the crus cerebri and, in T1-weighted MRI, appears a darker shade of gray (hypointense) than does the crus. The red nucleus and the periaqueductal gray are located in the midbrain, but do not border on the crus cerebri. The brachium of the inferior colliculus is found on the lateral surface of the midbrain, and the pretectal area is adjacent to the cerebral aqueduct at the midbrain–diencephalic junction. (pp. 175, 178–180)

13. Answer A: The combination of weakness on one side (corticospinal involvement) and a loss of pain sensation on the opposite side specifies components of Brown-Séquard syndrome. The motor loss is ipsilateral to the damage and the sensory loss is contralateral; second order fibers conveying pain information cross in the anterior white commissure ascending one to two spinal segments in the process. In this patient, the lesion is on the left side at about the T6 level; this explains the loss of pain sensation on the right beginning at the T8 dermatome level. Lesions at T8 or T10 would result in a loss of pain sensation beginning, respectively, at dermatome levels T10 or T12 on the contralateral side. (pp. 192–195, 206–209)

14. Answer B: A tap on the patellar tendon results is contraction of the quadriceps muscles of the thigh and the knee abruptly swinging forward; this is mediated through spinal levels L2–L4. This is a monosynaptic reflex with excitation of the extensor muscles of the leg and, through an interneuron, inhibition of leg flexors. The biceps reflex is mediated through C5–C6, and the triceps through C7–C8. The abdominal reflex is mediated through spinal levels T8–T10; level S1, with contributions from L5 and S2, mediates the ankle reflex. (p. 230)

15. Answer D: Lesions in the lateral portions of the brainstem damage descending projections from the hypothalamus to the ipsilateral intermediolateral cell column at spinal levels T1–T4, these being the hypothalamospinal fibers. The result is Horner syndrome on

the side ipsilateral to the lesion. Horner syndrome also may be seen following cervical spinal cord lesions. A contralateral hemiplegia is not seen in lesions in lateral areas of the brainstem. The other choices are syndromes or deficits specific to medial brainstem areas or to only a particular level. (pp. 120–121, 134–135, 146–147, 258–259)

16. Answer **D:** The afferent limb of the tearing (lacrimal) reflex is via the trigeminal nerve (pain receptors in the conjunctiva and cornea), and the efferent limb travels on the facial nerve; the preganglionic parasympathetic cells are in the superior salivatory nucleus, and the postganglionic cells are in the pterygopalatine ganglion. The dorsal motor vagal nucleus contains preganglionic parasympathetic cells that distribute to ganglia in the thorax and abdomen. The geniculate ganglion contains the cell bodies of somatic afferent (SA) and visceral afferent (VA) fibers that enter the brain on the facial nerve; the otic ganglion contains postganglionic parasympathetic cell bodies that serve the parotid gland. (pp. 266–229, 233)

17. Answer **D:** The paralysis of facial muscles on one side of the face (left in this case) with no paralysis of the extremities is a facial hemiplegia; this is also commonly known as *Bell palsy* or *facial palsy*. Hemifacial spasms are irregular contractions of the facial muscles, and a central seven (also called a *supranuclear facial palsy*) refers to paralysis of muscles on the lower half of the face contralateral to a lesion in the genu of the internal capsule. *Alternating hemiplegia* describes a motor loss related to a cranial nerve on one side of the head and motor deficits of the extremities on the contralateral side of the body. A similar pattern of sensory losses is called an *alternating hemianesthesia*. (pp. 226–229)

18. Answer **E:** Degenerative changes in the dopamine-containing cells of the substantia nigra pars compacta on the right side correlate with a left-sided tremor. The altered message through the lenticular nucleus and thalamus and on to the motor cortex on the side of the degenerative changes will result in tremor on the opposite (right) side via altered messages traveling down the corticospinal tract. The initial symptoms of Parkinson disease appear on one side in about 80% of patients and extend to bilateral involvement as the disease progresses. Bilateral changes in the substantia nigra correlate with bilateral deficits. The globus pallidus does not receive direct nigral input but rather input via a nigrostriatal-striatopallidal circuit. (pp. 250–251, 254–255)

19. Answer **A:** This inherited disease is Friedreich ataxia; it initially appears in children in the age range of 8 to 15 years and has the characteristic deficits described. Huntington disease is inherited, but appears in adults; olivopontocerebellar atrophy is an autosomal dominant disease and gives rise to a different set of deficits. The cause of Parkinson disease is unclear, but it is probably not inherited; the Wallenberg syndrome is a brainstem lesion resulting from a vascular occlusion. (pp. 238–239)

20. Answer **C:** A fracture through the jugular foramen would potentially damage the glossopharyngeal (IX), vagus (X), and spinal accessory (XI) nerves. The major observable deficit would be a loss of the efferent limb of the gag reflex and paralysis of the ipsilateral trapezius and sternocleidomastoid muscles (drooping of the shoulder, difficulty elevating the shoulder especially against resistance, difficulty turning the head to the contralateral side). Involvement of facial muscles would suggest damage to the internal acoustic or stylomastoid foramina; this would also be the case for the efferent limb of the corneal reflex. Diplopia and ptosis would suggest injury to the superior orbital fissure, as all three nerves controlling

ocular movement traverse this space. The hypoglossal nerve (which supplies muscles of the tongue) passes through the hypoglossal canal. (pp. 222–225)

21. Answer **C:** A relay nucleus is one that receives a specific type of information from a comparatively specific source, and sends this information on to an equally specific cortical target. The medial geniculate nucleus receives mainly auditory information from the cochlear nuclei and brainstem auditory relay nuclei and projects to the transverse temporal gyrus. The dorsomedial, centromedian and pulvinar are association nuclei; these receive input from diverse sources and project to equally diverse cortical targets. The thalamic reticular nucleus, while not specifically classified as either a relay nucleus or an association nucleus, basically functions as an association nucleus. (pp. 274–275)

22. Answer **E:** Dystonia is a movement disorder characterized by abnormal, sometimes intermittent, but frequently sustained, contractions of the muscles of the trunk and extremities that force the body into a twisted posture. Dystonia may be seen in patients with diseases of the basal nuclei. Dysmetria is the inability to judge the distance and trajectory of a movement. Dyspnea is difficulty breathing; this may result from heart and/or lung disorders as well as from neurological disorders. Dysphagia is difficulty swallowing, and dysarthria is difficulty speaking. (pp. 250–251)

23. Answer **D:** A prolactinoma, a tumor that produces excessive amounts of prolactin (a hypersecreting tumor), may result in milk production in females in the absence of pregnancy. In females, excess luteinizing hormone may disrupt the ovarian cycle but not result in milk production. Overproduction of corticotrophin results is Cushing disease; excessive growth hormone results in either gigantism (before growth plates close) or acromegaly (after growth plates close). Overproduction of vasopressin influences urine excretion. (pp. 290–291)

24. Answer **C:** These three involve the roots of the oculomotor and abducens nerve and the nucleus of the abducens nerve, all of which innervate extraocular muscles. Each of these patients would experience some form of diplopia, one of their complaints would be seeing "double." Aphasia and agnosia are usually associated with lesions of the forebrain. Dysarthria and dysphagia are frequently seen in medullary lesions, but may also be seen in patients with large hemispheric strokes. Hemianesthesia may be present in patients with lesions at many levels of the central nervous system, but rarely with medially located lesions as is the case with these three patients. (pp. 222–225)

25. Answer **B:** In most instances (approximately 80%–85%), the ophthalmic artery originates from the cerebral portion of the internal carotid artery just as this parent vessel leaves the cavernous sinus and passes through the dura. In a small percentage of cases, the ophthalmic artery may originate from other locations on the internal carotid artery, including its cavernous portion. This vessel does not originate from the petrous portion of the internal carotid or from anterior or middle cerebral arteries. (pp. 25, 294)

26. Answer **D:** The P₃ segment lies along the orientation of, and adjacent to, the parahippocampal gyrus as this part of the posterior cerebral artery courses around the midbrain. Branches of the P₃ segment serve the inferior surface of the temporal lobe, which includes much of the laterally adjacent occipitotemporal gyri. The lingual gyrus and the cuneus are in the territory of the P₄ segment and the orbital gyri are served by branches of the anterior and middle cerebral

arteries. The superior temporal gyrus is served by M_4 branches of the inferior trunk of the middle cerebral artery. (pp. 21, 29)

27. Answer C: Clipping the P_3 segment proximal to the aneurysm would block all blood flow to targets distal to this point. Distal portions of the posterior cerebral artery (the P_4 segment) serve the primary visual cortex. Somatosensory, somatomotor, and auditory regions of the cerebral cortex are served by terminal branches of the middle cerebral artery (M_4 in the case of motor and sensory, M_3/M_4 in the case of auditory). Blindness in one eye would result from a lesion rostral to the optic chiasm; in the case of a vascular cause, this may relate to damage to the ophthalmic branch of the internal carotid. (pp. 21, 29)

28. Answer C: Vestibular schwannomas larger than 2.0 cm in diameter may impinge on the root of the trigeminal nerve and cause numbness on the same side of the face. Although the other deficits listed are not seen in these patients, diplopia (involvement of oculomotor, abducens or trochlear nerves, singularly or in combination) may be present, but in fewer than 10% of these individuals. (pp. 48, 303)

29. Answer B: The internal acoustic meatus contains the vestibulo-cochlear nerve, the facial nerve, and the labyrinthine artery, a branch of the anterior inferior cerebellar artery. A vestibular schwannoma located in the meatus may affect the facial nerve and result in facial weakness. While certainly a potential complication, facial weakness is seen in only about 10% of patients with a vestibular schwannoma. The vagus and glossopharyngeal nerves exit the skull via the jugular foramen (along with the accessory nerve). The cerebellar arteries originate within the skull and distribute to structures within the skull. (pp. 48, 303)

30. Answer C: In this patient the weakness of the right lower extremity is related to a lesion of lateral corticospinal tract fibers on the right side of the spinal cord. The left corticospinal tract serves the left side of the spinal cord and the left lower extremity. Rubrospinal, reticulospinal, and vestibulospinal fibers influence the activity of spinal motor neurons; however, the deficits related to corticospinal tract damage (significant weakness) will dominate over the lack of excitation to flexor or extensor motor neurons in the spinal cord via these tracts. (pp. 98–101, 104–105)

31. Answer C: The loss of pain and thermal sensations beginning at the level of the umbilicus (T10 dermatome) on the left side results from damage to fibers of the anterolateral system at about the T8 level on the right. These fibers ascend one to two levels as they cross the midline. Damage at the T6 level would result in a loss beginning at the T8 level on the contralateral side and damage at the T10 level would result in a loss beginning at about the T12 level. (pp. 98–101, 104–105)

32. Answer C: Weakness of the muscles of the face, particularly when upper and lower portions of the face are involved, indicate a lesion of either the facial motor nucleus or the exiting fibers of the facial nerve; both are located in the lateral pontine tegmentum at caudal levels. The hypoglossal nucleus innervates muscles of the tongue, the trigeminal nucleus innervates masticatory muscles, and the abducens nucleus innervates the lateral rectus muscle, all on the ipsilateral side. The arcuate nucleus is a group of cells located on the surface of the pyramid. (pp. 126–129, 134–135)

33. Answer B: The fibers of the anterolateral system are located in the lateral portion of the pontine tegmentum anterior (ventral) to the facial motor nucleus; these fibers convey pain and thermal inputs.

The spinal trigeminal tract and the anterior trigeminothalamic tract also convey pain and thermal input but from the ipsilateral and contralateral sides of the face, respectively. The lateral lemniscus is auditory in function and the medial lemniscus conveys proprioception, vibratory sense, and discriminative touch. (pp. 52, 126–129, 134–135)

34. Answer D: Damage to the gracile fasciculus on the left (at the T8 level this is the only part of the posterior columns present) accounts for the loss of vibratory sensation (and discriminative touch). Injury to the gracile fasciculus on the right would result in this type of deficit on the right side. The level of the cord damage is caudal to the cuneate fasciculi and the anterolateral system conveys pain and thermal sensations. (pp. 98–101, 104–105)

35. Answer A: The loss of pain and thermal sensations on the right side of the body correlates with a lesion involving the anterolateral system on the left side of the spinal cord. A lesion of the right anterolateral system would result in a left-sided deficit. The gracile and cuneate fasciculi convey discriminative touch, vibratory sensation, and proprioception. The posterior spinocerebellar tract conveys similar information, but it is not perceived/recognized as such (consciously) by the brain. (pp. 98–101, 104–105)

36. Answer A: In this case the weakness of the upper and lower extremities on the right reflects damage to corticospinal fibers on the left side of the basilar pons. A lesion of these fibers on the right side of the pons would produce a left-sided weakness. Rubrospinal fibers are not located in the territory of paramedian branches of the basilar artery. Also, lesions of rubrospinal fibers and of the middle cerebellar peduncle do not cause weakness but may cause other types of motor deficits. (pp. 126–129, 134–135)

37. Answer A: The exiting fibers of the abducens nerve (on the left) are in the territory of the paramedian branches of the basilar artery and are laterally adjacent to corticospinal fibers in the basilar pons. Diplopia may result from lesions of the oculomotor and trochlear nerves, but these structures are not in the domain of the paramedian basilar branches. A lesion of the optic nerve results in blindness in that eye and damage to the facial root does not affect eye movement but may cause a loss of view of the external world if the palpebral fissure is closed due to facial muscle weakness. (pp. 52, 126–129, 135)

38. Answer D: At caudal pontine levels most, if not all, of the medial lemniscus is located within the territory served by paramedian branches of the basilar artery. Penetrating branches of the anterior spinal artery serve the hypoglossal nucleus. The other choices are generally in the territories of short or long circumferential branches of the basilar artery. (pp. 52, 126–129, 134–135)

39. Answer D: The vocalis muscle (this muscle is actually the medial portion of the thyroarytenoid muscle) is innervated, via the vagus nerve, by motor neurons located in the nucleus ambiguus. The gracile nucleus conveys sensory input from the body and the spinal trigeminal nucleus relays sensory input from the face. The hypoglossal nucleus is motor to the tongue and the facial nucleus is motor to the muscles of facial expression. (pp. 112–117, 120–121)

40. Answer A: Fibers comprising the anterolateral system convey pain and thermal sensations from the body, excluding the face. These fibers are located in lateral portions of the medulla adjacent to the spinal trigeminal tract; this latter tract relays pain and thermal sensations from the face. The gracile and cuneate fasciculi convey

proprioception, discriminative touch, and vibratory sense in the spinal cord and the medial lemniscus conveys this same information from the medulla to the dorsal thalamus. (pp. 112–117, 120–121)

41. **Answer E:** The loss of pain and thermal sensations on one side of the face correlates with damage to the spinal trigeminal tract; in this case the loss is ipsilateral to the lesion. The anterolateral system relays pain and thermal sensations from the contralateral side of the body, the solitary tract conveys visceral sensory input (especially taste), and the medial lemniscus contains fibers relaying information related to position sense and discriminative touch. The medial longitudinal fasciculus does not contain sensory fibers. (pp. 112–117, 120–121)

42. **Answer C:** The posterior inferior cerebellar artery (commonly called PICA by clinicians) serves the posterolateral portion of the medulla, which encompasses the anterolateral system, spinal trigeminal tract, and nucleus ambiguus. The anterior and medial areas of the medulla (containing the pyramid, medial lemniscus, and hypoglossal nucleus/nerve) are served by the anterior spinal artery and the anterolateral area of the medulla (the region of the olivary nuclei) is served by penetrating branches of the vertebral artery. The posterior spinal artery serves the posterior column nuclei in the medulla and the anterior inferior cerebellar artery (commonly called AICA) serves caudal portions of the pons and cerebellum. (pp. 112–117, 120–121)

43. **Answer B:** The uncus is at the rostral and medial aspect of the parahippocampal gyrus, and, in this position, is directly adjacent to the anterolateral aspect of the midbrain. The diencephalon is rostral to this point and the medulla, the most caudal part of the brainstem, is located in the posterior fossa. Late stages of uncal herniation may, but not always, result in damage to the rostral pons; this is especially so if the patient becomes decerebrate. The cerebellum is not involved in uncal herniation. (pp. 160–161)

44. **Answer D:** Uncal herniation compresses the lateral portion of the brainstem, eventually resulting in compression of the corticospinal fibers in the crus cerebri. Weakness on the patient's left side indicates damage to corticospinal fibers in the right crus. In situations of significant shift of the midbrain due to the herniation, the contralateral crus also may be damaged, resulting in bilateral weakness. Although all other choices contain corticospinal fibers, none of these areas are directly involved in uncal herniation. (pp. 146–147)

45. **Answer C:** The root of the oculomotor nerve conveys general somatic efferent fibers to four of the six major extraocular muscles and general visceral efferent (GVE) parasympathetic preganglionic fibers to the ciliary ganglion from which postganglionic fibers travel to the sphincter muscle of the iris. Pressure on the oculomotor root, as in uncal herniation, will usually compress the smaller diameter, and more superficially located GVE fibers first. Optic nerve damage results in blindness in that eye, injury to sympathetic fibers to the eye results in constriction of the pupil, and an abducens root injury results in an inability to abduct that eye. A lesion of corticonuclear fibers in the crus results primarily in motor deficits related to the facial, hypoglossal, and accessory nerves. (pp. 146–147)

46. **Answer C:** The absence of, or the aberrant development of, muscle around the oral cavity and over the cheek (muscles of facial expression, innervated by the facial [VII] nerve) indicate a failure of proper differentiation of the second pharyngeal arch. Arch 2 also gives rise to the stapedius, buccinator, stylohyoid, platysma, and

posterior belly of the digastric. Mesoderm of the head outside of the pharyngeal arches gives rise to the extraocular muscles and muscles of the tongue. The muscles of mastication (plus the tensor tympani, tensor veli palati, mylohyoid, anterior belly of the digastric) arise from arch 1, the stylopharyngeus from arch 3, and striated muscles of the pharynx, larynx, and upper esophagus from arch 4. (pp. 226–229)

47. **Answer C:** The best localizing sign in this patient is the paucity of eye movement and dilated pupil on the left; this indicates a lesion of the midbrain on the left at the level of the exiting oculomotor fibers. The red nucleus is found at the same level and, more importantly, immediately lateral to the red nucleus is a compact bundle of cerebellothalamic fibers. The ataxia and tremor are related primarily to damage to these cerebellar efferent fibers. The motor deficit is contralateral to the lesion because the corticospinal fibers, through which the deficit is expressed, cross at the motor (pyramidal) decussation. Lesions at the other choices would not result in a paucity of eye movement and, therefore, are not potential candidates. (pp. 244–247)

48. **Answer C:** The lesion on the exiting oculomotor fibers (on the left) damages the preganglionic parasympathetic fibers from the Edinger-Westphal Activation of these fibers produces pupil constriction; when their influence is removed the pupil dilates. Consequently, the intact postganglionic sympathetic fibers from the ipsilateral superior cervical ganglion predominate, and the pupil dilates. Choices on the right are on the incorrect side. Damage to hypothalamospinal fibers would remove sympathetic influence at the intermediolateral cell column, and the pupil would constrict (parasympathetic domination). (pp. 222–225)

49. **Answer B:** Cell bodies in the nucleus ambiguus innervate muscles of the pharynx and larynx, including what is commonly called the vocalis muscle. A lesion of this nucleus is one cause of dysarthria. The solitary tract and nuclei are concerned with visceral afferent information, including taste, and the spinal trigeminal tract is made the central processes of primary sensory fibers conveying general somatic afferent (GSA) information from the ipsilateral side of the face and oral cavity. Proprioceptive information from the ipsilateral upper extremity is transmitted via the cuneate nucleus; the vestibular nuclei are related to balance, equilibrium, and control of eye movement. (pp. 226–229)

50. **Answer C:** The area of the brainstem that contains the nucleus ambiguus is served by branches of the posterior inferior cerebellar artery (PICA). Occlusion of this vessel usually gives rise to the PICA (lateral medullary or Wallenberg) syndrome. The anterior inferior cerebellar artery (AICA) serves the lateral and inferior cerebellar surface and the superior cerebellar artery serves the superior surface and much of the cerebellar nuclei. The labyrinthine artery, a branch of AICA, serves the inner ear. The posterior spinal artery serves the posterior columns and their nuclei. (pp. 226)

51. **Answer B:** The lesion in this woman is in the medulla, and the sensory loss on the body (excluding the head) is on her left side; a lesion in the medulla on the right side, involving fibers of the anterolateral system (ALS), accounts for this sensory deficit. A lesion of the ALS on the left side of the medulla would result in sensory deficits on the right side of the body. The spinal trigeminal tract and nucleus convey pain and thermal sensations from the ipsilateral side (right side in this case) of the face, and the medial lemniscus conveys vibratory and discriminative touch sensations from the contralateral side of the body. (pp.192–195, 198–201)

52. Answer C: The woman is hoarse because the lesion involves the region of the medulla that includes the nucleus ambiguus. These motor neurons serve, via the glossopharyngeal (IX) and vagus (X) nerves, the muscles of the larynx and pharynx, including the medial portion of the thyroarytenoid, also called the vocalis muscle. Paralysis of the vocalis on one side will cause hoarseness of the voice. Hypoglossal nucleus or nerve, or facial nucleus lesions, may cause difficulty with speech but not hoarseness. The spinal trigeminal tract conveys sensory input from the ipsilateral side of the face. There are no historical or examination findings to support a diagnosis of upper respiratory viral findings (cold or flu). (pp. 52, 226–229)

53. Answer C: The posterior inferior cerebellar artery (PICA) serves the lateral area of the medulla that contains the anterolateral system, spinal trigeminal tract (loss of pain and thermal sensations from the ipsilateral side of the face), and the nucleus ambiguus. Many patients that present with a PICA (Wallenberg or lateral medullary) syndrome also have involvement of the vertebral artery on that side. The posterior spinal artery serves the posterior column nuclei in the medulla, and the anterior spinal artery serves the pyramid, medial lemniscus, and exiting roots of the hypoglossal nerve. The anterior inferior cerebellar artery and the superior cerebellar artery distribute to the pons and midbrain, respectively, plus significant portions of the cerebellum. (pp. 120–121, 192–195)

54. Answer E: Excessive eating (gluttony), which may include a propensity to attempt to eat things not considered food items, is hyperphagia. Dysphagia is difficulty in swallowing, and aphagia is the inability to eat. Hyperorality is the tendency to put items in the mouth or to appear to be examining objects by placing them in the oral cavity. Dyspnea is difficulty breathing. (pp. 278–281)

55. Answer A: The constellation of deficits experienced by this man is characteristic of the Klüver-Bucy syndrome; this may be seen following bilateral damage to the temporal poles that includes the amygdaloid complex. The Korsakoff syndrome is seen, for example, in chronic alcoholics, and senile dementia is a loss of cognitive and intellectual function associated with neurodegenerative diseases of the elderly (e.g., Alzheimer disease). Wernicke (receptive or fluent) aphasia is seen in patients with a lesion in the area of the inferior parietal lobule, and the Wallenberg syndrome results from a lesion in the medulla characterized by alternating hemisensory losses and, depending on the extent of the damage, other deficits. (pp. 278–281)

56. Answer B: Bilateral damage to the temporal lobes, as in an automobile collision, may result in damage to the hippocampus. While remote memory, the ability to recall events that happened years or decades ago, is intact, the man will have difficulty "remembering" recent or immediate events. That is, he will find it difficult, if not impossible, to turn a new experience into longer-term memory (something that can be recalled in its proper context at a later time). Dysphagia (difficulty swallowing) and dysarthria (difficulty speaking) are deficits usually seen in brainstem lesions. Bilateral

sensory losses of the lower portion of the body could be seen with bilateral damage to the posterior paracentral gyri (falcine meningioma) or to the anterior white commissure of the spinal cord. Dementia is a multiregional symptom that usually involves several areas of the brain, cortical as well as subcortical. (pp. 276–277)

57. Answer C: The Meyer-Archambault loop is composed of optic radiation fibers that loop through the temporal lobe; these fibers, on each side, convey visual input from the contralateral superior quadrant of the visual field. Consequently, a bilateral lesion of these fibers results as a bilateral superior quadrantanopia. Bilateral inferior quadrantanopia is seen in bilateral lesions that would involve the superior portion of the optic radiations. Right or left superior quadrantanopia is seen in cases of unilateral damage to, respectively, the left or right Meyer-Archambault loop. A bitemporal hemianopsia results in a lesion of the optic chiasm. (pp. 260–263)

58. Answer C: The combination of eye movement disorders and a contralateral hemiplegia localizes this lesion to the midbrain on the side of the ocular deficits (right side). This also specifies that corticospinal fibers on the right (in the crus) are damaged, and places the location of the cells of origin for these fibers in the somatomotor cortex on the right side. The right crus contains the axons of these fibers but not the neuronal cell bodies. The left somatomotor cortex influences the right extremities. The right precentral gyrus does not contain cells projecting to the left lumbosacral spinal cord (left lower extremity), and the right anterior paracentral gyrus does not contain the cells that project to the left cervical spinal cord (left upper extremity). (pp. 206–209, 210–213)

59. Answer A: The lesion in this man is central (brainstem) and involves the third nerve. Consequently, the damage is to the preganglionic parasympathetic fibers in the root of the oculomotor (III) nerve; this removes the parasympathetic influence (pupil constriction) that originates from the Edinger-Westphal nucleus. Fibers from the superior cervical ganglion are intact, hence the dilated pupil. Fibers from the geniculate ganglion and inferior salivatory nucleus distribute on the facial (VII) and glossopharyngeal (IX) nerves, respectively. Postganglionic fibers from the ciliary ganglion, although involved in this pathway, are not damaged in this lesion. (pp. 222–225)

60. Answer E: The loss of most eye movement on one side (oculomotor nerve root involvement) coupled with a paralysis of the extremities on the contralateral side is a superior alternating hemiplegia (this is also known as Weber syndrome): *superior* because it is the most rostral of three; *alternating* because it is a cranial nerve on one side and the extremities on the other; and *hemiplegia* because one-half of the body below the head is involved. A middle alternating hemiplegia involves the abducens (VI) nerve root and adjacent corticospinal fibers, and an inferior alternating hemiplegia involves the hypoglossal (XII) nerve root and corticospinal fibers in the pyramid. Alternating hemianesthesia is a sensory loss, and a Brown-Séquard syndrome is a spinal cord lesion with no cranial nerve deficits. (pp. 222–225)

Index

Note: Page numbers in italics denote figures; those followed by t refer to table; those followed by Q denote questions; and those followed by A denote answers.